Androgen Deficiency in the Adult Male

Causes, diagnosis and treatment

T0203938

Nomogram for Calculating Free Testosterone from Total Testosterone (TT) and Sex Hormone-Binding Globulin (SHBG)

The value for calculated free testosterone (CFT) is obtained by joining the value for TT to that for SHBG, and where the line intersects the middle curved scale is the value for CFT.

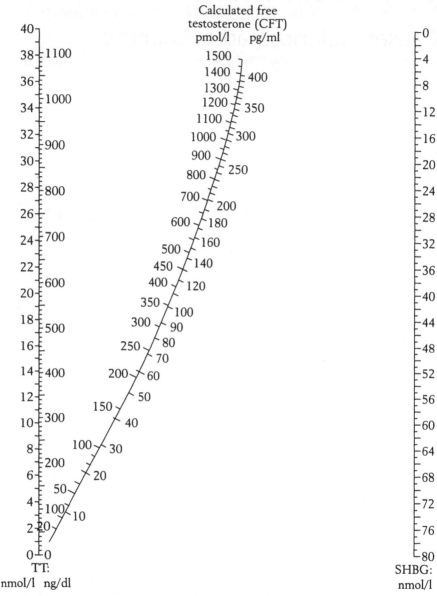

The figure is derived from the equation given by Vermeulen A, Verdonck L, Kaufman JM. A critical evaluation of simple methods for the estimation of free testosterone in serum. *J Clin Endocrinol Metab* 1999;84:3666–72. An average albumin value of 43 g/l is assumed, though unless there are markedly lower levels due to malnutrition or immobilization, changes in this variable make little difference.
© 2004 M Carruthers

Androgen Deficiency in the Adult Male

Causes, diagnosis and treatment

Malcolm Carruthers MD FRCPath MRCGP

Consultant Andrologist
Harley Street
London
UK

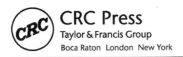

CRC Press
Taylor & Francis Group
Boca Raton London New York

CRC Press is an imprint of the
Taylor & Francis Group, an **informa** business

CRC Press
Taylor & Francis Group
6000 Broken Sound Parkway NW, Suite 300
Boca Raton, FL 33487-2742

First issued in paperback 2019

© 2010 by Taylor & Francis Group, LLC
CRC Press is an imprint of Taylor & Francis Group, an Informa business

No claim to original U.S. Government works

ISBN-13: 978-1-84214-032-1 (hbk)
ISBN-13: 978-0-367-39392-2 (pbk)

This book contains information obtained from authentic and highly regarded sources. While all reasonable efforts have been made to publish reliable data and information, neither the author[s] nor the publisher can accept any legal responsibility or liability for any errors or omissions that may be made. The publishers wish to make clear that any views or opinions expressed in this book by individual editors, authors or contributors are personal to them and do not necessarily reflect the views/opinions of the publishers. The information or guidance contained in this book is intended for use by medical, scientific or health-care professionals and is provided strictly as a supplement to the medical or other professional's own judgement, their knowledge of the patient's medical history, relevant manufacturer's instructions and the appropriate best practice guidelines. Because of the rapid advances in medical science, any information or advice on dosages, procedures or diagnoses should be independently verified. The reader is strongly urged to consult the relevant national drug formulary and the drug companies' and device or material manufacturers' printed instructions, and their websites, before administering or utilizing any of the drugs, devices or materials mentioned in this book. This book does not indicate whether a particular treatment is appropriate or suitable for a particular individual. Ultimately it is the sole responsibility of the medical professional to make his or her own professional judgements, so as to advise and treat patients appropriately. The authors and publishers have also attempted to trace the copyright holders of all material reproduced in this publication and apologize to copyright holders if permission to publish in this form has not been obtained. If any copyright material has not been acknowledged please write and let us know so we may rectify in any future reprint.

Visit the Taylor & Francis Web site at
http://www.taylorandfrancis.com

and the CRC Press Web site at
http://www.crcpress.com

Contents

Foreword

It is indeed an honor to be able to write a foreword for *Androgen Deficiency in the Adult Male*. This textbook represents the lifelong work of Dr Malcolm Carruthers, a true gentleman, for whom I have great respect. He is one of the early pioneers in the field of aging men's health and andrology. What is most remarkable is that his clinical research was performed in his private office, away from the traditional ivory towers of medicine. I had the wonderful opportunity of visiting Dr Carruthers' Harley Street clinic in 2002 and was particularly impressed with his detailed record keeping, which allowed a lot of the analysis to be presented in this work.

Androgen decline in aging males (ADAM), or andropause, is a very contemporary issue for several reasons. Firstly, the life expectancy is increasing for males, albeit not to the extent of females; but there may be some modifiable factors that can influence the quality of life of individuals. This would include not only hormonal replacement but also attention to diet and exercise. Secondly, there is increasing demand by baby boomers to achieve not only longevity but also quality-added lives.

This book will enlighten the inquisitive practitioner's mind on this subject. Hopefully, it will also silence critics about the nonexistence of the andropause. ADAM is often confounded by clinical depression, psychological disorders and side effects of medications, but its existence is real. Patients around the world can attest to this. The United Kingdom Andropause Study (UKAS) is probably one of the larger database sets in the study of aging men. The results are shared in this book, as well as techniques such as testosterone pellet implantation. This book will appeal to a wide medical audience including primary care physicians and specialists in men's health, urology, endocrinology, psychiatry, geriatrics, cardiology and others. An interesting aspect of the book is the historical journey of testosterone replacement, which has seen a tumultuous time; and I anticipate it will see further turmoil in the future. Like everything in medicine, there will be high and low tides, and I hope that with this book, the tides will rise in favor of men's health and the management of andropause.

Robert S Tan MD

Clinical Director, Geriatrics and Extended Care, Veterans Affairs Medical Center Houston, Texas

Associate Professor, Department of Family and Community Medicine, University of Texas

Division of Geriatrics, Department of Internal Medicine, Baylor College of Medicine, Houston, Texas

Advisory Board, Men's Health Network, Washington, DC, USA

Acknowledgements

Help is gratefully acknowledged in three areas.

Production of this book David Bloomer and Nick Dunton of Parthenon Publishing (now Taylor & Francis Medical Books) were unfailingly encouraging in both the inception and extended production of the manuscript. The whole publishing team have been a pleasure to work with throughout.

Professional advice Many kind colleagues have given advice during the writing of this book. In relation to the introduction, Professor Bruno Lunenfeld, President of the International Society for the Study of the Ageing Male (ISSAM), and Dr Alex Kalache, Chief of the WHO Ageing and Health Program, made clear the urgency and importance of measures designed to slow the onset of disability in the older male, and the contribution that carefully applied androgen treatment could make to the active aging program.

In the 'history' chapter, Dr Bruce Wilkin of Ely, Nevada, USA, has been endlessly kind, both in providing books on the history of testosterone and 'high-testosterone' men, and particularly in introducing me to the inspiring book by Paul de Kruif on *The Male Hormone*.

In the chapter on the 'Causes of androgen deficiency', Professor Roland Tremblay of Laval University, Quebec, Previous President of the Canadian Andropause Society, was very helpful in shaping my thoughts on testosterone transport in the blood. The three key conferences on 'Testosterone: Action, Deficiency, Substitution', held at Castle Elmau in Bavaria by Professors Eberhard Nieschlag and Hermann Behre, of Munster and Halle Universities in Germany, gave a wealth of information on all aspects of androgen metabolism. Particularly with the contributions of Dr Focko Rommerts of Erasmus University, Rotterdam, The Netherlands, on androgen receptors, Professor Alex Vermeulen of Ghent in Belgium, on hormonal changes in male senescence and Professor Louis Gooren of the Free University of Amsterdam in The Netherlands, on the metabolic effects of testosterone, the publications arising from these conferences have provided the pillars of wisdom in the field.

In the chapter on 'The diagnosis of androgen deficiency', there were important comments from Dr Lisa Tenover of Emory University in Atlanta, Georgia, USA, Dr Tom Trinick of the Ulster Hospital, Belfast, current

Chairman of the Andropause Society, and Dr Mike Wheeler of St Thomas's Hospital, London. Dr Neil Burman of the Monism Health Planning Foundation in Cape Town, South Africa, has contributed a wealth of fascinating material on the reference ranges of blood androgens and the pitfalls in their measurement and interpretation.

In the 'Androgen replacement therapy' chapter, Dr Gene Shippen of Reading, Pennsylvania, USA, was endlessly helpful in discussing the recommendations of the Andropause Consensus Committee of the American Endocrine Society, of which he was a member. These, together with the ISSAM Guidelines laid down by Professor Bruno Lunenfeld and Professor Morales, underlie the basic approach to androgen replacement therapy. Dr Farid Saad, Head of the Men's Health Care Program of Schering Berlin, was also most kind in providing information on transdermal testosterone treatment, and the metabolic syndrome. Mr Mark Fenely, Senior Lecturer in Urologic Oncology at the Institute of Urology in London, and Professor Aksam Yassin, of the Urology Department, Gulf Medical University School of Medicine, Ajman, UAE, have given great support and evidence to the idea that testosterone treatment is safe for the prostate. Dr Adrian Zentner, and Linda Byart, long-standing friends and colleagues in Perth, Western Australia, who have fought long and hard for the right of Australian men to have testosterone treatment, also provided the latest information on transdermal testosterone creams.

In the 'Sex steroids and the brain' chapter, Professor Sam Gandy, Director of the newly established Farber Institute for Neurosciences, of Thomas Jefferson University, Philadelphia, gave advice on earlier versions of the chapter, and introduced me to the key work of his colleagues in the field, Bruce McEwen, Professor of Neuroendocrinology at Rockefeller University in New York, and Ralph Martins, Professor of Neuroscience at the Univerity of Western Australia, Perth. Professor Andzej Gomula, University of Warsaw, Poland, showed new ways of treating androgen deficiency, and the amazing results this could provide in patients with Parkinson's disease. The encouraging advice and exciting work on andropause and testosterone treatment of memory disorders of Robert Tan, Associate Professor of Geriatrics in the Health Science Center at Houston, Texas, USA, was also invaluable. In the UK, Dr Eva Hogervorst and Stephan Bandelow of the Oxford Project to Investigate Memory and Ageing (OPTIMA) at the Radcliffe Infirmary, Oxford, advised on the role of different hormones in cognitive function, and suggested new lines of research which could be undertaken in exploring this field.

I would also like to thank my critics for continuing to stimulate my interest in androgens, and extending the learning experience.

Mr Hugh Welford, web-master extraordinary, has created brilliant and elegant computer programs to handle the mass of data coming from patients in the London Andropause Clinic, as well as the practice management system which organizes the whole thing, and makes audit of and research on the resulting clinical data possible. Mr Jim McGrew has, for many years, managed the practice, befriended the patients and recorded their data.

The medical research on which the UK Andropause Study is based was supported partly by grants from the European Organization for the Control of Circulatory Diseases (EOCCD) and the Sophus Jacobsen og hustru Astrid Jacobsen Fond and LBK Foundation in Copenhagen, Denmark. The work was also greatly helped by Dr Michael Hansen and Professor Jesper Mehlsen, good friends, and previous and current Presidents of these organizations. The pioneering work and forceful personality of the founder of these organizations, Dr Jens Moller, was the inspiration for this advocacy of testosterone treatment, particularly in relation to cardiovascular disease and the prevention of debility and dependency, with their tragic personal, social and economic consequences.

Personal My wife, Jean Coleman, has also been endlessly loving, kind and supportive throughout, and contributed much invaluable material to the 'Sex steroids and the brain' chapter. An important part of this has been her work as Secretary of the Andropause Society, helping this charity into existence, and organizing its conferences and training courses. Also on the personal level, my brother Dr Barry Carruthers influenced my choice of career and sparked my interest in andrology, and has maintained it over the past 40 years.

Preface

This book takes a practical approach to the causes, diagnosis and treatment of androgen deficiency. It aims to fill the gap between more general books on men's health and the specialist works on androgen metabolism and replacement therapy. The information contained will enable clinicians to make evidence-based decisions on whether to start testosterone treatment and how to plan safe regimens in line with the recommendations of the two major organizations in the field, the International Society for the Study of the Aging Male (ISSAM) and the American Endocrine Society.

Many of the ideas expressed in this volume are unconventional and are presented to stimulate debate and break up the logjam of entrenched beliefs based on theory, rather than practical clinical experience. Few are aware of how widespread and serious androgen deficiency is; it is the urgency of instigating treatment when needed, rather than any lack of convenient and safe testosterone preparations, that prevents androgen replacement being made far more widely available.

In an age of rapid scientific advance, it is all but impossible to write a completely up-to-date text – especially in the ever-widening field of testosterone research. In the 25 years since I began studying this area, androgens have been increasingly recognized as having an important role in the functioning of more and more body systems. In this introductory book, it has been impossible to cover all these new developments. Many topics, such as the effects of testosterone on the cardiovascular, musculoskeletal and immunological systems, as well as erectile dysfunction, need more detailed coverage to do them justice. It is hoped to do this in a more comprehensive volume at a later date.

The part played by environmental factors such as xenoestrogens and antiandrogens in creating 'hormonal havoc' would also benefit from much more analysis. This has been highlighted by recent reports that sperm counts appear to be falling quite rapidly in some countries, and hormone-related developmental abnormalities of the male urogenital system are increasing, emphasizing the importance of androgen–estrogen interactions.

Large amounts of information are accumulating from the ongoing UK Andropause Study (UKAS). Its results coincide closely with the findings of many of the published studies quoted, and underlie many of the ideas put forward in this book. Preliminary results of this work have been presented at several international congresses and in a number of articles over the last 10 years. Working with other specialists in each area, I intend to present and publish more detailed analyses of the principal findings in the near future.

There is also the case to be made for the use of testosterone treatment in preventive medicine – adding life to years as well as years to life for men. This is another rapidly expanding area of clinical, epidemiological and economic research that we hope to cover in more detail at a later date.

Malcolm E. Carruthers
m.carruthers@btconnect.com

1 Introduction

I keep six honest serving-men
They taught me all I knew;
Their names are What and Why and When
And How and Where and Who.
Rudyard Kipling

This book has been written for many reasons. The main one is a strong personal belief that androgen deficiency in the adult male is far more common than is generally realized by either the medical profession or the general public, and that its prevention and treatment are matters of great medical, social and economic importance.

The whole area is one of considerable controversy, and this book is unlikely to be an exception. However, it is reassuring that bodies such as the World Health Organization (WHO), the International Society for the Study of the Aging Male (ISSAM) and the Endocrine Society in America have over the past 10 years become much more interested in and supportive of studies of androgens and their importance. So, let us take a brief look at some of the questions frequently raised before going into detailed consideration of each one in the separate chapters of the book.

WHAT IS ANDROGEN DEFICIENCY?

Androgen deficiency can be defined as an absolute or relative deficiency of testosterone or its metabolites according to the need of that individual at that time in his life.

The definition is derived from that of diabetes mellitus, another endocrine disorder, which increases in frequency with age, may be associated with high hormone levels owing to the various factors causing insulin resistance and results in a characteristic pattern of symptoms. Androgen deficiency is comparable to the absolute or relative deficiency of insulin in diabetes, the low levels in juvenile diabetics being equivalent to the low testosterone levels due to non-descent of the testes, or mumps orchitis.

The maturity-onset diabetic resembles more the typical andropausal male in his 50s with insufficient testosterone to overcome the 'resistance' caused by rising sex hormone-binding globulin (SHBG) levels, stress, obesity and impaired androgen receptor function. Also, like diabetes, androgen deficiency is treated largely on the basis of the relief of these symptoms and the prevention of long-term complications, rather than endocrine assays. This principle will be referred to again when considering the application of androgen therapy.

Whatever its cause, androgen deficiency can either result in the characteristic group of symptoms termed andropause in the adult male, or silently and insidiously accelerate the aging process in organs as diverse as the heart, bones and the brain.

WHY IS ANDROGEN DEFICIENCY IMPORTANT?

The importance of androgen deficiency lies in its being a major and increasing cause of disease, debility and dependency in an aging male population.

While the good news is that men in the developed countries are living longer on average, the bad news is that as they age, they become more prone to a variety of degenerative diseases which result in debility and dependency, the medical, social and economic costs of which are vast and rising[1].

The Director General of the WHO has graphically illustrated this dilemma of 'Global Ageing: A Triumph and a Challenge'[2], the consequences of which are only gradually dawning on social scientists and politicians. Paradoxically, many members of the medical profession are ignoring it, seeming to hope it will go away, regardless of the fact that the challenges are likely to be far greater by the end of their own lives if they adopt the Doctor 'Do-little' or 'Do-nothing' options now.

The triumphal aspects have been two-fold. First, during the past 50 years, family planning combined with changing attitudes has decreased the birth rate dramatically in nearly all countries. Second, life expectancy has increased worldwide due to increased food production, public health measures and medical advances.

The challenges are related to the fact that although the 'population explosion' has been controlled, it is far from being avoided. The world population, which has risen from 1 billion people in 1800 to 1.6 billion in 1900 and 6 billion in 2000, is projected to increase to 9 billion by 2050.

This 50% increase is going to be mainly in older people, not only in the more affluent 'developed' countries, but also in 'developing' countries. This 'global graying', as it has been called, is clearly seen in Figure 1, taken from the United Nations Population Division report on 'World Population Prospects: The 2000 Revision'[1].

While most of Europe and the UK can expect a 50–70% increase in the over-60s population and the USA a doubling, in India, China and Malaysia, in particular, it will treble or quadruple. There are three factors which will increase the impact of this demographic shift in the Western world and Japan earlier than elsewhere:

(1) The post-Second World War population bulge in the USA and Europe, known as the 'baby boomers', have gone through their 50s, and are now rapidly advancing on the 60-year-old threshold. Not only that, but they are more likely to be obese, diabetic, hypertensive, hyperlipidemic, sedentary, stressed and heavily medicated for these conditions than their predecessors. They represent what could be called the 'Syndrome-X Generation', and are likely to be less healthy generally, and more prone to androgen deficiency and its multiple consequences because of these predisposing factors.

This generation is likely to be vocal and demanding. Already baby-boomers control more than half of discretionary income in America and three quarters of its wealth. Within 6 years the over-40s will spend $2.6 trillion each year against the $1.6 trillion spent by those under 40. A million baby-boomers will live to be 100.

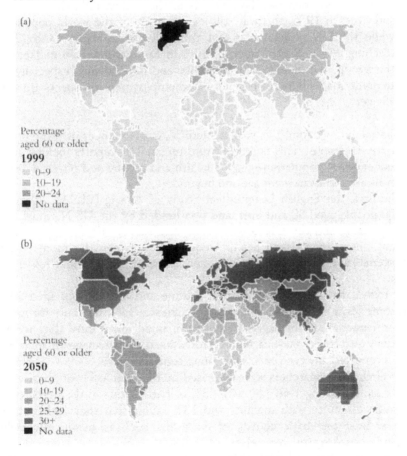

Figure 1 World map of 'global graying' over the next 50 years. Percentage of population aged 60 or older in (a) 1999 and (b) 2050. Reproduced with permission from reference 1

(2) The 'old-age dependency ratio' (the total population aged 60 and over divided by the population aged 15–60) is likely almost to double in most developed countries in the next 25 years, i.e. from 0.26 to 0.44 in the USA, from 0.36 to 0.56 in Europe, with Japan leading the way, going from 0.39 to 0.66[2]. This means that for the Japanese, who are leading the world in longevity at present, unless retirement ages rise, within a generation the number of dependent people over age 60 who will have to be supported by every 100 people in work will rise from 39 to 66. This will be a huge burden on the working population, especially in view of the deteriorating pension fund situation, and is likely to lead to demands for a 'work until you drop' culture.

(3) The official United Nations (UN) definition of 'older' refers to those aged 60 and above. The greatest proportional increase in the population of developed countries, however, is in the 'oldest old', those aged 80 and over. In 1975, this was still less than 1% of the world population, while the UN projection is that this will rise to about 4% by 2050, reaching 7% in North America, 10% in Europe and 15% in Japan. In this group, the incidence of disability and dependency, especially due to dementia, will increase rapidly, and employment prospects are virtually zero.

The social and economic, as well as medical, consequences of these predictions are enormous. This is seen in two recent UK reports looking at the consequences of population aging on health and mental and physical disability levels around retirement age and beyond.

The first, the English Longitudinal Study of Ageing (ELSA)[3], looked at 12000 people aged 50 and over, and was funded by the US National Institute on Aging and the UK Government. The survey showed that, even at present, there are marked health inequalities between the more well-off managerial and professional groups, and those in manual and lower-paid work.

It found that one-third of men in routine and manual jobs aged 50–59 had some form of limiting, long-standing illness, while the figure for men in the professional and managerial groups remained lower until they reached 75. Only just over one-quarter of professional and managerial men aged 60–74 reported any type of limiting, long-term illness.

Overall, the researchers were surprised by the high levels of physical disability among younger people, with 43% of participants in their 50s reporting some difficulty with mobility and 13% saying that they had problems with at least one basic activity of daily life, such as getting themselves dressed or cooking for themselves.

This should be combined with the fact that in the UK the proportion of people in work (as employees or self-employed) declined with age from 72% amongst those aged 50–54 to only 10% of people aged 65–69. Worldwide, less than 5% of men work past age 65. At all ages, men are more likely than women to be in employment. The so-called 'feminization of aging' resulting from the average 7-year-longer life expectancy of women is likely to magnify this employment discrepancy, and emphasizes the importance of keeping men healthy and independent for longer.

Similar inequalities emerged with mental ability. In cognitive tests, university graduates aged 75 and over performed as well as, and sometimes better than, younger academically unqualified people, particularly with numbers.

The second report is from the London School of Economics for the Alzheimer's Research Trust in the UK, and focuses on 'Cognitive impairment in older people: its implications for future demand for services and costs'[4]. It was based on the fact that the incidence of dementia, two-thirds of which is due to Alzheimer's disease, rises logarithmically from around 1% at age 65 to 10% aged 80, and to 50% aged 90.

The results of their model, based on official population projections for the increasing number of aging people, showed a 66% increase in the number of people with cognitive impairment over the next 30 years, rising faster than that with dependency due to physical causes (58%), and there would be an equivalent rise in institutionalized people from both causes. The economic consequence of this in England alone would be to raise the long-term health-care expenditure for older people with cognitive impairment from around £5 billion to £11 billion within a generation, with total long-term costs for older people amounting to more than twice this sum (Figure 2).

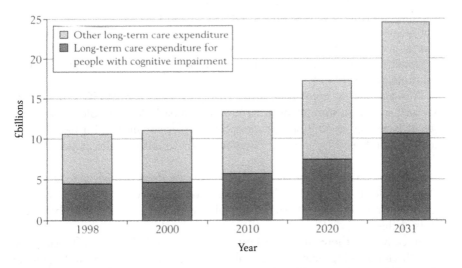

Figure 2 Projected long-term care expenditure for older people (in £billions) for England, to 2031

Extrapolating these figures to the approximately six times larger American population, this means an increase in the costs of dementia care from $50 billion to $110 billion.

If we couple that with deteriorating pension funds, and fewer people able or willing to care for dependent relatives, it indicates that, unless more effective treatments for cognitive impairment are developed and made widely available, substantial rises in formal services for their care will be required at a hugely increased financial and social cost. The implication from this study is that there is an urgent need to develop, and make widely available, better means of preventing and treating dementia from all causes, but particularly Alzheimer's disease.

WHEN SHOULD ANDROGEN DEFICIENCY BE TREATED?

In most countries, modern medicine has added years to life, but now we need to be able to add life to years. Prevention is certainly generally better than cure, particularly in the elderly patient where disease processes are more difficult to halt and reverse. Slowing the older man's progress towards the three Ds, debility, dependency and death, needs action in early and middle as well as late life. To help the individual limit the time spent in the first two of these stages involves skilled input from a variety of health professionals throughout the life cycle.

Our mental and physical functional capacity throughout life can be compared to a flight in a glider. Helped by the hormonal surge in puberty, we are catapulted to the peak of our trajectory in our teens and 20s, and then follow a variable glide path to death. The rate of descent varies according to our lifestyle, and social and medical history. As with androgens, the mainly anabolic 'thermal' up-currents of success at work or in love, relaxation or recreation can help us reach new heights. At other times, stress, physical or mental inactivity, or illness, can produce catabolic down-drafts which cause us to fall suddenly to lower levels or even into the cloud layer of function, the disability threshold.

This analogy is consistent with the policy of the WHO on 'Active Ageing', aiming to support optimal function in early life, middle age and old age. It is defined as 'the process of optimizing opportunities for health, participation and security in order to enhance the quality of life as people age' (Figure 3).

Although only part of the much broader medical, social and economic picture, the prevention and treatment of androgen deficiency has an important role to play at each stage of life in helping to bring about the goals of this policy.

In early life there are a variety of endocrine influences affecting the growth and development of the male. Xenoestrogens and antiandrogens in the environment can influence mental and physical development *in utero* and throughout childhood into adult life. The recognition and correction of

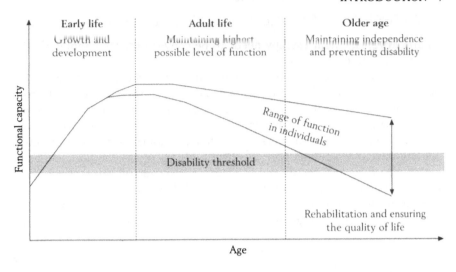

Figure 3 Maintaining functional capacity over the course of life[2]

varying degrees of testicular nondescent or malfunction can promote androgen levels sufficient to establish normal levels of fertility and male physique
and psychology at puberty and beyond. Good patterns of eating and physical activity in childhood can be carried into adult life and help to prevent
the hormonal disorders underlying syndrome X.

Similar principles, particularly in relation to a healthy lifestyle, apply in
adult life. As discussed later in the book, many factors, including stress, lack
of exercise, obesity, excess alcohol, and acute and chronic illness can all
result in impaired androgen production or activity. As well as being able to
recognize when these factors are impairing mental, physical and sexual
function, or contributing to premature aging, the physician should be able
to monitor androgen levels between the ages of 30 and 40 at a time when
these might be expected to be optimal. This would provide reference levels
for that man which might be target values for replacement in that individual
if he needs treatment later in life. Also, there should be awareness that
andropause symptoms, although they tend to peak around the age of 50,
can occur much earlier.

In older age, androgen deficiency becomes much more common. How
common depends on whether the diagnosis is made on the characteristic
andropausal symptoms, or on arbitrary laboratory norms, as will be argued
later. The latest controlled trials of androgen replacement are supporting
the uncontrolled studies going back over 60 years, reporting improvements
in musculoskeletal, cardiac, metabolic, sexual and even cognitive function
on testosterone. There does not appear to be any particular cutoff point in
age at which testosterone treatment may be beneficial.

HOW SHOULD ANDROGEN DEFICIENCY BE TREATED?

Androgen replacement therapy needs to be convenient, acceptable, physiological, safe and economical.

Since testosterone was first isolated and synthesized in 1935, there has been an intensive search for the ideal form of testosterone treatment. Convenience of application is essential if a potentially long-term form of treatment such as testosterone is to be widely taken up. This is one of the main reasons why testosterone pellet implants, although unphysiological, prone to rejection and primitive in execution, have the longest history of any method, and being highly effective, and requiring no effort on the part of the patient, have remained popular with patients who have used them over the past 60 years.

Conversely, although giving a good physiological pattern of testosterone levels, and representing great technological advances, testosterone patches were irritant and inconvenient to wear. Proving unacceptable to patients, they lasted only 2–3 years in the market before they were discarded as a method of treatment.

As discussed in Chapter 5, given the basic safety guidelines as laid down in the recommendations of the International Society for the Study of the Aging Male[5], androgen replacement therapy has established its place as a safe and effective form of treatment.

To be widely available, and realize its full potential in preventing and treating related disease, androgen treatment has to be more economical than it currently is. Partly because of the poor absorption of testosterone preparations given by mouth or the transdermal route, where over 90% of the administered dose is wasted, the parenteral route of implantation or the recently developed long-acting injections appear to offer the greatest potential for economy. However, with improved absorption through the scrotal skin, simple testosterone creams could also provide a low cost solution.

Also, rather than being the preserve of specialist andrologists or endocrinologists, it should be within the therapeutic armory of most primary-care physicians. To give the basic information needed to diagnose and treat androgen deficiency effectively is the main aim of this book.

WHERE DO THE PROBLEMS LIE?

To achieve its aims, this book seeks to remove the blocks to testosterone treatment. Some of these are:

(1) *Not understanding its importance* As described above, this form of treatment has the potential to make a major contribution to the ideal of 'Active Ageing' proposed by the WHO. To quote its Director General: 'In all countries, but in developing countries in particular, measures to help older people remain healthy and active are a necessity, not a luxury'. It is suggested that androgen treatment for deficient males is one such necessity.

(2) *Not diagnosing the condition*   There is overreliance on laboratory tests to diagnose androgen insufficiency. For reasons described in the chapter on diagnosis, it can be argued that andropause symptom checklists are a more reliable guide to the condition than blood tests. The latter are subject to a wide range of problems of sampling, analysis and interpretation which can largely invalidate them.

(3) *Not relating it to the causation of disease*   Partly because of the image of testosterone in both the medical and lay mind as being just a sex hormone, there is a lack of awareness of the part that testosterone deficiency can play in accelerating not only the aging process overall, but also diseases of the heart, bones and brain in particular. In some conditions such as heart disease, the simplistic reasoning that because, before the age of 50, men have more coronary thromboses than women testosterone is to blame, has created a pervasive myth. Only gradually is the work of British cardiologists such as Dr Peter Collins[6] and Dr Keith English[7] showing the antianginal and antithrombotic properties of testosterone.

(4) *Psychological blocks*   Patients in general, and male doctors in particular, often seem to feel that to be diagnosed as being 'hypogonadal' or having the 'male menopause', even if dignified by the term 'andropause', is unacceptable to their macho image of themselves, and that andropause does not constitute a real or serious illness.

(5) *Safety concerns*   This again is naturally uppermost in the minds of both doctors and patients when androgen treatment is being considered, even though the large majority of current evidence points to its being one of the safest forms of medication on the market.

(6) *Economic and political blocks*   Many state systems, although paying lip service to preventive medicine, see testosterone as a 'lifestyle drug' which they regard as being misused as well as abused, and therefore an unjustified burden on the health budget[8]. They choose to overlook the sometimes severe damage to a man's mental and physical well-being that androgen deficiency can cause, or the persuasive cost–benefit analysis that can be done in its favor in terms of slowing the aging process in accordance with the WHO policy. This is likely to be shown quite soon to be an expensive mistake in terms of the health and welfare of the aging male.

These concerns were highlighted by the recent Institute of Medicine report "Testosterone and Aging: Clinical Research Directions"[9], which came up with the following key considerations and conclusions:

Focus on the population most likely to benefit (i.e. men over 65)
Use testosterone as a therapeutic intervention, not as a preventative measure

Establish a clear benefit before assessing long-term risks
Focus on clinical outcomes in which there is a preliminary suggestion of
efficacy and for which therapeutic options are not currently available
Ensure safety of the research participants

As we shall see later in Chapter 4 on the diagnosis of androgen deficiency,
by limiting studies to men over 65 with "testosterone levels below the
physiologic levels of young adult men and with one or more symptoms that
might be related to low testosterone", this effectively blocks research on
the mass of men aged 40–65 who might have the most to gain from early
treatment of their symptoms, or be in need of preventing the many life-
threatening complications of syndrome X. It also disregards the mass of
evidence that total testosterone alone is an invalid marker for androgen deficiency when taken in isolation in a geriatric population. As Chapter 5 on
testosterone treatment records, both short-term and long-term safety for
periods of up to 10 years have been established, and risks have to be balanced against symptom relief and improvement in the quality of life in a
rapidly aging population.

Is there not enough evidence from 60 years of clinical experience, and
the placebo controlled trials that have been carried out with the newer
preparations, that following the recommendations of authoritative bodies
such as ISSAM and the Endocrine Society that are given in this book,
experienced clinicians can use their clinical judgement to decide who might
benefit from androgen treatment?

WHO SHOULD BE AWARE OF ANDROGEN DEFICIENCY AND BE WILLING TO PREVENT AND TREAT IT?

The primary-care physician who is alert to the condition, and willing to give
the patient the benefit of the doubt in the form of a therapeutic trial when
uncertain of the diagnosis, is likely to come soon to the conclusion that androgen replacement therapy is a powerful, effective and safe form of treatment.

The pediatrician may become aware of intrauterine influences and less
obvious inborn errors of testosterone metabolism which can affect male
health and development in childhood. The fertility and hormonal problems
presented by failure of the testicles to develop and descend, as well as
delayed puberty, all lead to questions requiring a long- as well as a short-
term solution.

I hope endocrinologists who read this book, while probably finding objections to many of the ideas raised, will find some of interest and use, and
supply mainly constructive criticisms of those they find unacceptable.

Diabetologists will find that where their work enters the field of metabolic syndrome, testosterone treatment can play a pivotal role in reversing
abdominal obesity, increasing lean body mass and reducing hyperlipidemia.
There is also encouraging work suggesting that androgens may be of benefit

in preventing and treating a variety of diabetic complications, including particularly peripheral vascular disease.

Cardiologists need to be aware of the part that androgen deficiency can play in the causation of coronary heart disease and atheromatosis.

Urologists will be reassured to know that there is now a great deal of evidence that androgen replacement therapy, if correctly applied and monitored, is safe in relation to benign enlargement of the prostate, and does not appear to cause malignancy. Also, they will appreciate the important role that androgen deficiency can cause in erectile dysfunction.

Sexologists should find that this book helps them to recognize when the problems with desire and erectile function in their patients are due to underlying androgen deficiency, rather than psychological factors.

Psychiatrists will be encouraged to consider the part that androgen deficiency can cause in two of the most common problems they see in their adult male patients, depression and dementia. Testosterone treatment opens up new therapeutic frontiers in the prevention and treatment of these distressing and increasingly prevalent disorders.

Neurologists may be interested in the possibility of treating Parkinson's disease with androgens, and the ways in which anticonvulsant medication can bring on the andropause.

Pathologists and biochemists will be interested in the ways in which clinicians use and misuse the androgen assays they provide, and in which measures provide the most valid information on androgen activity and which are misleading.

Epidemiologists and social scientists will come to appreciate the important part that androgen deficiency in the aging male can play in present and future patterns of diseases that look set to cripple older men and the economies in which they live. They will have more information on which to base interventions to help stem the rising tide of disability in this rapidly increasing population group.

Geriatricians will find that testosterone can greatly influence many of the degenerative disorders they see in their daily practice, and will realize the potential of testosterone treatment in achieving the overall physical and mental welfare of their male patients.

In general, the more we learn about the multifaceted role that testosterone plays in male health and disease, the more difficult it becomes to think of a group of physicians who would not benefit from the detailed appreciation of the consequences of androgen deficiency and its treatment which this work sets out to provide.

References

1. Kalache A. Gender-specific health care in the 21st century: a focus on developing countries. *Aging Male* 2002;5:129–38

2. Brundtland GH. Report of the World Health Organisation; Active ageing: a policy framework. *Aging Male* 2002;5:1–37

3. Marmot MG, *et al. The English Longitudinal Study of Ageing.* London: Department of Epidemiology and Public Health, Institute for Fiscal Studies and Department of Economics, UCL, 2003

4. Comas-Herrera A, Wittenberg R, Pickard L, Knapp M, and Medical Research Council-Cognitive Function and Ageing Study. *Cognitive impairment in older people: its implications for future demand for services and costs.* PSSRU 1728. London: Alzheimer's Research Trust, 2003:1–7

5. Morales A, Lunenfeld B. Investigation, treatment and monitoring of late-onset hypogonadism in males. Official recommendations of ISSAM. International Society for the Study of the Aging Male. *Aging Male* 2002; 5:74–86

6. Collins P. Coronary artery function and androgens. *Aging Male* 2001; 4:38–9

7. English KM, Mandour O, Steeds RP, Diver MJ, Jones TH, Channer KS. Men with coronary artery disease have lower levels of androgens than men with normal coronary angiograms [see Comments]. *Eur Heart J* 2000; 21:890–4

8. Conway AJ, Handelsman DJ, Lording DW, Stuckey B, Zajac JD. Use, misuse and abuse of androgens. The Endocrine Society of Australia consensus guidelines for androgen prescribing. *Med J Aust* 2000;172: 220–4

9. Liverman CT, Blazer DG. Institute of Medicine Committee on Assessing the Need for Clinical Trials of Testosterone Replacement Therapy. *Testosterone and Aging: Clinical Research Directions.* Washington, DC: The National Academies Press, 2004.

2 History of testosterone

Hormones have a long, exciting and checkered history, and that of testosterone is the longest, most exciting and most checkered. However, its history is part of the problem in androgen deficiency being accepted as a common and important condition, so it is worth looking back to see where the maze of myths surrounding testosterone started.

The word 'hormone' was introduced in 1905 by a British physiologist, Professor Ernest Starling, in a lecture he was giving at the Royal College of Physicians in London. It was derived by two scholarly dons in Cambridge from the Greek verb *hormao*, meaning to put into quick motion, to excite or to arouse. He used it to describe the 'chemical messengers' that were released into the bloodstream by the body's ductless, or endocrine glands (*endo*, internal, plus *krino*, secrete), such as the testis, thyroid and adrenals, compared with the external (*exo*, outside) secretions of glands with ducts, the exocrine glands, such as those that produce saliva or tears. This heralded the birth of the science of hormones, or endocrinology, which lived up to its prophetic name by making rapid advances that excited both the public and the medical imagination and often aroused great passion and controversy.

Typically, the history of any one hormone goes through four stages. First there is the observation that a gland or organ produces an internal secretion that has a general effect on the body. Second, methods of detecting the internal secretion and measuring its effects are developed. This is usually initially by biological assay, seeing what action the preparation containing the hormone has on an animal or organ lacking it. Later, chemical methods of measurement can be found. Third, the hormone is extracted from the gland or organ, and isolated in a pure form. Fourth, chemists define its structure and synthesize it.

We will see how testosterone was unique in being the first hormone to be recognized and measured, but because of the complexity of its molecule, it was relatively slow to be isolated and synthesized.

ANTIQUITY

The observation that castration makes the eunuch, properly credited to primitive man, ushered in the dawn of hormone research. The fact that the testes are so easily removed in many species, including man, with dramatic, obvious and widespread consequences, has caused them to be described as the oldest key to the treasure-trove of knowledge about hormones. To para-pharase one of Sir Winston Churchill's most famous sayings: 'Never in the field of human science was so much learned by so many by the removal of so little.'

As the journalist Paul de Kruif wrote in his excellent book on *The Male Hormone – A New Gleam of Hope for Prolonging Man's Prime of Life*, printed in 1945[1]: 'From the beginning of human record, priests, saints, medicine men, farmers and sultans had been demonstrating how clear-cut, sure and simple it was to take the vigour of animals and men away. How? By removing their testicles.'

He went on to put the important question: 'Why didn't they reason that older men, losing their youth gradually, might also be suffering a slow, chemical castration taking place invisibly with the passage of time?' He then documented the slow march of the 'hormone hunters' towards their goal of the 'rescue of broken men', providing them with a 'new lease on life' by iso-lating and then synthesizing testosterone. However, his message has had to wait another 50 years to be heard.

Castration carried out on young boys was always recognized as prevent-ing the onset of puberty, with lack of body hair or beard, more feminine fat distribution and a high-pitched voice much valued in singing. This was thought to be worth the sacrifice by some Italian singers, the 'castrati', or at least their managers, as graphically shown in the film *Farinelli, Il Castrato*. Eunuchs were also known not to develop the male pattern of baldness, and to be less muscular.

Depending on how long after puberty it was performed, castration, as well as making the eunuch infertile, reduced his sexual and other drives, but did not invariably make him lose erectile power. The more potent were used by Roman women, particularly when their husbands were away fight-ing for the empire, for recreation without procreation. This suggests that in the younger male, erections can be achieved at much lower than average levels of testosterone. However, as other physical factors such as a reduc-tion in the number of steroid receptors and vascular damage occur, and psy-chological factors such as stress and familiarity set in, the required testosterone threshold is likely to rise.

Eunuchs were also known to be less competitive and aggressive. In the Byzantine period, for the 1000 years from about AD 400, the empire was run increasingly by eunuchs, who were efficient, but predictably unadven-turous and did what they were told. Similarly, they played an important part in the administration of the Imperial Court. They presumably knew their place, and posed no threat to the Emperor or those vying for power.

Likewise, farmers of antiquity knew that castration could be used to fatten pigs, bullocks and cockerels to produce capons. The taming of wild animals for domestic purposes, and tempering the fiery nature of both horses and dogs, made the psychological effects of castration in other species equally apparent.

About 4000 years ago the *Pen Tsao*, the Chinese 'Great Herbal', recommended use of the semen of young men for the treatment of sexual weakness in the elderly, a remedy no doubt popular with the wives of impotent potentates.

In India, the Hindu Ayervedic system of medicine, which developed from 1400 BC onwards, suggested the consumption of testicular tissue to treat impotence and obesity. It was also known at that time that hot baths could reduce fertility, which is still news over 3000 years later.

The great physician Hippocrates, who is said to have created medicine as both an art and a science, lived during the golden age of Greek culture, being born in 460 BC and dying at the age of over 90. His contemporaries included Socrates, Plato, Aristophanes, Euripides and Sophocles, and yet, of all these, his reputation is probably the greatest. His is the moral medical code still used as the basis of medical ethics.

In the many classic writings noted by his pupils, he observed that gout does not appear before puberty, and that eunuchs do not develop it at all. Modern theory would suggest that the high levels of uric acid needed to cause this exquisitely painful condition of the joints, characteristically of the feet, come from breakdown of the protein in the large muscle masses which testosterone produces in the postpubertal male. Another interesting observation he made was that women did not suffer from it until after the menopause.

He also knew that mumps could be followed by inflammation of the testes known as orchitis, and then sterility. As described later, this, together with other viral illnesses such as glandular fever which cause testicular damage, can contribute to early onset of the andropause.

Nearly 2000 years ago, the Greek physician Pliny recommended eating animal testicles to improve sexual function. This remedy is still popular in many countries, especially Spain, where cooked bulls' testes are served as the delicacy known as 'cojones'. Not coincidently, this is also the Spanish word for 'courage'. Unfortunately, any benefits obtained from eating such dishes are likely to be more morale-boosting than hormone-boosting, because although most of the body's supply of testosterone is made in the testes, it is rapidly exported to the rest of the body in the bloodstream, and there is little on site at any one time.

For example, when chemists first extracted the hormone from bulls' testes in the early 1930s, it took several tons to produce a few hundred milligrams, the dose currently used as 1 day's supply for a patient. To make things worse, testosterone taken by mouth, unless it is in a special easily absorbed and stable form, is broken down in the liver, and never gets into the general circulation. This makes Pliny's treatment, although it must have seemed a theoretically good idea at the time, practically useless apart from the doubtlessly strong placebo effect of many exotic remedies.

Later, the Graeco-Roman physician Aretaeus, who gave the first detailed description of sugar diabetes, wrote: 'For it is the semen, when possessed of vitality, which makes us to be men, hot, well braced in limbs, well-voiced, spirited, strong to think and act'. He added the rider: 'For when the semen is not possessed of its vitality, persons become shrivelled', which is a good description of the wrinkled skin and wasted muscles of the testosterone-deficient male.

The message in Judaic medicine derived from the Old Testament is that health is the gift of God, and disease His wrath. This can therefore only be prevented by submission, atonement, prayer, moral reform or sacrifice, which are still unpopular remedies, and may be ineffective if left too late. It was also recognized that stress, disease, fatigue and starvation could reduce the amount of semen, which are all factors now known to lower testosterone levels, particularly in older men.

The Bible differentiated between those who developed eunuchoid features because of diseased or undescended testes, known in Egypt as those 'castrated by Ra', the sun-god, 'sun-castrates', and those castrated by man, 'man-castrates'. When castration was performed for religious reasons, the penis was often removed as well, a mutilation now only seen in some transvestites.

This differentiation is described in Matthew, Chapter 19, Verse 12, and Jesus is quoted as saying: 'For there are some eunuchs, which were so born from their mother's womb: and there are some eunuchs, which were made eunuchs of men: and there be eunuchs which have made themselves eunuchs for the kingdom of heaven's sake.' In the last category, he appears to be referring to priests who achieved celibacy without going to such extreme measures.

In India, those who renounce sexual activity because they believe it dissipates their spiritual energy are known as 'bramacharya'. In Hindu tradition, it is one of the requirements of becoming a monk or swami. A vegetarian diet may help them to make this difficult sacrifice and keep from straying from the spiritual path by decreasing the amount of cholesterol available for testosterone production.

This was confirmed in 1984 when a Swedish study showed that switching from a high- to a low-fat diet, particularly one high in polyunsaturates, lowered blood testosterone levels by 10%. This makes sense in evolutionary terms, as the aggressive killer-instinct of the hunter, red in tooth and claw, would be enhanced by the higher level of testosterone produced by having a higher-fat, higher-cholesterol diet than that of his more placid herbivorous prey.

The beadle of the parish in Dickens' story *Oliver Twist*, Mr Bumble, rebuked the undertaker who employed Oliver until he got into a fight, with the words: 'You never should have given the boy meat. Meat heats the blood.'

Recent research has shown that diets high in protein and fat can raise total testosterone, and lower the testostosterone-binding protein, sex hormone-binding globulin (SHBG), which has a double effect in raising the free testosterone in the blood[2]. Perhaps the old man who for many years used to wander up and down Oxford Street in London with sandwich boards denouncing the 'passion proteins' in meat, declaring that they led to war, may have stumbled onto an important truth.

Also, the estrogens present in many plants, phytoestrogens, can antagonize the effects of testosterone and give a more female type of fat distribution. The plants richest in these phytoestrogens are soy, particularly tofu and miso, citrus fruits, wheat, liquorice, alfalfa, fennel and celery, which may be why some vegetarian yogis have enlarged breasts, a condition known as gynecomastia, and large abdomens. Pliny recorded 2000 years ago that 'Hempseed and chondrion make men impotent'. Also, heavy beer drinkers, because of the phytoestrogens in hops, as well as the calories from the alcohol, and its damaging effect on the testes and liver, can show enlarged breasts and a 'beer-belly', as well as the erection problems described as 'brewer's droop'.

The most influential physician of Roman times was Galen (AD 130–200), who is considered the greatest medical man of antiquity after Hippocrates. He wrote more than 100 books, whose influence carried on for more than 1500 years, well into the Renaissance period and beyond. However, he could also be thought of as the founding father of medical dogmatism, in that his system was so authoritative and rigid that it almost completely stifled fresh ideas throughout that time.

In spite of this, Galen could be thought of as the forerunner of sex hormone theory and research. He describes how the 'maleness' of men could cease with castration, and the 'femaleness' of women with disease or aging of the ovaries. He noted that these sexual characteristics were generalized throughout the body in all the species he studied, and were not purely genital, being seen, for example, in the lion's mane, the cockscomb and the boar's tusk. These remote and widespread effects are the characteristic features of hormonal action.

He also raised a key question of great importance to our thinking in relation to the reduction in vitality as well as virility seen in the andropausal male, when he asked in his book *Peri spermatos* ('On the Seed'): 'What is, therefore, the cause, that castrates slow down in their whole vital capacity?' He remarks in this book that castrated animals lose not only the power to procreate, but also the desire to do so, as well as undergoing the characteristic changes in normal male fat and hair distribution well recognized in eunuchs. In modern medical parlance, they show all the signs of testosterone deficiency.

RENAISSANCE PERIOD

It was only with the wave of radical new thinking that swept through Europe at the beginning of the 16th century that medicine broke free of the bondage imposed on it by Galen's words. This rebirth in both the arts and the sciences was precipitated by two events. One was the fall of Constantinople in 1453, which ended the Byzantine Empire and caused many scholars to move from there to Italy. As a result, there was a revival of Greek medical thought in terms of the ideas and observations of Hippocrates, rather than the unquestionable dogma of Galen.

The other was the information revolution started by the printing of the Gutenberg Bible in 1454, which soon led to the production of medical texts. Let us hope that the new information revolution produced by the computer and the Internet, which is starting to give us access to medical databases all over the world, will produce even greater advances in freedom of thought on all medical subjects, including the andropause.

One of the most remarkable physicians from this period was Paracelsus (1493–1541), or to give him his full title, Aureolus Theophrastus Bombastus von Hohenheim, the most important medical thinker of the 16th century. As his name suggests, he was a Swiss, a swashbuckling physician and chemist, who not only had the audacity to challenge Galen's ideas, but also publicly burned his books. He revived Hippocratic thought and ideals in medicine and introduced many new ideas of his own, especially in relation to thyroid disease. He died unloved and unrecognized by the medical establishment of his day, but left a legacy of original thought which became part of the active ferment that led to fresh medical thinking and experimentation on hormonal factors in health and disease. It influenced Charles Darwin, who appealed to scientists to abandon intellectual 'idolatry'.

Paracelsus introduced a new vision of disease as a distinct, explicable entity which could and should be treated, rather than the Galenic view that most conditions were untreatable, which encouraged the population to bear with fatalistic resignation. For example, he successfully introduced mercurials for the treatment of syphilis, the most feared disease of the 16th century, which was viewed in the same light as autoimmune deficiency syndrome (AIDS) is in the present day.

How did the intelligent public view aging in the male at that time? With his usual intuitive clinical accuracy, Shakespeare, about 400 years ago, described in his play *As You Like It* the seven ages of man, and we can now recognize how each age is influenced by the effects of testosterone:

At first the infant,
Mewling and puking in the nurse's arms.

In the infant there is no real difference between testosterone levels in the male and the female, although intrauterine differences have left their physical and emotional imprints.

And then the whining schoolboy, with his satchel,
And shining morning face, creeping like snail,
Unwillingly to school.

The surge of testosterone at puberty generates the rebellious male nature, as well as the increase in skin oil or sebum, which makes the skin shine and later in excess causes acne. The sexual characteristics of the adult male appear.

And then the lover,
Sighing like furnace, with a woeful ballad
Made to his mistress' eyebrow.

With the libido driven by the peaking levels of testosterone in the 20s going full blast, and rampant priapic power available, mating and procreating activities normally tend to predominate.

Then a soldier,
Full of strange oaths, and bearded like the pard,
Jealous in honour, sudden and quick in quarrel,
Seeking the bubble reputation
Even in the cannon's mouth.

High levels of testosterone in the 30s still make him belligerent and drive him through what is often a period of questing and hasty decisions, the 'midlife crisis'.

And then the justice,
In fair round belly with good capon lin'd,
With eyes severe, and beard of formal cut,
Full of wise saws and modern instances.

In the 40s and 50s, with testosterone levels declining and SHBG rising, the scene is set for the andropause to appear along with the fatty degeneration shared with the capon, showed by weight gain and the muscle deterioration seen first in the Elizabethan 'couch potato's' expanding waistline. Extremes of this condition are now recognized as the 'metabolic syndrome' which is beginning to become more common in this age group.

The sixth age shifts
Into the lean and slipper'd pantaloon,
With spectacles on nose and pouch on side,
His youthful hose well sav'd a world too wide
For his shrunk shank; and his big manly voice,
Turning again towards childish treble, pipes
And whistles in his sound.

In the 60s and 70s, the decreasing free testosterone levels and lack of phys-ical activity fail to maintain muscle mass, particularly in the legs, so that the calves and thighs shrink. Osteoporosis of the spine can cause loss of height and kyphosis at this age, as well as death from a fractured hip. Extreme lack of testosterone can also result in thinning of the vocal cords, which return to their prepubertal state, giving a higher pitch. This can terminate an opera singer's career, when his vocal cords, like his skin, become more easily damaged, and can no longer sustain the great roles.

> *Last scene of all,*
> *That ends this strange eventful history,*
> *Is second childishness, and mere oblivion,*
> *Sans teeth, sans eyes, sans taste, sans everything.*

The old saying that what you do not use you lose comes sadly true at this stage of life, and there is considerable evidence to suggest that testosterone treatment can slow the rate of physical and mental deterioration in the final stages of life, and help men to maintain both the will and the ability to continue active life until they drop.

Shakespeare also wrote: 'Is it not strange that desire should so many years outlive performance?', a question which taxes the minds of doctors and their patients to this day. The answer could well be that lower levels of testosterone are needed to maintain libido than are required for potency, and there are many complex circulatory factors involved in obtaining an erection, and well as the hormonal drive. The spirit is often still willing long after the flesh has weakened, although following repeated erectile failures the desire tends eventually to fade also.

EIGHTEENTH AND NINETEENTH CENTURIES

The dominant figure in experimental medicine in the 18th century was the British surgeon John Hunter (1728–1793). Among his amazing range of original studies were experiments supporting his view that sexual characteristics 'depend on the effects that the ovaria and testicles have upon the constitution'. He obtained evidence for this statement in a variety of ways.

An interesting experiment on how the testes were enlarged in the mating season in a variety of animals was carried out by killing and preserving a series of London cock sparrows at monthly intervals from midwinter to spring. His students later reported Hunter's demonstration that 'The one killed in December has testes not bigger than a small pin's head, the rest are gradually larger, the testes of the last, killed in April, are as large as the top of your little finger.' It is now known that this seasonal growth of the testes, with its accompanying surge in testosterone, is due to longer days triggering the pineal gland at the base of the brain to switch off production of its 'hibernation hormone' melatonin. This in turn causes the pituitary gland to produce more of the gonadotropins, luteinizing hormone (LH) and follicle-stimulating hormone (FSH), which rouse the dormant testes to spring-fever pitch, increasing both testosterone and sperm production. It seems, however, that the bright city lights are now suppressing this seasonal cycle, and causing mating activity in cosmopolitan sparrows all year round. Although in humans there is a slight surge in conception rates around holiday periods such as Christmas, there is a larger rise in late spring and early summer, so we retain this link between sunshine and sex.

What has not been sufficiently recognized is that Hunter carried out transplantation experiments which showed that if the spur of a hen was transplanted to a cock, it would grow to the size of a cock's spur. He went on to demonstrate that if the small spur of a young cock was transplanted to a hen, it failed to grow at all. In 1771 he also transplanted cocks' testicles into their abdomens, and observed that they continued to grow there, and into the same site in hens, with some evidence of a masculinizing effect.

However, he failed to publish his results, illustrating the truth of that old medical dictum 'publish or perish'. It was not until over 70 years later, in 1849, that a German professor at the University of Göttingen, Adolf Berthold, who knew of Hunter's work, repeated the experiment, showing that capons could grow into normal cocks following testicular transplants. He wrote: 'They crowed quite considerably, often fought among themselves and with other young roosters, and showed a normal inclination to hens.' In particular, the transplants prevented atrophy of the comb, restoring this dramatic red crowning glory of the male of the species which signals his sexual maturity.

This was clear proof that the testis produced a substance which traveled in the blood to maintain the sexual characteristics of the adult male animal. This first well-documented successful hormone replacement therapy inaugurated a century of attempts to use testicular extracts or implants to rejuvenate men. However, most of these attempts were either of doubtful effectiveness, mainly relying on the placebo effect of giving patients a novel form of treatment, or fraudulent confidence tricks based on the instinctive wish for a long and active life. It is difficult to this day to decide whether doctors offering rejuvenation treatments are 'leading-edge pioneers' or 'medical buccaneers' who navigate 'this poorly charted sea of medical research'. This is still hotly debated today. Time, experience and future research will tell.

One who must certainly be regarded as a pioneer was the eminent neurologist and physiologist Charles Edouard Brown-Séquard (1817–1894). He had a distinguished career in France, where he had been the successor of the celebrated physiologist Claude Bernard at the Sorbonne in Paris, and had held posts in Britain and America, as well as being the first to demonstrate that the adrenal glands are essential to life.

However, his colleagues became critical of his ideas when, in 1869, he suggested that 'the feebleness of old men is in part due to the diminution in function of the testicles'. He also said that 'if it were possible to inject, without danger, sperm into the veins of old men, one would be able to obtain with them some manifestations of rejuvenation at once with respect to intellectual work and the physical powers of the organism'.

They were even more skeptical when, in 1889, still actively researching his ideas at the age of 72, he announced at a learned gathering in Paris that he had mentally and physically rejuvenated himself with subcutaneous injections of extracts of the testicles of dogs and guinea pigs. Within 3 weeks the *British Medical Journal* had published a report on his lecture criticizing his ideas and the manner of their presentation. Under the heading of 'The pentacle of rejuvenescence', it said sarcastically that 'The statements he made – which unfortunately attracted a good deal of attention in the public press – recall the wild imaginings of mediaeval philosophers in search of an elixir vitae.' Similar responses to reports of the benefits of treating the andropause are still prevalent over 100 years later. Looking back, Brown-Séquard's ghost might well comment, 'plus ça change, plus c'est la même chose'.

In Britain and America his results were said to be due to autosuggestion, or even hypnosis, which was very fashionable in France at the time. He tried to counteract this notion by not giving the patients any idea of the results he was expecting, although any treatment by such a distinguished and imposing professor must have had some placebo effect. He also sent his extracts to sympathetic colleagues in Britain and America, and although some reported good results, the general medical reaction in Britain to what rapidly became known as one type of 'organotherapy', treatment with glandular extracts or transplants, was hostile. However, some of the critics were given pause for thought by work going on at the same time on the more obvious, reproducible and clear-cut benefits of treating thyroid deficient, myxedematous, patients with thyroid extracts.

In America, however, the reactions to Brown-Séquard's work were over-enthusiastic, and the testicular extract was widely inflicted by charlatans on a gullible public as 'the elixir of life' for every type of ailment from senility to tuberculosis. This and other 'organotherapies' became even more fashionable because of the simultaneous introduction of 'serotherapies', the use of sera and vaccines of animal origin for the prevention and treatment of infectious diseases.

Particularly in Victorian Britain, studies in matters relating to sexual activity were considered unsuitable topics for research. Brown-Séquard died a discredited man, he who 'made the blunder that put the male hormone in the scientific dog-house', as Paul de Kruif points out[1]. Moralists were quick to jump on this failure in therapy, and as he documents, the ridicule that it brought to the whole field of research into the hormonal functions of the testis has lasted to the present day, and is an unfortunate legacy. Brown-Séquard's mistake at the end of a long and innovative career in research is still being used by opponents as evidence against the existence of the andropause to this day.

Even learned and very influential physiologists such as Sir Edward Schafer, who wrote many papers and a book on *Endocrine Organs*, had a Freudian block about reproductive hormones, and in a lecture on 'Internal Secretions' given to the British Medical Association in London in 1895, he denied that the testes had any endocrine actions. It is amazing that so great a pioneer in other areas of endocrinology could have had so complete a blind spot to the millennia of evidence to the contrary. However, we hear

echoes of this disapproval of research into the effects of testosterone treatment in relation to slowing the aging process even now

What also had a bad but unforeseen long-term result in relation to the acceptance of testosterone treatment by doctors and the general public was an experiment by two Austrian doctors in 1896, who claimed that testicular extracts of
bulls' testicles could improve the strength of their hand muscles. They concluded that: 'The training of athletes offers an opportunity for further research
in this area.' This report foreshadowed the damaging influence of steroid abuse
by athletes on the medical and public image of testosterone treatment.

TWENTIETH CENTURY

Although 'organotherapy' using extracts of different glands, particularly the
thyroid and adrenal, continued to be the subject of much speculation and
experimentation, it soon became clear that testicular extracts were not sufficiently powerful to have the hoped-for and much publicized effects originally claimed. This was because the minute amount of testosterone produced
in the testis is continuously being swept away into the bloodstream, and is
not stockpiled in the gland.

Remembering the work of Hunter and Berthold, doctors attempted what
would be a difficult feat even nowadays, that of transplanting testicles from
man to man. In 1912 and 1913 there were reports of the first two apparently successful operations in America. The second of these was performed
by a Dr Victor D. Lespinasse of Chicago, who reported full restoration of
libido and sexual function over a 2-year period in a man previously without
desire, and impotent from the loss of both testes.

Although the First World War delayed endocrine research and stopped
communication between doctors working in different European countries
for many years, there was an interesting report that the famous Danish
surgeon Thorkild Rovsing carried out an experiment which seemed to indicate that testicular function might be important in relation to the circulation, as indeed Brown-Séquard had claimed. After a young soldier had been
killed in battle, Rovsing transplanted his testicles into an old man with gangrene, which then, according to the case report, healed completely.

In 1918 the resident physician in San Quentin Prison in California, Dr
Leo L. Stanley, who had access to many fresh testicles 'donated' by
executed prisoners, started transplanting them into other inmates of various
ages. Some of these regained their sexual potency, although how this was
measured in the prison is unclear, and freedom is a great aphrodisiac. Two
years later, because of 'the scarcity of human material' even in that situation, he moved on to transplanting into his rapidly expanding patient population the testes of rams, goats, deer and boars, which, perhaps suspiciously,
seemed to be equally effective. Interestingly, as with Rovsing, gangrene was
among the wide range of conditions from senility to diabetes which he
claimed to benefit.

In the early 1920s, a flamboyant Russian-French surgeon called Serge Voronoff, working in Algiers, made his fame and fortune by transplanting chimpanzee and baboon testicles into humans, and claimed they had powerful rejuvenating effects. This work naturally attracted great medical and public interest, and international deputations of doctors as well as patients from many countries made the pilgrimage to Algiers to investigate his 'monkey gland' treatment.

If Voronoff was just fooling people, he did so with a lot of detailed evidence and seemingly convincing results for at least a decade. Even one of the leading professors of physiology of his time, Samson Wright, described Voronoff's work in detail in his standard textbook of the day in 1926[3]: 'In successful cases it is claimed that very striking results are obtained from this operation. Old people, with marked signs of senility, are claimed to be thus transformed into vigorous energetic individuals. Previously castrated persons may regain their secondary sex character – e.g. growth of beard and moustache may occur.'

The same writer obviously took this work seriously because he went on to say: 'While Voronoff's operation appears quite justifiable in young subjects in whom the testes have been damaged or destroyed by injury or disease, the treatment of senility by this method is more questionable. We have no proof whatever that senility is solely due to atrophic changes in the testis; it is almost certain that many other factors are concerned. Though the testicular graft may stimulate physical activity and sexual desire, it cannot restore the worn heart, arteries and essential organs to their normal state. There is a grave danger that excessive strain may be put on damaged structures, with disastrous results.'

Similar lines of argument are used up to the present day by doctors who urge that testosterone deficiency is a natural part of aging, and to reverse it in an elderly patient must automatically be dangerous.

ISOLATION AND SYNTHESIS OF TESTOSTERONE

As the war clouds cleared in Europe after the First World War, a great pharmacological arms race developed, with three drugs firms competing to be the first to produce the active ingredient of the testicles in pure chemical form. It is an amazing story of synchronicity that, after a search for the essence of manhood lasting over 4000 years, the three different groups passed the finishing post within 4 months of each other.

First past the post on 27 May 1935 was Ernst Laqueur, a professor of pharmacology in Amsterdam, who led an excellent research team for the Organon drug company, and emerged triumphant with a few precious crystals from a veritable mountain of bulls' testicles. He submitted a paper called 'On crystalline male hormone from testicles' and coined the name 'testosterone' for it.[4]

Second was a formidable, dynamic German chemist with a dueling scar on his left cheek, Professor Adolf Butenandt. He was working for the Schering Company in Berlin, and had succeeded in collecting 25 000 l of policemen's urine, enough to fill an Olympic size swimming pool. From this, Butenandt, with bravery clearly above and beyond the call of duty, extracted 15 mg, a few crystals, of a relatively inactive urinary breakdown product of testosterone called androsterone.[5]

He then decided that the method of preparation was too much like hard work, and thought up the much more commercial way by which testosterone is made to this day. He methodically worked out its structure and then produced it, as does the body, from cholesterol, its natural precursor. He sent his paper on this process and the structure of testosterone itself to the German *Journal of Physiological Chemistry* on 24 August 1935[6].

Just 1 week later a Swiss chemical journal received a paper from Leopold Ruzicka[7], a Yugoslavian chemist working for the Ciba company in Zurich, announcing a patent on the method of production of testosterone from cholesterol. For this work, he and Butenandt received the Nobel Prize in 1939.

Within 2 years of these momentous discoveries a variety of testosterone preparations were in clinical use. It had soon been found that, because it was an oily substance which did not dissolve readily in water, in the pure form it could not be absorbed by mouth. A slow-release form that could be given by injection, testosterone propionate, was one of the most widely used, and proved very successful in patients whose testes were insufficiently active for a variety of reasons. Rather like the insulin injections for diabetics which had been introduced 15 years earlier, it was dramatically effective in relieving symptoms of the 'male climacteric'[8]. Now that you could 'get it in a bottle', testicular transplants and extracts went out of the window.

Case reports and small series of patients in the late 1930s and throughout the 1930s and 1940s showed a wide range of benefits in a wide range of conditions, ranging from heart and circulatory problems, including even gangrene, to diabetes.

Although the injections lasted about 3 days, another form of testosterone, as compressed crystals fused together to form tablets and later small cylindrical pellets, which under local anesthetic could be implanted under the skin of the buttock or abdomen, was introduced. This was both effective and convenient, as the implant continued to act for 6 months[9]. Sixty years later this is still one of the best methods of giving long-term testosterone treatment. There are few medical preparations, particularly in endocrinology, which have stood the test of time so well.

A third type of preparation which was also made in the early years was a water-soluble form called methyltestosterone. Unfortunately, although effective in relieving symptoms, this proved very toxic, especially to the liver. As it was so widely used for over 50 years, and was included in a wide range of under-the-counter, gold- and silver-covered pills, attributed with almost magical powers in the sexual arena, it has done a great deal of harm to the safety image of testosterone in many doctors' minds. Although still available in the USA, it has been taken off the market throughout the rest of the world, where several safe oral forms have been introduced[10].

TESTOSTERONE TREATMENT

From 1940 onwards, largely because of the obvious improvements brought about by testosterone, it was generally accepted by many doctors that there was a group of symptoms commonly experienced by men in their 50s that were similar to the female menopause or 'climacteric', from the Greek word *klimakter*, meaning the rung of a ladder, and hence a critical period in life at which the vital force begins to decline.

Dr August Werner

Rating scales for diagnosis of the andropause have evolved since the earliest descriptions of the symptoms of 'the male climacteric' by Dr August Werner from 1939 onwards[8]. This is probably because not only was he working with menopausal women, and consistently pointed out the similarity of symptoms in the two sexes, but also, since the first synthetic testosterones and estrogens had become available in the mid-1930s, he could clearly show how the symptoms could be relieved in both by hormonal treatment.

Interestingly, in his collected works and autobiography published in 1952[11], he recounts how at the age of 54 he experienced the same symptoms as his female menopausal patients had been describing:

> *About 1937 Dr Werner, almost suddenly, developed all of these symptoms in a severe form, which left no doubt in his mind that the male of the species is also subject to this condition. A perusal of his reports on the male climacteric should be convincing.*

Indeed, doctors who have experienced these symptoms of the andropause, the impact that it can have on all aspects of their lives and the relief which testosterone treatment rapidly provides are amongst the most dedicated practitioners of the art and science of androgen replacement.

Dr Werner was Assistant Professor of Internal Medicine at St Louis University School of Medicine. His series of key papers detailing his experience with the 'male climacteric' were published between 1939 and 1946, describing its symptomatology and the effects of treatment with testosterone in prestigious journals such as the *Journal of the American Medical Association*, and the *Journal of Urology*.

In his first article in 1939 he made several key points[8] based on his observations of a few cases studied in his practice. In his opening sentences he states:

It seems reasonable to believe that many if not all men pass through a climacteric period somewhat similar to that of women, usually in a less severe but perhaps more prolonged form ... The average age of onset for women is about 40.8 years and for men approximately 48 to 50 years ... Again, because of the prevalent belief that men do not have a climacteric period (which has been based on cessation of menstruation in women) the condition has probably been overlooked or ignored in men.

The most prominent symptoms he described were loss of potency and libido, but in addition he mentions that, as with women, he observed:

intense subjective nervousness, definite emotional instability characterised by irritability, sudden change in mood, decreased memory and ability for mental concentration, decreased interest in the usual activities, a desire to be left alone, and depression and crying. There may be tachycardia ... palpitation even on moderate effort, vertigo with or without change of position, scotomas, tinnitus, numbness and tingling of the extremities, fatigability and disturbed sleep ... The neurocirculatory symptoms such as hot flushes and suddenly increased perspiration ... occur irregularly. The symptoms which are mental and psychic ... are usually more constant. The climacteric disturbance may be so severe in some men that they become despondent and develop a psychosis with thoughts of self destruction. It is very probable that many men have committed suicide and no one could understand the reason for their having done so.

Of the effects of treatment with 10 mg of testosterone propionate (Perandren®; Ciba) in 1 ml oil given intramuscularly three times a week, he wrote:

Adequate clinical treatment with testosterone propionate was causally associated with remarkable clinical improvement characterised by a marked increase in erectile capacity and sensitivity of the penis, in the strength of the sex urge and in the capacity to respond with the proper emotions not only to intercourse but also to other acts such as kissing or embracing ...

Also normal sex function and motivation were accompanied by great changes in the entire mental attitude of all patients ... Their previous despondency gave way to definite elation ... [They were] less broken in spirit and were more spontaneous in their interests and activity ... They exhibited more rational aggressiveness and less irrational irritability and sullen brooding. Nervousness and emotional instability were replaced by greater stability and control. Abnormal physical and mental fatigability disappeared. Energy and stamina returned.

These early clinical observations are quoted in length because they were not only confirmed by his subsequent careful study and documentation of several hundred 'male climacteric' patients over the subsequent 7 years, but also remain the common experience of all those involved in testosterone treatment of the andropause to this day.

His second paper on the subject in 1943 reported a more detailed study of 37 patients diagnosed as having the 'male climacteric'[12]. It gave for the first time an analysis of the frequency of the various symptoms, reporting 'nervousness' in 100%, decreased potency in 94.9% and libido in 89.2%, depression in 89.4%, decreased memory and concentration in 86.5% and fatigability and lassitude in 75.7%.

In this paper, he reported that increasing the dosage of testosterone propionate to 25 mg given on alternate days was more effective than the 10-mg doses given in his previous study. Although other symptoms were consistently relieved, he adds 'a word of caution' at the end of the paper about patients who are disappointed when their potency is not restored:

> It is questionable whether androgens should be administered to promote potency; at least, the return of potency should not be promised to the patient, and he should be advised that decrease in potency is a normal consequence of age and that the chief objective of treatment is relief of the symptoms.

These remarks coincide with the observations from the UK Andropause Study (UKAS) that, while complete remission of the majority of andropausal symptoms routinely occurred, potency was restored in only 67% of the cases treated with testosterone alone. This could be increased to over 95% by combining the testosterone with sildenafil, which further makes the point of the complex and multifactorial etiology of erectile dysfunction in men over the age of 40.

In a third and final paper written in 1946[13], reporting his experience in what by then were 273 cases diagnosed as 'male climacteric', he confidently asserts in his opening paragraph:

> That man is subject to varying degrees of sexual function and does have a climacteric is now an established fact.

There is still great argument about this statement over half a century later.
Concerning the age of onset of the condition, he writes:

> Hypogonadism produces a definite syndrome when it occurs during the period of active sexual life regardless of the age of the patient, except that the syndrome is less apt to occur or is apt to be less severe before the age of approximately 25 years ... The most prevalent time for this decline of gonadal function to occur in man is in later life, approximately from the ages of 45 to 55.

This is still the case at the beginning of the 21st century, the age range at which symptoms began in the 1500 patients in the UKAS being 31–88 years, mean 54.2 years, with 68% in the 45–55 age range (Appendix 3). Usually, as Dr Werner described in this report, those cases occurring in men under the age of 40 have a predisposing cause, such as primary hypogonadism from late or poor testicular descent, or damage due to severe mumps orchitis or following herniorrhaphy.

The paper is an excellent summary of his clinical experience in this field over the previous 8 years, and Dr Werner's list of symptoms became the standard means of diagnosing the andropause, or 'male climacteric' as it was then called, throughout the 1940s, and was routinely quoted by other physicians for diagnostic and treatment purposes[14,15]. The incidence of symptoms which Werner reported closely coincides with the Aging Male Symptom (AMS) scale, developed and validated over 50 years later by Prof Heinemann[16]. It is a significant body of practical clinical experience, carefully gathered throughout the 1940s, and should not be overlooked even by clinicians armed with the latest laboratory tests.

Drs Heller and Myers

An outstanding paper of this time, which used testosterone as definitive proof of the existence of the andropause, was published in the prestigious *Journal of the American Medical Association* in 1944. It was called 'The male climacteric: its symptomatology, diagnosis and treatment', and was by two American doctors, Carl G. Heller and Gordon B. Myers. It is well worth looking at this paper in detail, as the case has seldom if ever been better made[14].

The symptoms which they attributed to the male climacteric were exactly as described in Chapter 4 on diagnosis, i.e. nervousness, depression, impaired memory, the inability to concentrate, easy fatigability, insomnia, hot flushes, sweating and loss of libido and potency. They began by listing all the points raised by those who were skeptical of the existence of this condition, and then used their clinical studies to answer them one by one.

The majority of these queries were based on the general view that no objective evidence had been put forward to prove it was an actual clinical entity, or to differentiate it from neurosis or impotence of purely emotional origin. Also, many men remained fertile to an advanced age, and did not show the marked physical changes in body form that women showed in the days before hormone replacement therapy (HRT) became commonplace.

To study these points, they developed a measure of testicular function based on the hormonal feedback mechanism which exists to control the production of testosterone by the testis in men, and estrogen by the ovary in women. When the level of testosterone in the former or estrogen in the latter drops, the pituitary releases more gonadotropins, LH and FSH. When the level of testosterone is adequate for the body's needs, the gonadotropins fall to a low level.

Lacking sensitive blood assays, they had to extract a 12-h overnight sample of each man's urine, inject the extract into immature female rats and measure the increase in weight of their ovaries caused by the gonadotropins in the sample. This simple biological test gave surprisingly clear-cut results. The urine of normal men, or those whose symptoms were due to anxiety or neurosis, showed virtually no gonadotropin activity in the urine. Those whose symptoms were due to a true male-climacteric syndrome showed high levels of urinary gonadotropins, as demonstrated by the ovaries of the test rats doubling or trebling in size.

This carefully performed and detailed study gave unequivocal evidence that the andropause was a physical fact, and not just a fiction created by the emotionally disturbed and neurotic. Also, when a therapeutic test was carried out on samples of both groups of men by giving injections of testosterone propionate, the neurotic group 'experienced little, if any, improvement in potency or in well-being'. By contrast, in the andropause group:

> *Definite improvement in the symptomatology was noted by the end of the second week in all of the twenty cases treated. Complete abolition of all vasomotor, psychic, constitutional and urinary symptoms was accomplished by the end of the third week in 17 of the 20 cases treated. In the remaining three cases vasomotor and urinary symptoms were abolished but the psychic and constitutional symptoms persisted in spite of continuation of treatment for several months and doubling the dosage for brief periods. It was concluded that these three persons were suffering from involutional melancholia [depression of old age].*

The same study also answered a frequent criticism of testosterone treatment to this day, that it will restore libido but not help problems with erections, leaving the patient more frustrated than before. The Heller and Myers experience coincides with my own when they stated: 'Sexual potency was restored to normal with these doses in all but two cases, in one of which involutional melancholia was present.' They go on to remark that with increased dosage, 'sexual vigour in both previously refractory cases exceeded that of normal men'.

They further gave evidence that this is a real response to testosterone treatment and not just a placebo effect:

> *In 14 cases therapy was subsequently withheld for from four to fourteen weeks and in all instances the symptoms returned and sexual potency was again lost. On resumption of the therapy with testosterone propionate, relief of symptoms was again afforded and sexual potency returned. Thus the specificity of therapy was established.*
>
> *To investigate further the possibility that the improvement may have been due to suggestion, placebo injections were administered. Ampoules containing 1 cc of sesame oil, packaged similarly to the original testos-*

terone propionate, were substituted without the patient's knowledge in several cases. No improvement was noted in any case.

As well as recommending pellet implants for long-term treatment, they made two final important points in this historic paper. These were that 'the male climacteric is not confined to middle and old age but may occur as early as the third decade', and they concluded that 'whereas in the female the menopause is an invariable and physiologic accompaniment of the ageing process, in the male the climacteric is an infrequent and pathologic accompaniment of the ageing process.' We will see later why the andropause may have become more common over half a century and yet remains under-recognized and -treated.

Dr Tiberius Reiter

Starting in 1950, a German physician who trained in Berlin, Edinburgh and Glasgow, but set up in private practice in London's Harley Street, used testosterone pellet implants to treat men in their 40s, 50s, 60s and 70s suffering what he called IDUT syndrome. These initials indicated the main features of the condition, which were impotence, depression, urinary disturbances and thyroid overactivity, and he attributed all these to testosterone deficiency. Included in the last term were irritability, headaches and attacks of rapid heartbeat, particularly at night, which just about completes the classic picture of the andropause.

Over 20 years he treated about 500 patients with very good clinical results. These he wrote up in considerable detail in five eloquent articles, and carefully documented the improvements in each symptom on his own rating scale. He also wrote a monograph describing his method of implanting testosterone pellets into the buttocks for Organon, the company who made the implants, and this is the same method used to this day and described in the chapter in this book on treatment.

I have spoken to his medical colleagues, several of his patients and his widow Nancy Reiter, and an interesting picture emerges of this remarkable man. He was a dynamic, charismatic individual who delighted in the improvements he saw in his patients' condition. He, too, believed in a broad approach to treatment, and would sometimes take his patients to his favorite fish restaurant to teach them at a pleasant practical level of the benefits to virility of eating oysters, because of their high zinc content.

As Nancy put it, he was regarded with 'plenty of scepticism from the medical world – but the patients kept coming!' A prophet unrecognized in Britain, he was well received in America, where he published articles in the *Journal of the American Geriatrics Society* in 1963, 1964 and 1965, and in the last year lectured at their 22nd Annual Meeting in New York City, receiving considerable interest and approval. He died much loved by his patients, but unrecognized by the medical profession, in 1972.

Dr Jens Moller

The Danish doctor Jens Moller was one of the great pioneers of testosterone treatment. With all the fire and tenacity of his Viking ancestors he fought a 30-year war for its use against the medical establishment in Denmark and throughout Europe. I had the privilege of working with him during the last 10 years of that war, and it was he who in 1977 first interested me in testosterone.

At the time I had been working as Senior Lecturer in Chemical Pathology at St Mary's Hospital Medical School in London. Although my office and research laboratory were located within the Department of Professor Vivian James, an eminent steroid biochemist, I was more excited by the stress hormones such as epinephrine and norepinephrine, which appeared to be more directly related to my theories on stress, tension and heart disease, my main area of research at the time.

However, I was very much interested in the benefits of exercise as a means of balancing the effects of stress and a way of protecting the heart from its effects. As part of this program of research, I was taking part in a study set up by the Medical Research Council at the City Gymnasium at Moorgate in London. The founder and owner of this gymnasium was an ex-Olympic weight lifting coach called Alistair Murray, who with tremendous energy and enthusiasm originated the use of vigorous but not violent exercise in the form of circuit training in both the prevention and treatment of heart disease in London businessmen. We later wrote a book together called *F40 – Fitness on Forty Minutes a Week*, based on his ideas and reporting this research[17].

One day while I was at the gym he called me into his office to meet a tall Dane with an interesting story. Although friendly, this doctor had a military bearing and the charm of a diplomat, which he could switch on or off at will, and when it was off he could be what he described as 'very direct'. He was in his 70s, but with the brisk manner and energy of a man 20 years younger, and I learned later that he had had a varied career which involved an amazing tale of how the subject of testosterone treatment could arouse extreme passions in the minds of medical men.

Born in North Jutland in 1904, he left home at the age of 16, and, even without a university education, became a successful entrepreneur, working in turn in Paris, London and Berlin. Even with money to burn he found his business career meaningless, and at the end of the Second World War he enrolled at the university medical school in Copenhagen, getting his entry qualifications in 3 months rather than the usual year. He qualified 5 years later at the age of 50, and began his medical career, which was to be as unusual and turbulent as his previous one in business.

After a variety of work in hospitals and the pharmaceutical industry, he decided he wanted to be a neurosurgeon and worked in Sweden for a time. As neurosurgical jobs were few and far between, he took a locum job with

Dr Tvedegaard, a private physician working in Copenhagen, a decision which was to alter the course of the rest of his career.

Dr Tvedegaard was already a controversial figure in Danish medicine because of his use of testosterone to treat severe arterial disease, particularly in the legs. He had studied the use of this hormone by German doctors and seen surprisingly good results, even in the most severe cases with gangrene spreading from the toes to the rest of the leg, especially in diabetic cases.

The typical history given by his patients was one of painful cramps in the calves of the legs on walking, especially uphill on cold days, classical intermittent claudication. As the blood supply became worse, this gradually progressed to more continuous pain even at rest, and in bed at night, so that the patient would have to hang his leg out of bed to ease the intense discomfort. Eventually the limb would stay cold and blue most of the time, and an otherwise trivial injury to the foot would turn into an infection leading to gangrene of one or more toes. According to conventional practice at the time, these would then have to be amputated, and the surgeons would start on what often turned out to be a series of amputations, 'nibbling' their way up one or both legs to above the knee.

Testosterone injections, often in considerably higher doses than generally prescribed, seemed to have halted or in some cases even reversed the otherwise inexorable process at almost any stage. Walking distances would be prolonged because the cramps in the calves would come on later and later, and even disappear. Night cramps would also go, greatly improving the quality of sleep. Cold, blue painful feet and legs would become pink and comfortable as the circulation mysteriously improved.

Even gangrene would heal without surgical intervention, much to the relief and delight of the patients and their relatives. Although this did not necessarily prolong their lives indefinitely, it did give them a much better quality of life and could prevent their becoming crippled by their circulatory problems. Many were the patients who went happier to their graves with two whole legs rather than one or none as a result of this testosterone treatment.

Although the medical establishment in Denmark generally remained hostile to the 'Dr Tvedegaard treatment', which they used to tell their students was 'hormonal humbug', Dr Moller's practice flourished.

As is traditional with native prophets, he began to receive much more recognition from the many distinguished doctors from America, Britain and all over Europe who came to visit his clinic, and it became his mission for the rest of his life to hammer home the message of the effectiveness and safety of testosterone.

To this end he established the 'European Organization for the Control of Circulatory Diseases' or EOCCD, at a meeting of the European Parliament in Strasbourg in 1976, and enlisted many prominent politicians as well as doctors in his fight against what he called 'the international enemy' of these disorders.

From 1977 onwards I made many visits to his clinic in Copenhagen, and saw for myself the dramatic benefits of testosterone treatment to the circulation, especially in the legs. Also, I went with him as he went round Europe in his capacity of President of the EOCCD, holding meetings in London, Luxembourg, Strasbourg, Bonn, Berlin and Munich. We visited many eminent authorities throughout Europe, and he achieved a great deal of scientific support for his ideas. It was difficult to keep up with him even when he entered his 80s, and it soon became apparent that he certainly took his own medicine, which was as effective for him as for his patients.

When he finally died in 1989, active to the last, he left thriving national and international organizations which are carrying on his work under the direction of his successor, Dr Michael Hansen, in Copenhagen. This seems a fitting guarantee that Dr Jens Moller's heroic work in the service of testosterone will continue to bear fruit.

The Favorable Forties

Even though the work of pioneers, such as Dr August Werner in St Louis[13], and Drs Heller and Myers[14] in Vancouver, Washington and Detroit, set an early lead throughout the 1940s in the recognition and treatment of what was then called the 'male climacteric', interest in the condition then seemed to fade from sight.

A book written in 1948[15] by Dr Elmer Sevringhaus, Director of Endocrine and Nutritional Clinics at the Gouverneur Hospital in New York, represented the peak of the 1940s' enthusiasm for treating the 'male climacteric'.

This book gave a clear and logical account of the condition and its treatment as seen by the American pioneers in the field nearly half a century before. It quoted the previously reported view of the editor of the *Journal of the American Medical Association* that 'there is no longer clinical doubt of the existence of a male climacteric'.

This was echoed by the widely reported views of the writer and pathologist, Paul de Kruif. In the last chapter of his book *The Male Hormone*[1], having taken methyltestosterone for 4 years following the abrupt onset of his classic andropausal symptoms, he remarks that:

> *Now I'm fifty-four years old, and there's so much left to do. I've grown old much too quick and smart much too late ... I feel that testosterone has already helped me. Of course the male hormone isn't the whole story. I'll watch my nutrition and go on supercharging myself with vitamins ... I'll stick to long hard walking in the dunes and along Lake Michigan in the wind and rain and sun. All this – plus methyl testosterone.*
>
> *I'll be faithful and remember to take my twenty or 30 milligrams a day of testosterone. I'm not ashamed that it's no longer made to its old*

degree by my own aging body. It's chemical crutches. It's borrowed manhood. It's borrowed time. But, just the same, it's what makes bulls bulls. And, who knows, maybe tomorrow, they'll hit on a simple dietary chemical trick that will, to a degree, bring back the power of the glands that make my own natural male hormone.

Meanwhile I'll keep taking the methyl testosterone that now gives me the total vitality to go on working and waiting for such a not impossible discovery. Here's hoping.

The nearest thing to the dietary supplement of his dreams to come along during the half-century since he wrote so eloquently about the slow 'chemical castration of men' is dehydroepiandrosterone (DHEA). Although much used in the USA, probably because of the still limited availability of safe testosterone preparations, it only raises testosterone levels a small amount. It may also boost estrogen production, adding to the harmful effects of these hormones in food and water, which can also contain other hormone disruptors such as antiandrogens, present in a wide and increasing variety of agrochemicals, preservatives and plastic containers.

Overall, the environmental factors affecting men's hormonal balance may well have got worse rather than better since de Kruif's day, and androgen antidotes are only just becoming more readily available again.

The dark ages of testosterone treatment

The years between the end of the 1940s and the beginning of the 1990s could be called the dark ages of testosterone treatment.

As reported earlier in the book, this was largely due to the negative image of the hormone which developed in both medical and lay minds because of its abuse by athletes and bodybuilders, as well as the prohibition by the Food and Drug Administration (FDA) in the USA of the safe and convenient preparations which were allowed onto the market elsewhere in the world. Meanwhile, the adverse side-effects of methyltestosterone, particularly its toxic effects on the liver and cardiovascular system, were being emphasized in the textbooks.

Also, when immunoassays of testosterone and the gonadotropins became available, they failed to show any consistent relationship to the symptoms of the andropause.

Because the climate of medical opinion was against the concept of the andropause, even when safer oral preparations such as testosterone undecanoate and mesterolone became available in the 1970s, only limited clinical trials were carried out. These lacked the double-blind, placebo-controlled design that became the norm for pharmaceutical research in the 1980s and 1990s, and so were largely ignored.

TWENTIETH CENTURY: DAWN OF THE TESTOSTERONE REVOLUTION

There were a wide range of factors emerging in the 1990s which led to what I have called 'the testosterone revolution' starting in the year 2000[18].

Largely because of the availability of safe oral androgen preparations, and the pioneer work of Professors Ebhard Nieschlag and Hermanne Behre in Germany[10], who determined the pharmacokinetics and safety parameters of these preparations and both the older injectables such as testosterone enanthate and the newer ones like testosterone buciclate, there was a resurgence of interest in androgen therapy throughout Europe.

This was given fresh impetus by the interest in androgen treatment as a form of male contraception, which resulted in the World Health Organization (WHO) steroid synthesis program, and the search for the ideal long-acting testosterone preparation to suppress spermatogenesis.

This coincided with more detailed work on the androgen receptor and its polymorphic variations underlying the principle of androgen resistance, and more detailed understanding of age-related changes in different androgens.

One of the most important of the workers in this field is Professor Alex Vermeulen at the University of Ghent, who from the early 1970s to the present day has conducted invaluable studies on the decline in testosterone levels in aging males. Working with his colleague Dr Jean Kaufman, he has recently produced evidence confirming that it is the free active testosterone level which falls more from age 25 to 75 (50%) than the total testosterone (30%)[19,20], because of the increased binding protein in the blood.

Using the current view that it is the drop in a man's present androgen levels compared with the high levels he had in his youth which determines whether he can be regarded as testosterone deficient, they found that more than 20% of men over age 60 had low total, and a slightly higher percentage but nevertheless low free, levels of the hormone.

A recent study by a German, Dr Leifke, in a large group of healthy non-obese men aged 20–80, showed a mean lifetime fall of 51% for total testosterone, 64% for free testosterone and 78% for bioavailable testosterone. These changes started in the third decade, and of the 60–80 age group, in relation to these different fractions of testosterone, 25%, 40% and 60%, respectively, could be considered androgen deficient by comparison with the lowest levels seen in the 20–29 age group[21].

Professor Louis Gooren of the Free University Hospital in Amsterdam confirmed these falls, and completed a 10-year study of oral testosterone treatment with Restandol®, showing it to be both effective and safe[22]. More recently, in a discussion of quality-of-life issues in the aging male, he raised the interesting question of why the halving of a man's youthful testosterone levels of 35 nmol/l to 17 nmol/l should be regarded as insufficient to bring on andropausal symptoms[23].

Meanwhile, other researchers during the 1980s and 1990s produced detailed evidence of the safety of even high doses of testosterone in relation to the heart and prostate, and defined the pharmacology and clinical uses of a wide variety of preparations[24].

First World Congress on the Aging Male, 1998

The First World Congress on the Aging Male in February 1998 was organized by a very dynamic and far-sighted Israeli physician and gynecologist, Professor Bruno Lunenfeld, president of the International Society for the Study of the Aging Male and editor in chief of *The Aging Male* journal, which he started that year. This journal has rapidly become the key reference source, and is compulsive reading for all those interested in the world view of men's health, and the important part testosterone can play in treatment and preventive medicine.

As he said in a call to arms at that first conference:

> *The conventional approach of the medical, behavioural and social sciences to the problem of male aging has been for a long time, the subject of oversight, absence of focusing, disconnection and, most of all, lack of interdisciplinary collaboration.*

To correct these failings he assembled for the first time at any international conference a mixture of andrologists, gynecologists, urologists, gerontologists and general physicians from 35 countries who presented over 120 papers on a wealth of subjects. As could be seen from the conference proceedings, many of the speakers were either ultracautious or even hostile to the concept of the andropause. They also expressed fear of the possible side-effects of testosterone treatment, especially in relation to possible problems with the prostate, and were unsure about the indications for its use.

Despite this tone of the conference, the assembled delegates, again skillfully steered by Professor Lunenfeld towards the broader view, drafted a 'Centennial Prospective – Healthy Aging for Men'. This predicted a rapid rise in the number of men over the age of 65 in many parts of the world, to over 25% of the male population in some countries within the decade. It considered that this would raise major social, economic and ethical issues worldwide, and might strain to the limit the health, socioeconomic and even political infrastructures of many countries.

Therefore, it was suggested, the promotion of healthy aging and the prevention, or drastic reduction, of morbidity and disability of the elderly must assume a central role in the formation of the health and social policies of many, if not all, countries in the next century. The report included in its recommendations that, as interventions such as HRT may favorably influence many of the diseases associated with male aging, as had been shown in women, there was an 'urgent need' to obtain such information in men.

Second World Congress on the Aging Male, 2000

The climate of opinion at the Second World Congress was very different, especially towards the andropause and its treatment. Symbolic of this change was that there were several additional sponsors of the congress, including not only five major pharmaceutical companies who were waking up to the huge potential market in male HRT, but also academic bodies, including the European Association of Urology, the World Association of Sexology, and the European Menopause Society, which had just changed its name to the European Menopause and Andropause Society.

Again, the emphasis was on the WHO 'Ageing and Health Programme', with the stated goal of promoting 'health and well-being throughout the life span, thus ensuring the attainment of the best possible quality of life for as long as possible, for the largest possible number of older people'. As an important part of this drive, there were many more papers directly supporting testosterone treatment, and reporting good results and a high level of safety with it.

The best overall view of this was probably given by the interactive voting session organized and sponsored by the Ferring AG Pharmaceutical Company. The jury, 400 leading experts in the field, mainly urologists, endocrinologists, gynecologists and research scientists from all over the world, invited to a symposium called 'Testosterone Deficiency as a Real Clinical Issue in the Aging Male Population', came out overwhelmingly in favor of testosterone treatment being important and beneficial. The questions put to them, and the answers they gave, are reported in detail because they show a huge change in medical views on the theory and practice of diagnosis and treatment of the andropause.

Given electronic vote recorders for instant analysis of their views, they were asked the following ten questions.

What do you consider a subnormal testosterone level?

Given a choice of 4, 8 and 12 nmol/l, the vote was split evenly between the three levels, with a slight preference for the highest. Any clinician who could recognize the units would never have chosen the lowest level, as that would be grossly subnormal, the only real area of debate being between the upper two. This confusion may have resulted from the schism between units of measurement used in different countries. Many of the large contingent of US and Canadian delegates were unable to equate 12 nmol/l total testosterone, the more favored lower limit of normal in Europe, with the level of 350 ng/dl used by doctors trained in North America.

What are the most important symptoms of testosterone deficiency in men over 50?

The symptoms rated by the delegates as being most common were, in decreasing order of importance, loss of libido, erectile dysfunction, depression, reduced cognitive function, osteoporosis and reduced muscle strength. It is interesting that this vote by an authoritative body of expert opinion from all round the world should recognize exactly the same frequency of characteristic symptoms of androgen deficiency as found in a detailed comparison of these in studies ranging from that of Dr August Werner in 1939[8] to those reported in the latest AMS[16] questionnaire. This consistency of the clinical features of the andropause, as observed by doctors all over the world for more than 60 years, further validates the importance of low testosterone levels in causing the condition[25], and the validity of this questionnaire in its diagnosis.

What is the most appropriate way of diagnosing testosterone deficiency?

A large majority of the experts felt that characteristic symptoms must be present as well as subnormal testosterone levels, rather than reduced levels alone, with raised pituitary gonadotropins being the least essential. This is a most important point, as the purpose of testosterone treatment is to relieve symptoms, and this is why men with andropausal symptoms, even with borderline laboratory findings, should be offered a therapeutic trial with adequate doses of the hormone for at least 3 months.

Do you prescribe testosterone replacement to men over 50?

Over 80% were currently prescribing testosterone to their male patients, and that presumably did not include gynecologists, who are also increasingly using small doses of testosterone in addition to HRT with estrogens in their female menopausal patients, to boost libido and well-being.

Which testosterone therapy do you prescribe to men over 50?

Oral treatment was used by around 60%, intramuscular injections by over 50%, transdermal body or scrotal patches by only about 10% and pellet implants by less than 5%. This suggests that men find patches inconvenient and irritant, and injections are the main form of testosterone treatment in the USA, where, unlike in Canada, Europe and most of the rest of the world, safe oral forms of testosterone are not yet available, although hopefully this will soon change.

Which testosterone therapy do these patients prefer?

Oral treatments followed by injections were by far the most favored forms of treatment. This coincides with my clinical experience that scrotal and body patches are inconvenient to use, can easily fall off and tend to irritate the skin. They also seem to deliver a lower testosterone dosage, and suppress the body's own production more than oral treatments, but not as much as injections or implants. Also, compared with the 60-year experience of the safety and convenience of pellet implants of testosterone, these newer methods have relatively little 'track record' in terms of safety and efficiency in relieving andropausal symptoms long term. All these reasons may be why Ferring AG stopped actively marketing their patches after this symposium, although we must be grateful to them for the interesting information gained from the ballot they sponsored at this conference.

What are the most important considerations when choosing which type of testosterone treatment to prescribe?

Effective symptom relief was most highly rated at nearly 35%, ease of use, convenience and examination for pre-existing disease at around 25% each, and cost, lifestyle and availability at less than 10% each. While recognizing the overriding importance of the first of these, because in most state medical systems availability is limited by cost, most of the patients describe the high price of most testosterone preparations as being the limiting factor in the uptake of this form of treatment.

Where do you stand on concern about potential risk of prostatic disease?

The responses to this question were most reassuring to doctors and patients alike. Over 75% of delegates said they would start treatment but carefully monitor the level of prostate-specific antigen, 15% thought the potential benefits outweigh the potential risks, 6% would await the outcome of stringent risk versus benefit analyses and only 2% would not consider prescribing it because of the concerns about prostatic disease. These views coincided with good news from other speakers at the conference about prostate safety. These included papers by Professor Herman Behre from Germany and Stefan Arver from Sweden reporting detailed clinical studies of a variety of testosterone treatments, without adverse effects of the prostate[24,26,27].

Where do you stand on concern about potential risk of cardiovascular disease?

This was again reassuring, especially for doctors who had been told from medical school onwards that testosterone was bad for the heart. Nearly

70% were confident that the potential benefits outweighed the risks, less than 30% wanted to await the outcome of more stringent risk/benefit analysis and only 3% would not consider prescribing it because of concerns about cardiovascular disease. The safety of testosterone treatment in relation to the circulation was reinforced by two other speakers at the conference, both from London, Dr Peter Collins[28], who reported that testosterone dilates the coronary arteries, and Dr David Crook[29], who reviewed the data on its relationship with heart-attack risk factors, and found evidence of benefit rather than harm.

Do you consider there is sufficient evidence to initiate testosterone therapy for decreased bone mineral density in aging men?

Nearly 75% did think there was sufficient evidence to initiate treatment for osteoporotic aging in males. This view was supported at the conference by another speaker, Dr Jean Kaufman from Ghent, Belgium, who reported studies suggesting a beneficial effect of reducing osteoporosis in men with low testosterone by giving HRT[20].

These views represented a dramatic shift of opinion in favor of testosterone treatment even over the 2 years since the First World Congress on the Aging Male held in Geneva. At the first conference, opinions had been much more evenly divided between those in favor and those wishing for a lot more evidence before they would consider treating their patients with testosterone.

The most important point about the second congress is that the majority of experts seemed to think that evidence had been produced to their satisfaction, and they now felt confident about beginning treatment. The jury of international experts had considered the extensive evidence, and returned a verdict very much in favor of testosterone treatment.

Testosterone treatment: an idea whose time has come

The year 2000 was a turning point in the history of testosterone treatment for several reasons, as well as because of the evidence presented at the Second World Congress on the Aging Male held in Geneva in February.

In March, my colleague at the London Andrology Clinic, Dr Duncan Gould, coauthored a paper in the British Medical Journal which helped turn the tide of medical opinion to favor recognition of the andropause[30].

This was regarded as so important for American physicians that it was reprinted in its entirety as 'Editor's Choice' in the Western Journal of Medicine in August 2000[31].

The year ended with another important event, the launch conference of The Andropause Society (TAS) at the Royal Society of Medicine on 6 December. This is a new web-based international charity with the aims of encouraging research, education and training about the andropause and its treatment.

Meanwhile, in Canada, where Organon had just launched its oral testosterone treatment, testosterone undecanoate (Andriol®), the company funded a most telling survey of the attitude of both doctors and the general population in Canada to the andropause concept.

This poll, coordinated by the Angus Reid organization, was presented at the second International Society for the Studies of the Aging Male (ISSAM) conference by Dr McCready of Scarborough, Ontario, working with Organon Canada. The questions were put to a random sample of equal numbers of laymen and -women, 1500 in total, and 200 doctors. Analyzed separately, 70% of the lay group had heard of the term 'andropause', 80% believed it existed and about half thought it could affect the quality of a man's life and might lead to more serious problems.

Of the doctors, 80% believed it existed, 70% thought that it could affect the quality of life and 90% thought that low testosterone was a contributory factor. When asked what conditions might be related to low testosterone, other than sexual problems, 45% mentioned osteoporosis and 25% heart disease.

Overall, there was a surprisingly high degree of awareness in both groups of the andropause and its effects, especially amongst women. With the usual attitude of high denial, however, few men in either group thought the diagnosis might apply to them, although they could nearly all think of friends or patients it might apply to. Most of the physicians were aware of the condition, but vague about its diagnosis and treatment.

On the basis of this survey, and the confident assessment of the national and international scene by the society, the home page of the Canadian Andropause Society (CAS) website starts with the encouraging statement that: 'The existence of andropause is now recognized by the medical world – including the Canadian Andropause Society – and by Canadians alike.'

How has this victory in the worldwide testosterone revolution been won in Canada? As I saw when visiting the then President of the Canadian Andropause Society, Dr Tremblay, in Quebec in the autumn of 2000, he encouraged public awareness of the andropause and its treatment by press and television interviews. He also traveled tirelessly around Canada, as did Dr Alvaro Morales and several other members of his committee, attending and speaking at meetings of andrologists, endocrinologists and general physicians. This high level of activity in making the case for treatment of the andropause inside and outside the medical profession bore the fruit of a high level of acceptance in both.

Combined with an ongoing research and teaching program, this made the Canadian Andropause Society a model for organizations with similar goals around the world[25].

Asia and the Pacific area

From the very limited interest and activity 10 years ago, this whole area has become a hive of interest in the health of the older man and the potential for male HRT. As was made clear at the historic First Asian Meeting of ISSAM held in Kuala Lumpur, Malaysia, in March 2001, the meeting focused very much on 'Managing aging populations – a global challenge'.

Typical of the many excellent papers from delegates from every country in the region was a message from the organizing chairman, Dr H. M. Tan[32]:

> In the developed countries, the percentage of the population of around 65 years of age will increase by more than 50% by the year 2025. The greatest rate of increase will be for the age group of above 80 years. With declining unsustainable birth rates, the traditional working population (age group 18–65 years) will face a huge burden if they have to fully support this aged population. Similarly, developing countries like China and Indonesia will experience the highest increase in the number of people above the age of 65 years. Their aged populations will more than double in size in the next 25 years. The sheer immensity of numbers will certainly strain the developing economies and their related social and political infrastructures.
>
> Thus the problem of the aging population is universal, and in Asia where the majority of the countries are in the developing status, these problems may well be insurmountable if policy makers do not implement urgent and drastic steps well before this phenomenon occurs.

This sense of urgency was also conveyed by other speakers from every part of Asia, and one felt that each was ready and eager for the testosterone revolution to happen in their country.

Indonesia was facing the most severe problem, with a forecast increase of over 414% in its aged population in the years 2000–2025. Next came Kenya with 347%, Brazil with 255%, China with 220% and Japan with 129%, compared with the relatively modest increases in developed countries such as Germany with 66% and Sweden with 33%. The contrast was stark, and the thirst for knowledge on how to apply male HRT to maintain physical and mental activity, health span rather than just life span, was great.

While the knowledge of the nine invited speakers from the West was much sought and appreciated, there appeared to be less concern about the theory of testosterone treatment than about the urgent need to apply it. Generally, while there was stronger support from the health authorities than is seen in most Western countries, who generally lack this sense of urgency, it fell to urologists to provide this form of HRT. The guidelines the Asian doctors recommended, however, closely followed the diagnostic and treatment criteria developed in the West. As indicated in the Introduction, it is the pressure of aging populations which is creating the change in the climate of medical opinion needed to produce greater awareness of androgen deficiency and its treatment.

References

1. de Kruif P. *The Male Hormone*. New York: Harcourt, Brace and Company, 1945
2. Longcope C, Feldman HA, McKinlay JB, Araujo AB. Diet and sex hormone-binding globulin. *J Clin Endocrinol Metab* 2000;85:293–6.
3. Wright S. *Applied Physiology*. London: Oxford Medical Publications, 1926
4. David K, Dingemanse E, Freud J, Laqueur E. Ueber krystallinisches maennliches Hormon aus Hoden (Testosteron), wirksamer als aus Harn oder aus Cholesterin bereitetes Androsteron. *Hoppe-Seyl Z Physiol Chem* 1935;233:281–2
5. Butenandt AFJ. Ueber die chemische Untersuchung der Sexualhormone. *Z Angew Chem* 1931;44:905–8
6. Butenandt FJ, Hanish G. Uber Testosteron. Umwanlung des Dehydro-androsterons in Androstendiol und Testosteron; ein Weg zur Darstellung des Testosterons aus Cholesterin. *Hoppe-Seyl Z Physiol Chem* 1935;237:89–98
7. Ruzicka L, Wettstein A. Synthetische Darstellung der Testishhormons, Testosteron (Androsten 3 on 17-ol). *Helv Chim Acta* 1935;18: 1264–75
8. Werner AA. The male climacteric. *J Am Med Assoc* 1939;112:1441–3
9. Deansley R, Parkes AS. Further experiments on the administration of hormones by the subcutaneous implantation of tablets. *Lancet* 1938;2:606–8
10. Nieschlag E, Behre HM. Pharmacology and clinical uses of testosterone. In Neischlag E, Behre HM, eds. *Testosterone: Action, Deficiency, Substitution*. Heidelberg: Springer, 1990:92–114
11. Werner AA. *Research in Endocrinology*. St Louis, MO: Von Hoffman Press, 1952
12. Werner AA. Male climacteric: additional observations of thirty-seven patients. *J Urol* 1943;49:872–82
13. Werner AA. The male climacteric: report of two hundred and seventy-three cases. *J Am Med Assoc* 1946;132:188–94
14. Heller CG, Myers GB. The male climacteric: its symptomatology, diagnosis and treatment. *J Am Med Assoc* 1944;126:472–7
15. Sevringhaus EL. *The Management of the Climacteric*. Springfield, IL: CC Thomas, 1948
16. Heinemann LAJ, Zimmermann T, Vermeulen A, Thiel C, Hummel W. A new 'aging males' symptoms' (AMS) rating scale. *Aging Male* 1999;2:105–14
17. Carruthers M, Murray A. *F/40: Fitness on Forty Minutes A Week*. London: Sports Council and Futura Books, 1976
18. Carruthers M. *Testosterone Revolution*. London: Thorsons, 2001
19. Vermeulen A, Stoica T, Verdonck L. The apparent free testosterone concentration, an index of androgenicity. *J Clin Endocrinol Metab* 1971;33:759–67
20. Kaufman JM, Vermeulen A. Androgens in male senescence. In Nieschlag E, Behre HM, eds. *Testosterone: Action, Deficiency, Substitution*, Berlin: Springer-Verlag, 1998:437–71

21. Leifke F, Gorenoi V, Wichers C, Von Zur MA, Von Buren E, Brabant G. Age-related changes of serum sex hormones, insulin-like growth factor-1 and sex-hormone binding globulin levels in men: cross-sectional data from a healthy male cohort. *Clin Endocrinol (Oxf)* 2000;53:689–95

22. Gooren LJ. A ten-year safety study of the oral androgen testosterone undecanoate. *J Androl* 1994;15: 212–15

23. Gooren LG. Quality-of-life issues in the aging male. *Aging Male* 2000; 3:185–9

24. Behre HM. Testosterone effects on the prostate. *Aging Male* 2000;3:5

25. Tremblay RR, Morales AJ. Canadian practice recommendations for screening, monitoring and treating men affected by andropause or partial androgen deficiency. *Aging Male* 1998;1:213–18

26. Meikle AW, Arver S, Dobs AS, et al. Prostate size in hypogonadal men treated with a nonscrotal permeation-enhanced testosterone transdermal system. *Urology* 1997; 49:191–6

27. Sinha-Hikim I, Arver S, Beall G, et al. The use of a sensitive equilibrium dialysis method for the measurement of free testosterone levels in healthy, cycling women and in human immunodeficiency virus-infected women. *J Clin Endocrinol Metab* 1998;83:1312–18

28. Collins, P. Coronary artery function and androgens. *Aging Male* 2001; 4:38–9

29. Godsland IF, Wynn V, Crook D, Miller NE. Sex, plasma lipoproteins, and atherosclerosis: prevailing assumptions and outstanding questions. *Am Heart J* 1987;114: 1467–1503

30. Gould DC, Petty R, Jacobs HS. For and against: the male menopause – does it exist? *Br Med J* 2000;320: 858–61

31. Gould DC, Petty R, Jacobs HS. The male menopause – does it exist? *West J Med* 2000;173:76–8

32. Tan HM. First Asian ISSAM Meeting: managing aging populations – a global challenge. *Aging Male* 2001;4:7–12

3 Causes of androgen deficiency

INTRODUCTION

The key question is: what constitutes androgen deficiency in the adult male? In answer to this question, it is proposed to define it as:

> an absolute or relative insufficiency of testosterone or its metabolites in relation to the needs of that individual at that time in his life[1].

The definition is derived from that of diabetes mellitus, another endocrine disorder which increases in frequency with age, may be associated with high hormone levels due to the various factors causing insulin resistance and causes a characteristic pattern of symptoms. It is comparable to the absolute or relative deficiency of insulin in diabetes, the low levels in juvenile diabetics being equivalent to the low testosterone levels due to non-descent of the testes or mumps orchitis. The maturity-onset diabetic more resembles the typical andropausal male in his 50s with insufficient testosterone to overcome the 'resistance' caused by rising sex hormone-binding globulin (SHBG) levels, stress, obesity or androgen receptor (AR) changes. Also, like diabetes, it is treated largely on the basis of the relief of these symptoms and the prevention of long-term complications, rather than endocrine assays. This principle will be referred to again when considering the application of androgen therapy.

How do we determine the androgen requirements of an adult male at a given time in his life? As discussed in the next chapter, normal or reference ranges in different body fluids, usually plasma or serum, are the most commonly used diagnostic markers, but may not be the best indicators of optimal hormonal levels. Clinicians tend to adopt arbitrary laboratory ranges rigidly; these are often obtained by unknown methodology, from unspecified reference populations of various ages and degrees of mental, physical and sexual functioning, with statistical cutoff points of doubtful biological significance. Each of these factors needs to be recognized and taken into consideration in the diagnosis and treatment of individual cases.

To make matters more complex, there may well be different thresholds of action for different androgens and their metabolites, individually and in combination, influencing various physical and psychological functions at various ages, and individual thresholds of action, as in the 'high-testosterone male' (see next chapter). The case will be argued that each man has his own 'normal range' for androgens, within which he feels and functions well, and when levels fall below this optimal range, characteristic symptoms appear or there is related physical or mental impairment of function.

BIOSYNTHETIC PATHWAYS

In the normal adult male, 95% of the testosterone circulating in the blood is synthesized in the 500 million Leydig cells in the testes, a total of 6–7 mg per day. The remainder is produced in the adrenal glands.

The precursor of steroids, including testosterone, is cholesterol. Leydig cells have a large capacity for the synthesis of cholesterol from acetate, and circulating low-density lipoproteins are the main extracellular store. Activated by luteinizing hormone (LH), the mobilized cholesterol is converted to androgens by a series of oxidative enzymatic steps which shorten its side chain from 27C to 19C. These stages progressively increase the androgenic activity of the molecule from pregnenolone (C21), produced in the mitochondria, which is inactive, mainly via dehydroepiandrosterone (DHEA), or to a lesser extent progesterone, which are both weakly active, to testosterone, which is fully active (Figure 1). Although itself inactive, the pregnenolone can also be oxidized to Δ^{16} androgens, which can be further metabolized to the pheromones androstenone and androstenol.

CONTROL OF BIOSYNTHESIS

Testosterone biosynthesis has a complex and carefully regulated biofeedback control mechanism which is affected by a wide range of physiological and pharmacological factors. For the sake of future discussion it is useful to consider the different parts of this in detail at the present stage.

Gonadotropin-releasing hormone (GnRH)

GnRH is a decapeptide released into the pituitary portal circulation from neurons in the hypothalamus. Unlike other neurons in the hypothalamus, these have migrated during development of the embryo from the olfactory bulb towards the basal forebrain. They are located over a wide area of the anterior hypothalamus, preoptic area, septum and other parts of the forebrain. They synapse with cells producing melanocortin-related peptides, and those linked with the metabolism of norepinephrine and γ-aminobutyric acid (GABA), all substances known to affect GnRH secretion[2].

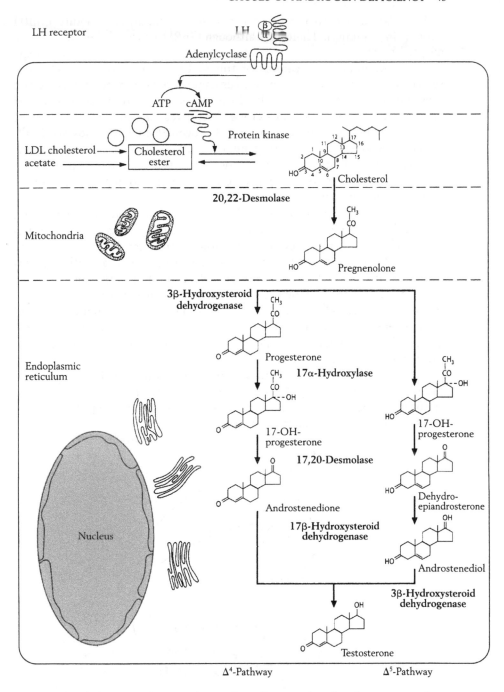

Figure 1 Steroid biosynthesis in the Leydig cell. Reproduced with permission from reference 3. LH, luteinizing hormone; ATP, adenosine triphosphate; cAMP, cyclic adenosine monophosphate; LDL, low-density lipoprotein

It is also known that behavioral and social stimuli can modify GnRH neurons in mammals. Therefore, although GnRH neuronal mechanisms are adapted to meet species-typical variations in environment and physiology, some of the important features of this system appear to be widely conserved amongst both fish and mammals. Associations between olfactory and reproductive systems are well documented in behavioral studies of pheromones, themselves testosterone derivatives, and in clinical studies of disorders including hypogonadotropic hypogonadism with anosmia (Kallmann's syndrome) or olfactory–genital dysplasia. This raises the intriguing possibility that through this 'ancient hormone' the sense of smell is one of the earliest regulators of sex hormone production, and at the same time a potent sexual stimulant.

GnRH has a short half-life of less than 10 min, and is retained and broken down in the pituitary by several peptidase systems. Therefore it is the frequency and amplitude of its pulsatile release that determine the type of LH and follicle-stimulating hormone (FSH) secretion, as both are produced in the same cells of the pituitary gland. GnRH is the sole releasing factor for both gonadotropins, although the frequency of the pulse generator in the GnRH cells depends on stimulation from surrounding cells and noradrenergic activity, and inhibition from circulating androgens and estrogens, and dopaminergic, serotonergic and GABAergic neurons. Opioid peptides reduce the negative feedback of gonadal steroids.

In man, both testosterone and dihydrotestosterone (DHT) act mainly at the hypothalamic level by decreasing the frequency of GnRH pulses, while estrogens reduce gonadotropin secretion by reducing the amplitude of LH and FSH peaks at the pituitary level (Figure 2).

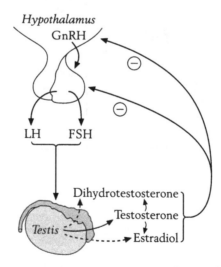

Figure 2 The negative feedback control of androgen secretion. GnRH, gonadotropin-releasing hormone; LH, luteinizing hormone

Gonadotropins

LH and FSH are structurally similar in that they have two polypeptide chains, the α subunit being identical to that of all the glycoprotein hormones, while the β subunits, although structurally very similar, have differences which give their specificity of action.

However, the latter subunits in LH and human chorionic gonadotropin (hCG) are very similar, and they act on the same receptor in the Leydig cell. Although the two gonadotropins are synthesized in the same anterior pituitary cells, they are stored in different secretion granules. The pattern of release is also different, with more constant secretion of FSH, and its preferential release with lower frequencies of GnRH pulses.

Their half-lives are also very different because of differing terminal glycosylation. That of LH is only 20 min because it is rich in glucosamine sulfate and quickly removed by the liver; that of the sialylated FSH is about 2 h[4]. Therefore, although they are both secreted simultaneously following a GnRH pulse, LH appears to be much more pulsatile than FSH.

Testicular synthesis

In the Leydig cells, biosynthesis of testosterone is controlled at several levels. First, there is the availability of cholesterol at the level of the outer membrane of the mitochondria, and its rate of transfer to the inner membrane under the control of the steroidogenesis activator protein (StAR). This labile protein, also present in the adrenal gland and ovary, produces transient 'contact sites' between the inner and outer mitochondrial membranes, allowing cholesterol to be transferred from one to the other for conversion to pregnenolone, at the start of the 'steroidogenic cascade' to the active C19 steroids.

The initial rate-limiting conversion is catalyzed by one of the oxidative enzymes, many of which are heme-containing proteins called cytochrome P450. Like the other cytochromes regulating each step in the cascade, this side-chain cleavage enzyme (P450scc) located on the inner mitochondrial membrane is induced by LH, but a complex interaction of other hormones and locally produced autocrine and paracrine factors also plays a part.

Most of the pregnenolone produced is then transported back into the cytoplasm, and converted to a variety of C19 steroids by enzymes in the endoplasmic reticulum, principally by P450c17, so called because it oxidizes the side chain at the 17 carbon atom. This is also under the control of LH.

METABOLISM OF ANDROGENS

Testosterone has a short half-life of only 12 min in the bloodstream. The steady state reached depends on the rate of production balanced against breakdown in the liver to inactive metabolites that are excreted in the urine

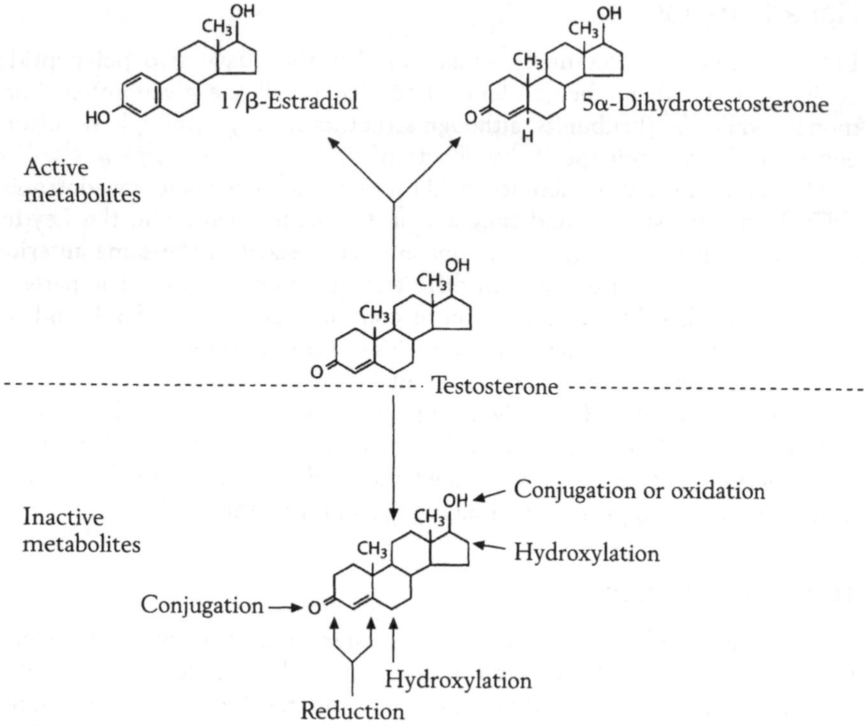

Figure 3 Testosterone metabolism. Reproduced with permission from reference 5

and skin, and conversion to active derivatives, mainly DHT and estrogens (Figure 3).

Many of the actions of testosterone are dependent on its conversion to DHT under the action of the two types of 5α-reductase. Type I is present in the skin, liver and brain, and type II is found in the prostate. The activity of the DHT formed is in turn limited by its rate of breakdown, and back-conversion from testosterone via androstenedione depending on the enzyme profile of the target cell.

In estrogen-dependent tissues, such as fat, liver and hair follicles, the aromatase cytochrome P450 enzyme (P450arom) converts testosterone to estrogen, which is then converted to inactive estrones. Alterations in the rate of breakdown and clearance of testosterone and its metabolites in disease, aging and drug treatments can therefore be as important as changes in the rate of synthesis.

TRANSPORT OF ANDROGENS

Testosterone cannot be stored in the testis, and is therefore immediately exported in the blood via the spermatic vein. In the plasma, only 2% is in

Capillary exchange

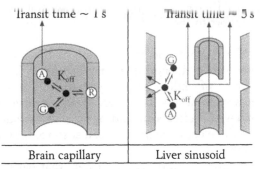

| Brain capillary | Liver sinusoid |

Figure 4 The 'free intermediate' model for the transport of protein-bound substances into tissues depends on transit time, net rate of dissociation (K_{off}) from plasma protein (albumin, A, or globulin, G) and rate of diffusion through membrane. Reproduced with permission from reference 7

the 'free' form (FT), about 54% is weakly bound to albumin (ABT) and the remaining 44% is bound to its specific transport protein, sex hormone-binding globulin (SHBG). The affinity of SHBG for DHT is 1.2–1.3 times higher than that for testosterone and four times higher than that for estradiol. The affinity of SHBG for the steroids decreases with increasing temperature[6].

Transport of steroids into various tissues in the body is dependent on their binding to transport proteins, their rate of dissociation from these proteins, their membrane permeability and their capillary transit time through an organ[7] (Figure 4). Steroids dissociate slowly from their specific binding proteins, and as transit time through most organs is rapid, being less than a second, apart from the free testosterone, only the albumin-bound fraction might theoretically make a significant additional contribution to tissue levels.

Protein binding of androgens is considered to be important in slowing their uptake and breakdown by the liver cells, but it has important clinical implications in regulating the amount of free, biologically active, androgens available to enter the target cells. Again and again, we see that it is the free testosterone which is the clinically most important fraction in both the diagnosis and treatment of androgen deficiency.

SEX HORMONE-BINDING GLOBULIN (SHBG)

Introduction

SHBG transports androgens and estradiol in the blood and regulates their bioavailable fraction and access to target cells. SHBG has a higher binding affinity for androgens over estrogens. The recent advances in the knowledge of its structure and gene expression, and notably the demonstration of a specific receptor (SHBG-R) located on membranes of sex steroid-responsive cells, gave support to the thesis that SHBG has much more sophisticated functions at cellular level.

In particular, the receptor-mediated action of SHBG, which uses as a second messenger cyclic adenosine monophosphate (cAMP), has been linked to the effects of androgens and estradiol. It is thought that the SHBG/SHBG-R system works as an additional control mechanism that inhibits or amplifies the effects of androgens and estradiol in cells. The system consists of three components, an agonist steroid, SHBG and a membrane receptor SHBG-R.

SHBG is a well-characterized plasma protein that has two binding sites: one binds certain estrogens and androgens, and the other binds to SHBG-R. The characteristics of this novel signal transduction system, from the interaction of SHBG with SHBG-R, to the intermediacy of G-proteins, to cAMP generation, to downstream effects of the second messenger, have been clearly characterized[8].

Structure and function

SHBG is a multifunctional protein that acts in humans to regulate the response to steroids in several ways. It was originally described as a protein, secreted by the liver, that is the major binding protein for sex steroids in plasma, thereby regulating the availability of free steroids to hormone-responsive tissues.

However, it has been found that SHBG also functions as part of a novel steroid-signaling system that is independent of the classical intracellular steroid receptors. Recent research has shown that SHBG is a modular protein, which comprises an N-terminal steroid-binding and dimerization domain, and a C-terminal domain containing a highly-conserved consensus sequence for glycosylation that may be required for other biological activities, such as cell-surface recognition.

Unlike the intracellular steroid receptors that are ligand-activated transcription factors, SHBG mediates androgen and estrogen signaling at the cell membrane by way of cAMP (Figure 5). That this is a separate pathway of steroid action is shown by the fact that inhibitors of the transcriptional activation of the androgen receptor (AR) and estrogen receptor (ER) do not affect the cAMP response[9].

In the prostate, it has been suggested that the estradiol-activated SHBG/SHBG-R complex cross-talks with the androgen receptor, and is able to activate AR even in the absence of DHT[10]. These factors may be of importance in relation to the actions of androgens and estrogens in the causation and treatment of both benign and malignant prostatic conditions.

A recent review of research into the localized expression of SHBG in hormone-responsive tissues by Rosner's group at Columbia University, New

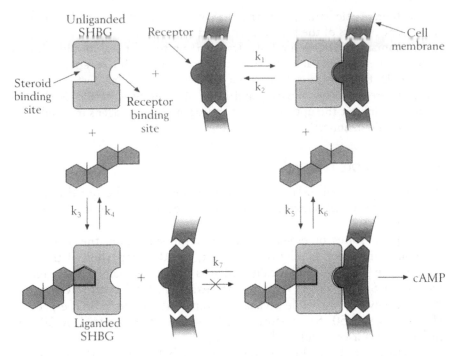

Figure 5 The steroid sex hormone-binding globulin (SHBG)/SHBG-R signaling system. Reproduced with permission from reference 11. cAMP, cyclic adenosine monophosphate; k_{1-7}, kinetic constants

York, raised the following interesting questions in relation to sex-steroid deficiency and replacement in both sexes:

(1) Does locally expressed SHBG affect intracellular steroid signaling pathways, or act in an autocrine or paracrine manner through SHBG-R?

(2) Does SHBG participate in cross-talk between epithelial and stromal cells, since SHBG is predominantly expressed in the former and SHBG-R in the latter?

(3) Do perturbations of SHBG expression in cancer cells, through allelic deletions, contribute to the malignant phenotype and, if so, can agonists or antagonists of SHBG-R signaling serve as useful therapeutic agents?

An example of such potential clinical applications is the observation that in estrogen-dependent breast cancer, SHBG, through SHBG-R, cAMP and protein kinase A (PKA), specifically inhibits the estradiol-induction of cell proliferation. This antiproliferative, antiestrogenic effect of human SHBG not only has increased our understanding of the molecular mechanisms involved in the biology of breast cancer, but also could be exploited as a future therapeutic strategy in the managing of androgen- and estrogen-dependent tumors of the breast, uterus and prostate[12].

In summary, SHBG is not just a transport protein for sex steroids. It also regulates their bioavailable fraction and access to SHBG receptor cells in sex steroid target organs throughout the body, including testes, ovaries, prostate, breast, bone, muscles and brain. In this way SHBG is able to enhance or inhibit the uptake of both androgens and estrogens in a cell- and tissue-specific manner[13].

Transport protein function

As stated above, only 2% of androgens circulating in the blood are free, approximately equal amounts being loosely bound to albumin, and firmly bound to SHBG.

Except in states of pregnancy and extreme starvation, the amount of albumin in the blood is relatively constant, and the proportion of the total testosterone which is biologically active is therefore mainly regulated by changes in SHBG levels. With age, for example, total testosterone levels decrease only slightly, while because of a rapid increase in SHBG, especially after the age of 50, free testosterone levels are often reduced by 50% or more from their youthful levels (Figure 6).

In plasma, SHBG also controls the metabolic clearance rate of sex steroids. The influence of danazol in altering both the transport and cellular actions of SHBG will be discussed in detail in the chapter on treatment of androgen deficiency.

As discussed later in this chapter, there are a large number of factors which can cause changes in SHBG levels. This makes it one of the key regulators of free testosterone levels and action.

Cellular actions of SHBG

While the androgen dependence of the prostate gland has long been accepted, the participation of estrogen, mediated via the stroma in the production of benign prostatic hyperplasia (BPH), has only recently been recognized. Its mode of action is still uncertain. It has become clear that the necessary phosphorylative activities, which transmit signals to nuclear receptors and thence transcription of target genes, can be performed by steroids or mimicked by proxy molecules and by cross-talk between discrete pathways. The character and concentration of the available estrogen are determined by the extent of its biosynthesis, its penetration of the cell and its subsequent metabolism. In addition, the estrogen affects its own access through stimulation of facilitating peptide hormones, prolactin and SHBG. Finally, the induction of BPH is determined by the androgen/estrogen ratio and the change in stromal/epithelial balance accompanying aging.

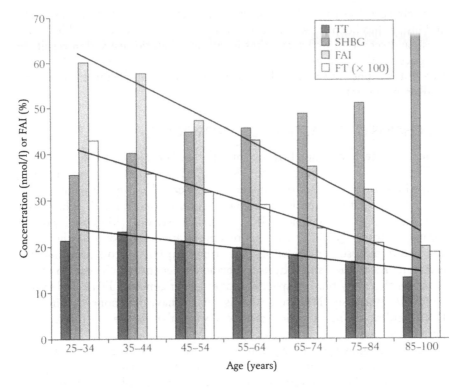

Figure 6 Decline in total testosterone (TT), free testosterone (FT) and free androgen index (FAI) with age, according to the figures of Vermeulen. Reproduced with
permission from reference 14

In this way, it has been proposed that estrogen, mediated by SHBG, par-
ticipates with androgen in setting the rate of prostatic growth and function.
It is suggested that the estrogen not only directs stromal proliferation and
secretion, but also, through insulin-like growth factor-I (IGF-I), conditions
the response of the epithelium to androgen[15].

Regulation of SHBG production

Plasma SHBG concentrations are affected by a number of different diseases, high values being found in hyperthyroidism, androgen insensitivity
and hepatic cirrhosis in men. Low concentrations are found in myxedema,
hyperprolactinemia and syndromes of excessive androgen activity. Concentrations are also affected by drugs such as androgens, estrogens, thyroid hormones, danazol and anticonvulsants.

Also, there is evidence that insulin may be the humoral mediator of the
weight-dependent changes in SHBG. Serum SHBG concentrations are

inversely correlated with both fasting and glucose-stimulated insulin levels, and insulin has been shown to have a direct inhibitory effect on SHBG synthesis and secretion by hepatocytes in culture. Calorie restriction results in a reduction of serum insulin followed by an increase in SHBG and a fall in free testosterone, but an isocaloric, low-fat diet has no significant effect on SHBG concentrations[16].

MECHANISMS OF ACTION OF ANDROGENS

When free testosterone diffuses into the target cells, the first step in androgen action is binding to the AR on the DNA of the X chromosome, located on the long arm close to the centromere. This receptor belongs to the closely related 'steroid hormone receptor superfamily', which also includes the glucocorticoid (GR), mineralocorticoid (MR) and progesterone receptors (PR). These four receptors are a subgroup of the larger and more diverse family of nuclear transcription factors that include estrogen receptors and thyroid hormone receptors. These have in common that they bind to specific sequences of genomic DNA and stimulate RNA synthesis. Members of this family have hormone-binding and DNA-binding domains which are closely similar, while the N-terminal domains are not.

This last, highly specific region makes up over half of the AR protein, and has the transcription initiation site at its end, containing a cAMP response element. It is the most variable in size and least homologous in sequence among members of the steroid receptor family. It contains three main regions of polymeric amino acid stretches (Figure 7).

First in line from the N-terminal end is the region that normally contains an average of 21 ± 3 CAG triplet repeats, coding for glutamine. This repeat region is highly polymorphic, with variation in the average repeat size between 18 in the black population and 21 in the white, and it is a useful genetic marker for AR defects. Next comes a stretch of nine proline residues, which does not vary in size, and nearer the DNA-binding domain is a polymorphic region with two predominant alleles of 23 or 24 GGN triplets coding for glycine. Since the CAG and GGN repeat regions both have significantly more amino acids than the polyproline region, they are more likely to undergo mutation, with important consequences in terms of AR function. It seems as though the recently established chromosomal abnormalities in the AR gene responsible for the androgen insensitivity syndromes and resulting changes in eternal genitalia and secondary sexual characteristics are only the tip of the genetic iceberg.

This suggestion is supported by findings within the normal range of CAG repeat length that show the clinical importance of the genetic mutations in the AR. These have been shown to affect prostate tissue, spermatogenesis, bone density, hair growth, cardiovascular risk factors, psychological factors and even testosterone levels. These key influences of

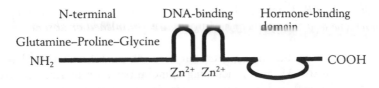

Figure 7 The androgen receptor protein with different functional domains

the CAG and GGN repeater genes are discussed in more detail in Chapter 4.

The DNA-binding domain is characterized by two zinc 'fingers', sticking up like the middle and index fingers of the hand, joined to the hormone-binding domain represented as the thumb by a hinge region (Figure 7). The hinge region changes the conformation of the AR during binding of androgens and antiandrogens. The more specific part of the receptor is called the hormone-binding domain, which has a 50% affinity with GR, MR and PR. Its main function is specific, high-affinity binding of androgens, but in the absence of androgen molecules it is kept inactive by a chaperone protein known as heat-shock protein 90 (HSP90).

Depending on 5α-reductase activity in the target cell, either the testosterone or the DHT molecule is the active agent in binding to the AR, and reconfigures the AR, unmasking its functional domains. These changes cause receptor dimers to form, which are transported to the cell nucleus, and interact with target DNA. The androgen–AR complex can either induce or suppress the androgen-responsive target genes. So far, more than 30 androgen target genes have been characterized, the majority of which are induced by androgens.

Although the AR has the highest affinity for DHT, followed by testosterone, it normally has low affinity for adrenal androgens such as DHEA and androstenedione, and nonandrogenic steroids such as estradiol and progesterone. However, some mutations of the AR show increased affinity for nonandrogenic steroids and antiandrogens.

An important point on the physiology and pathophysiology of the AR is made by Charmian Quigley in a discussion of androgen insensitivity syndromes which can arise through mutations of the AR gene[17]:

AR are found ubiquitously throughout mammalian tissues, implying that androgens have diverse roles not only in the development and maintenance of male sexual function, but also in many other sexually dimorphic processes, from modulation of immune function to development of neural tissues. Defective function of the AR results in a state of androgen resistance – the androgen insensitivity syndrome (AIS). AIS represents an archetypal example of a hormone resistance disorder: Androgens are secreted by the testes in normal or increased amounts; however, due to defective AR function there is loss of target organ response to the hormone and the effects of androgens are diminished or absent.

As examples of this she reports that more than 250 mutations have now been found in the AR gene, including spinobulbar muscle atrophy (SBMA, Kennedy's disease) and prostate cancer. In the first of these, there have been observations of pathologically elongated AR CAG repeats in patients showing marked hypoandrogenic traits[18]. In prostate cancer, especially in metastatic or recurrent disease, the AR undergoes somatic mutation in the tumor itself, but is normal in the genomic DNA. In many cases, the development of prostatic AR gene mutations coincides with the loss of hormone responsiveness of the tumor.

Functional differences have also been reported according to the number of repeats in the polglycine region of the AR. A study of infertile men in Sweden showed that those with 24 GGN repeats had lower testicular volumes and decreased seminal prostate-specific antigen (PSA) and zinc, compared with those with 23 repeats. These differences could not be explained by differences in CAG lengths and were not found in a normal control group[19]. The same Scandinavian group also found that, unlike normal men, boys with hypospadias more often have an AR gene with 24 rather than 23 repeats[20]. Again, it seems that, providing it is within critical normal limits, the lower the number of repeats of either glutamine or glycine units, the greater is the AR sensitivity.

It has also been reported that in aging men with a smaller number of CAG repeats, testosterone levels decrease more rapidly than in men with a larger number[21]. This could explain the increased sensitivity to sex hormone feedback at the hypothalamo-pituitary level seen with aging[22]. The clinical effects of this lowering of androgen levels would be made worse when combined with the reported decrease in the number of AR in several organs in elderly men.

The statement by Zitzmann and Nieschlag[18] that: 'The highly polymorphic nature of glutamine residues within the AR protein implies a subtle gradation of androgenicity among individuals within an environment of normal testosterone levels providing relevant ligand binding to ARs. This modulation of androgen effects may be small but continuously present during a man's lifetime and, hence, exerts effects that are measurable in many tissues as various degrees of androgenicity and represents a relevant effector of maleness'. With the inclusion of variations in glycine residues, this leads to a theory of the overall regulation of androgen levels within a particular individual.

As in diabetes mellitus, in the regulation of androgen action, it is the balance between hormone levels and tissue sensitivity or resistance that decides whether homeostasis is maintained or dysfunction results. Minor variations in the AR gene can have major consequences in deciding the structure and function of androgen-responsive tissues throughout life. Genetic, racial and individual variations in androgen resistance can render even the most accurate measurements of androgen and gonadotropin levels in the blood largely irrelevant in deciding whether or not a particular patient is androgen deficient and would benefit from testosterone treatment.

THE MULTIFACTORIAL CAUSES OF ANDROGEN DEFICIENCY IN THE ADULT MALE

The often multiple and interrelated causes of androgen deficiency can conveniently be considered by looking at every level of the cascade of events which regulates their production and action (Table 1). NB: age plays a major role at each and every level.

The cerebral cortex

Aging

Advancing years take their toll on the brain as the biggest sex organ in the body in many ways. Psychologically, sexual stimuli tend to be less frequent and less intense. Feedback of sensory impulses from the wrinkled skin and flaccid penis creating arousal are similarly reduced. The reduced penile sensitivity has been shown to be because of lower testosterone levels, and reduction of the number of AR in the penis.

Physically, apart from neuronal dropout in the cortex and various brain nuclei mediating sexual activity, there can be insidious cognitive impairment, leading in extreme cases to dementia. Lowered testosterone levels have been found in Alzheimer's disease[23], stroke[24] and Parkinson's disease[25]. Retirement, boredom, bereavement and illness lead to stress.

Table 1   The multiple causes of androgen deficiency

Cerebral cortex	Age, stress (underload and overload), drugs
Hypothalamus and pituitary	Age, GnRH decreased, and more sensitive to feedback, prolactin, drugs
Testes	Age, impaired development, infections, alcohol, diet, diabetes, temperature, trauma, drugs
Target organs	Age, receptor anomalies, reduction and down-regulation, connective-tissue thickening, drugs

GnRH, gonadotropin-releasing hormone

Testosterone and stress

There is a wealth of evidence from both primate and human research that a male's testosterone level changes when his status changes, rising when he achieves or defends a dominant position, and falling when he is dominated. Results of studies of men in various competitive stressful situations suggest that when a man achieves a rise in status through his own efforts, and has an elation of mood over the achievement, he is likely to have a rise in testosterone.

Both excessive and unpleasant physical and mental stress can activate the hypothalamic–pituitary–adrenal axis and reduce either the amount or activity of androgens. For example, extreme endurance training in military cadets, involving psychic stress and deprivation of food and sleep, resulted in a marked drop in testosterone levels, as have intensive on-duty periods in resident physicians.

Less acute psychological stress, such as financial problems, serious quarrels and loss of close friends or relatives, has also been shown to lower androgen levels. Physical illnesses ranging from life-threatening trauma to a variety of chronic diseases have also been related to reduced testosterone levels, although it is always difficult to establish which came first[26].

In general, there is a constantly shifting balance between mainly catabolic sympathetic activity, the fight–flight system mediated by norepinephrine, epinephrine and adrenal corticoids, and the mainly anabolic parasympathetic, rest–digest–restore relaxation system mediated by androgens, growth hormone and insulin. As shown by the lower pulse rate and blood pressure, together with higher androgen levels, according to 'Sleep that knits up the ravell'd sleave of care', the parasympathetic is normally dominant by night, and the sympathetic by day.

The endocrine and metabolic activity of both divisions of the autonomic nervous system tend to be reciprocal and antagonistic. If there is sustained overactivity of the sympathetic system, which is the usual response to stress, then androgen levels tend to drop as their rate of production decreases, and resistance to their action increases.

This is seen during foreplay and intercourse, where under the action of parasympathetic activity, soft lights, sweet music, a relaxed mood and sexual thoughts stimulate the secretion of testosterone[27] and local production of nitric oxide, which together induce erection and lubrication. Intercourse itself swings the balance towards sympathetic activity, with a rise in blood pressure and pulse rate, peaking in orgasm and ejaculation under noradrenergic stimulation, and followed by detumescence. By contrast, stress and performance anxiety-induced epinephrine release can inhibit erectile function almost completely, particularly in the older man.

Drugs

Psychotropics   A wide variety of drugs can reduce libido centrally, particularly in older patients who metabolize them slowly. The oldest of these is bromide, which is rarely used today, but is reputed to have reduced the libido of troops in the two World Wars, although some veterans may feel that it should be wearing off by now.

The modern equivalent in terms of a wide range of psychotropic drugs can have adverse effects on libido, erectile function and ability to ejaculate, so it is always worth determining whether the patient is taking any of these, or whether his problems began when he was taking them. These include virtually all antidepressant, anxiolytic, antiepileptic and antipsychotic drugs, although it is often unknown whether they work at the cortical or hypothalamic level, or peripherally by anticholinergic or antinoradrenergic effects[28,29].

Antihypertensives   Again, any of a wide range of antihypertensive drugs can cause erectile dysfunction by either central or peripheral action, especially the commonly prescribed diuretics and beta-blockers. One notable exception to this is doxazosin (Cardura®), which does not impair, and may even enhance erections. It also has the advantage that, being a potent and selective post-junctional α_1-adrenoreceptor antagonist, it can lessen urinary symptoms in men with benign prostatic hypertrophy. A final bonus is that it has been shown to produce a slight reduction in total cholesterol, low-density lipoprotein (LDL) and triglyceride, so that it can be of multiple benefit to patients with a combination of hypertension and hyperlipidemia.

Hypothalamus and pituitary

Detailed studies of the gonadal axis in older men have shown disappearance of nyctohemeral variation in testosterone levels, increased sensitivity of the gonadostat to sex hormone feedback and decreased opioid tonus, suggesting altered regulation at the hypothalamo-pituitary level[14]. The loss of circadian rhythmicity of LH and, hence, testosterone with age has been attributed to a reduced number and size of LH pulses.

Although there tend to be higher gonadotropin levels in older men, this response is insufficient to maintain declining androgen levels. The rise in FSH tends to be greater than that in LH, and also falls with testosterone treatment. It is known that both these gonadotropins are required for the development and maintenance of testicular function, and while LH is the most important hormone for control of Leydig cell function, other hormones and locally produced factors also play a role.

Reductions in testosterone production may also occur with raised production of prolactin. This may result from stress, but rarely goes over 500 pmol/l due to this. This hormone may be regarded as 'nature's contraceptive', suppressing the libido and fertility in both sexes at times when procreation might detract from the immediate chances of survival, as well as during lactation in women.

Larger rises in prolactin, usually to over 1000 pmol/l, are seen with prolactinomas, and can cause marked suppression of testosterone levels. Although these tumors are rare, occurring in about 0.4% of andropausal patients, they are eminently treatable, and should be considered in younger patients with very low testosterone levels and no other obvious cause.

A wide variety of drugs can also raise prolactin levels, including dopamine antagonists such as phenothiazines and imipramine, those which interfere with dopamine synthesis, e.g. α-methyldopa, depletion of dopamine stores, e.g. reserpine, or the direct stimulation of prolactin production, e.g. H_2-blockers and estrogens. As well as inhibiting GnRH secretion, chronic renal failure and hypothyroidism can cause hyperprolactinemia, and, like the other causes, may be associated with gynecomastia. Opiates such as heroin, morphine and methadone all markedly suppress LH and testosterone secretion by suppressing GnRH release.

Testes

Impaired development

Men with non-descent, or late descent, of one or both testes are often hypogonadal throughout their lives, and when testosterone treatment is stopped they develop typical andropausal symptoms. Even when there has been anatomical correction of the defect by orchidopexy, testicular function may well still be impaired, in terms of both sperm and testosterone production. Sometimes there is no overt history of testicular problems, but when the patient presents in middle age or later, there may be a lifelong history of low sex drive and activity, unexplained infertility and poor secondary sexual characteristics. Physical examination may show small, easily retractile testes in a poorly developed scrotum, with a penis of reduced size.

This is a reminder that testosterone is active in promoting development of the male urogenital tract from the ninth week of intrauterine life onwards, and reaches a peak in the first few weeks after birth which is not reached again until puberty. If the levels of this hormone are insufficient *in utero*, or are opposed by estrogens, then not only may penile development be impaired, with resulting micropenis or hypospadias, but the active part played by the gubernacula in steering the testes towards the developing scrotum is also retarded, which can impair their function for life.

Minor degrees of these developmental disorders can, surprisingly often, be missed, and predispose to hypogonadism appearing in later life. This is seen in about 2% of andropause cases, where the scrotum may be poorly developed, or there is a history of the testes retracting along the inguinal canal during intercourse. Even though non-descent of one or both testes has been surgically corrected prior to or during puberty, normal function in terms of either testosterone production or fertility may not be achieved. Sometimes there is evidence of lifelong androgen deficiency associated with micropenis.

Heredity and familial influences

Studies of monozygotic and dizygotic twins[30] have shown that familial factors accounted for twice as much of the concordance in total and free testosterone and DHT as genetic factors, and virtually all SHBG and aromatase activity. In all these factors, nurture appeared more important than nature. Only in estradiol and LH levels did heredity have a slightly greater influence. It is suggested that similar diet and physical activity levels in families may explain most of these factors in determining androgen levels, and hence liability to andropause.

Infections

Mumps is the classic example of an infection causing an endocrine disorder. The resultant orchitis, first described by Hippocrates, occurs in 25–35% of postpubertal cases, and like many testicular disorders, may affect its endocrine function as well as sperm production.

This potential for testicular damage to be caused by a wide variety of viruses may be linked to damage to the immunological defense system of the testes, which is established only at puberty. The testis has unique 'immune privilege' in three ways. First, diploid spermatogonia in the infant testis begin to divide and differentiate into haploid spermatozoa at puberty, causing the production of so-called 'novel antigens'. At the same time adjacent Sertoli cells form complex networks of tight junctions that cause isolation of the tubular contents from the blood vascular compartment. This 'blood–testis barrier' seals off the spermatogenic cells from the body's immunological defense mechanism, and largely prevents the production of autoantibodies to them.

What autoantibodies do arise seem to be dealt with by two other mechanisms regulating immune function within the testis. The endothelial cells of the testicular microvasculature, which develops at puberty under androgenic stimulation, selectively limit the diffusion of antigenic material into the circulation. Also, Leydig cells are able to adhere to lymphocytes and suppress their proliferation, bringing about local immunosuppression.

As in the female, there is an increasing tendency for puberty to occur earlier in males, and so it is worth enquiring about a history of mumps after the age of 10.

Other viruses, including those causing glandular fever (infectious mononucleosis) may also be associated with clinical or subclinical orchitis and damage. This has also been reported with herpes, Coxsackie, arbo-, dengue and Marburg viruses. The testes can also be affected by nephritis, prostatitis, vesiculitis and epididymitis, especially with gonorrhea, chlamydia and other causes of nonspecific urethritis, all of which should be excluded in the routine history.

It should be recognized, however, that quite often these infections may be asymptomatic, or obscured by other prostatic or urinary symptoms, so that the relevant history may not be reported. The clinician should have a high index of suspicion in patients who have been sexually very active with multiple partners, especially where there is unexplained testicular atrophy or epididymal cysts.

Nonspecific granulomatous orchitis is uncommon, and thought to be caused by an autoimmune response.

During the acute phase of orchitis the testis is usually swollen, hard and tender, but in the chronic stage the testis may be atrophied and soft. It is of interest that during the acute stage testosterone may be reduced, and FSH raised as a marker of damage to the germinal epithelium.

Ultrasound examination can provide a more accurate assessment of the condition of the testis, and can exclude testicular cancer, which is fortunately rare after the age of 40.

Age

Although there is no abrupt cessation of function in the aging testis, as there is with the ovary, there is a highly variable degree of atrophy, and both 'spermatogenic efficiency' and 'testicular reserve for testosterone secretion' tend to decrease with age[31]. The long-established reduction in the number of Leydig cells, with vascular changes underlying the measured decrease in testicular perfusion, and decrease in concentration of testosterone in the spermatic vein, make it probable that the decreased androgen production with old age is mainly of testicular origin. This is confirmed by the rising gonadotropin levels, and the reduced ability of the aging testis to produce more testosterone after human chorionic gonadotropin (hCG) stimulation. Production of androgens is reduced further by the increasing influence of other diseases associated with aging, and the drugs used to treat them.

Alcohol

Although excess alcohol intake is well recognized as a cause of infertility, its short- and long-term effects on testosterone production are often overlooked.

Short-term, low-dose alcohol intake has been found to increase testosterone levels in both women and men. In premenopausal women studied by Sarkola and colleagues[32], this effect was also seen in the free testosterone fraction. The effect on testosterone was more prominent among subjects taking oral contraceptives. Androstenedione levels were significantly lowered and the testosterone/androstenedione ratio significantly elevated by alcohol. No effect of alcohol on DHEA or DHT levels was observed.

The results also indicated that the testosterone effect is the result of an increased androstenedione to testosterone conversion in the liver caused by the alcohol-mediated elevation in the [NADH]/[NAD(+)] ratio (reduced/oxidized nicotinamide–adenine dinucleotide). These findings were thought to be relevant to the development of hyperandrogenism and loss of female sexual characteristics associated with heavy alcohol consumption.

In men[33], the same research group found similar results. Acute administration of a low dose (0.5 g/kg, 10% w/v) caused an increase in plasma testosterone (from 13.5 ± 1.2 nmol/l to 16.0 ± 1.6 nmol/l, mean $\pm$ SEM; $p < 0.05$), a significant decrease in androstenedione and an increase in the testosterone/androstenedione ratio. As with women, it was concluded that alcohol intake affects the androgen balance in men through an effect mediated by the alcohol-induced change in the redox state in the liver.

Long term in men it has been found that moderate levels of stable alcohol intake (non-binge drinking) had no adverse effects on gonadal function, as estimated by testosterone levels and the free testosterone index[34].

In contrast, excess alcohol intake, short- or long-term, has a variety of adverse effects on androgen status in men. Acutely, high doses cause a decrease in androgen levels by a variety of mechanisms. Partly, these are related to a direct inhibition of testicular testosterone production by acetaldehyde derived from the metabolism of alcohol[35]. Also, alcohol suppresses LH-releasing hormone (LHRH) release, by stimulating β-endorphinergic neurons that inhibit the production of norepinephrine, which drives the nitric oxide (NO)-mediated release of LHRH[36].

However, the majority of the endocrine effects of alcohol are probably indirect, resulting from either the stress of intoxication (stimulation of cortisol, catecholamines and possibly GH and prolactin), changes in the level of intermediary metabolites (e.g. a fall in circulating free fatty acids (FFA) stimulating GH secretion) or changes in the metabolism of hormones (e.g. catecholamines, estrogens and androgens) resulting from an alteration in the intracellular redox state or tissue damage[37].

Physical stress immediately before alcohol administration has been found to prolong the reduction in testosterone secretion. This seems to be mainly a consequence of direct inhibition at the testicular level, even though the role of LH as a contributory regulatory factor cannot be totally ruled out.[38]

This is certainly the case in prolonged excess alcohol intake, where there is multiorgan damage, with a variety of adverse effects on androgen status. Depending on the duration and degree of the overdose, many of these persist, even when alcohol has been withdrawn and liver function tests may have returned to normal. This is why in any andropausal patient it is important to take a history of previous as well as present alcohol consumption. The liver forgives and forgets, but the testes harbor grudges.

As well as the liver, damage has been shown to occur to testis, thyroid and adrenal function in male alcoholics. Lowered total testosterone and thyroxine, together with raised estradiol and tri-iodothyronine (T_3), have been found in this group. These changes were still present even after 20 days of total alcohol abstinence as part of a rehabilitation program[39], and are commonly found in alcoholics who have been dry for many years.

Similarly, the persistent elevation of FSH in cirrhotic men may be due to a deficient testicular secretion of inhibin as a result of alcohol toxicity to the testes[40].

The long-term effect of high doses of alcohol on increasing estrogen production, and possibly greater intake of phytoestrogens in some forms of alcohol, especially beer, can affect androgen metabolism in two ways. Raised estrogen levels, particularly as seen in cirrhosis with increased aromatization in the greater adipose tissue stores and in the liver, both inhibit gonadotropin release and increase the production of SHBG. This combination of low testosterone and high SHBG further reduces the availability of free testosterone.

It has also been found that nitric oxide synthase (NOS) inhibitors can antagonize alcohol-induced suppression of testicular steroidogenesis, and that NO is involved in mediating alcohol's testicular and reproductive effects[41]. There are some interesting corollaries to this idea, which are suggested by the work of several researchers in relation to not only the short- and long-term effects of alcohol on the brain and liver but also the causation of coronary disease.

First, raised NO concentrations inhibit alcohol narcosis, supporting the hypothesis that interference with NOS systems causes part of both the impaired erection and sedative–hypnotic effects of alcohol[42]. Also, it has been suggested that overconsumption of alcohol impairs NOS-dependent dilatation of large cerebral arteries[43].

This may explain the hangover effect of impaired brain function on the morning after the night before, loss of short-term memory of what happened in the intoxicated state and the pounding migraine-like headache, which is due not just to the congeners in the alcohol, but to dilatation of the cerebral blood vessels following norepinephrine-mediated vasoconstriction[44]. It may also underlie the cerebral anoxia which together with vitamin deficiency may contribute to delirium tremens, and some of the damage to the cerebral cortex seen with long-term alcoholism.

It has also been suggested that impaired reactivity of cerebral blood vessels to neuronal activation may contribute to the pathogenesis of cerebrovascular disorders observed during chronic alcohol consumption[45].

Second, these results suggest that endogenous NO acts as a vasodilator which reduces ethanol-induced vasoconstriction, thus reducing the disturbance of the hepatic microcirculation by ethanol[46].

Third, a great deal of epidemiological evidence indicates that the consumption of moderate amounts of alcoholic beverages, and in particular red wine, results in a reduction in cardiovascular risk factors and decreases mortality, while large amounts increase it. For the reasons discussed above, small amounts of alcohol increase testosterone in both sexes, and large amounts reduce it. A review article by Parks and Booyse discussed evidence to suggest that NO plays a critical role in cardiovascular protection and that NOS is the responsible cardioprotective protein[47]. However, there is also evidence to suggest that antioxidant polyphenols in red wine may play a beneficial part.

Epidemiologically it has been shown that myocardial infarction is associated with low testosterone levels[48], but there is a threshold of 15 nmol/l (438 ng/dl) above which there is no further decrease, according to Swartz and Young[49]. Among the 21 formerly heavy drinkers in their series, 62% showed testosterone levels less than 10 nmol/l (300 ng/dl). These authors conclude that formerly heavy drinkers should be routinely considered for serum testosterone determination[49].

Such considerations might suggest further research into whether drugs such as sildenafil (Viagra®), vardenafil (Levitra®) and tadalafil (Cialis®) might reduce the toxic effects of alcohol on the brain, liver and heart, in both the short and the long term.

For all the reasons outlined above, there is a highly variable decrease in both total testosterone and more particularly free testosterone (FT) with age. This is seen in Figure 6, which is derived from the extensive work of Kaufman and Vermeulen[14].

Diet, xenoestrogens and antiandrogens

Strict low cholesterol diets have been shown to lower total and free testosterone levels by 14%[50]. Vegetarian diets, especially if low in protein, can increase SHBG, further reducing FT. However, men put on a low-fat, high-fiber, vegetarian diet have a 18% reduction in both total testosterone and FT, which is reversed when they go back on a normal diet. This parallel reduction in both androgen measures would seem to indicate that, in this situation, the decrease is primarily in testosterone[50]. Conversely, high-protein, low-carbohydrate diets, such as the fashionable weight-reduction Atkins diet, may partly exert their slimming action by raising total testosterone and lowering SHBG.

Treated diabetes is one of the best predictors of reduced androgen levels according to the self-administered screener developed by Smith, Feldman and McKinlay[51]. This is one of the contributing factors to the metabolic syndrome.

Insulin-resistant diabetics therefore tend to have low SHBG levels, as the serum concentration of SHBG is inversely related to weight, and hence insulin levels. Using data from the Massachusetts Male Aging Study,

McKinlay and colleagues examined cross-sectional relationships between dietary components and SHBG levels in 1552 men (aged 40–70 years) for whom these factors were known. Age ($p < 0.001$) and fiber intake ($p = 0.02$) were positively correlated to SHBG concentration, whereas body mass index ($p < 0.001$) and protein intake ($p < 0.03$) were negatively correlated.

They conclude that age and body mass index are major determinants of SHBG concentrations in older men, and fiber and protein intake also significantly affect SHBG levels. Thus, diets low in protein in elderly men may lead to elevated SHBG levels and decreased testosterone bioactivity. The decrease in bioavailable testosterone can then result in declines in sexual function and muscle and red cell mass, and contribute to the loss of bone density[52]. Low-carbohydrate weight-reducing regimes can also have a similar effect by lowering insulin resistance, reducing insulin levels and allowing SHBG to rise[31].

Obese subjects have lower SHBG, FT, total testosterone and DHEA levels, but higher estradiol and insulin levels than the non-obese[53]. However, Longcope and colleagues[52], on the basis of Massachusetts Male Aging Study data, report that 'The intakes of calories, fat (animal or vegetable), and carbohydrate were not related to SHBG concentration', a finding which appears paradoxical.

Thus, when present in physiological amounts in the blood as a result of endogenous synthesis, there is a positive relationship between SHBG concentrations and testosterone and, to a lesser extent, FT and albumin-bound testosterone, but age and body mass index appear to be more important in predicting the SHBG concentration[54].

Both androgen and estrogen may be affected by diets rich in xenoestrogens, whether in the form of phytoestrogens such as soy products, or other compounds with estrogenic or antiandrogenic effects, such as agrochemicals. These compounds may considerably affect endocrine balance, and contribute to both the onset of the andropause and impaired fertility, without themselves being directly measured by the routine laboratory methods for androgens or estrogens.

Many conditions which damage the testis and affect fertility, from non-descent to mumps, can also affect the production or action of testosterone. There is currently concern about environmental influences on fertility, particularly in relation to xenoestrogens and antiandrogens. We need to consider the evidence in relation to the impact of such 'hormonal havoc' on endocrine balance in both the developing male fetus, and in men throughout their lives. Farmers are at particular risk, as often they may be exposed from an early age to a variety of growth-promoting hormones used to caponize chickens and turkeys, and increase the yield of meat from cattle.

Drugs

As well as the previously mentioned psychotropic drugs which interfere with GnRH and LH production, there are many drugs which can directly reduce the production of androgens at the testicular level or alter their metabolism. The commonest of these is alcohol, which in large amounts is a well-known cause of infertility and can irreversibly damage the Leydig cells, which lack the regenerative power of hepatocytes. It also promotes the conversion of testosterone to estrogen, which explains the beer-belly and gynecomastia often seen in patients with a history of alcohol abuse.

Other drugs, such as aminoglutethamide and ketoconazole, can inhibit steroidogenic enzymes, causing rapid and dramatic reductions in testosterone levels. Some act as AR antagonists, such as cimetidine, spironolactone and cyproterone acetate. Both herbal preparations, including saw palmetto, and pharmaceutical drugs such as finasteride (Proscar®), used to treat benign prostatic hypertrophy and hair loss, act as 5α-reductases, lowering DHT levels and in some cases contributing to reduced libido and erectile dysfunction.

Drugs which affect the level of SHBG also influence the levels of both total testosterone and FT. These include barbiturates, anticonvulsants and other hepatic enzyme-inducers, which have been shown to raise SHBG, which both reduces the clearance of testosterone and lowers the level of FT, causing one of many examples of iatrogenic androgen deficiency.

A reverse effect, which is likely to have the therapeutic potential of restoring a more youthful androgen profile, is shown by the ethisterone derivative danazol (Danol®). This drug can be used to raise FT by lowering the high level of SHBG seen in many andropausal men, as it reduces the hepatic synthesis of this carrier protein even when used in minimal doses, and also displaces testosterone from the binding sites on the molecule[55]. This appears to be associated with the relief of andropausal symptoms in patients with raised SHBG, and means they can be treated with lower doses of testosterone, especially oral preparations such as testosterone undecanoate (Andriol®).

Temperature

Varicocele and hydrocele are also considered to impair the temperature regulation function of the scrotum, which normally keeps the testes 3–4 °C cooler than core body temperature, and about 1.5–2.5 °C below the temperature of scrotal skin[3].

This remarkable feat, performed for presumably good evolutionary reasons, is achieved by two mechanisms. The first is the transfer of heat through the thin and fat-free scrotal skin, aided by the relaxation of the cremasteric muscle, which increases the surface area of the scrotum and lowers the testes, at higher environmental temperatures.

The second is by a refined countercurrent heat-exchange mechanism, whereby the incoming blood in the testicular arteries in the pampiniform plexus is cooled by the surrounding venous blood. This reduction of testicular temperature below that of the body core is crucial to the maintenance of both fertility and testosterone production. It explains why non-descent of the testis causes both hypogonadism and lifelong infertility. Also, it is one of the reasons why many andrologists interested in both infertility and the andropause encourage scrotal cooling measures such as the wearing of loose-fitting boxer shorts, and avoidance of tight jeans[6] and prolonged periods of driving[56].

Trauma

Testicular trauma as a cause of andropause is not always obvious from the history. It can include hernial repair at any age, but particularly in infancy when it may be an aspect of partial non-descent of the testes, and impaired development of the inguinal canal. Direct blows to the testes, sufficient to cause bruising, may cause unilateral testicular atrophy, as can torsion, even when surgically corrected at an early stage. This may be due to either a breach in the immunological defenses of the testis, or a prolonged sympathetic spasm that can affect both sides.

Similar mechanisms could account for testicular atrophy or hypofunction which may follow any operation on the testis, particularly when it involves trauma to the capsule, as in removal of a varicocele, or damage to the vas, particularly vasectomy[57]. Other operations on the prostate, particularly transurethral resection, may also damage the vas or its outflow, as shown by retrograde ejaculation of semen into the bladder, and possibly cause autoimmune orchitis.

Vasectomy

Although this is a controversial cause of possible damage to the testis, there are many theoretical reasons, and considerable clinical and experimental evidence that vasectomy may contribute to impaired testicular function, often 10–20 years after the operation. It is a major insult to a sensitive and complex endocrine and exocrine organ. It has been estimated that currently 500 000 Americans, 20 000 British and 10 000 Irish have the operation each year.

Anatomical and immunological changes after vasectomy   The vas deferens is just one of the structures in the spermatic cord which may be damaged by the operation and the bruising, infection and scarring which can follow. Running alongside it in the cord is a sheath of fine blood vessels, nerves and lymph vessels which nourish the testis, control its temperature to within very critical limits and drain fluid away from it.

Temperature control of the testis has been shown to be impaired after vasectomy, as has the drainage of fluid from around it, so that hydrocele occasionally results. As described above, this 'water-jacketing' tends to raise its temperature, which can have a harmful effect on the testes' ability to produce both sperm and testosterone. Also, there are nerve connections between the two testes, and damage to one can affect the other in a variety of ways. This is seen in experimental animals undergoing unilateral vasectomy[58], and in men with testicular torsion[59].

In relation to the immunological changes, it has been suggested that: 'Vasectomy can be considered a particular form of experimental autoimmunisation'[60]. This is because testicular tissue is highly antigenic, and from puberty onwards is immunologically isolated from the rest of the body. Since the antigenic properties of spermatozoa change during passage through the epididymis, the antigens detected by antisperm antibodies from men with vasectomy are mostly related to epididymal passage[61].

Although men with primary infertility also show a raised incidence of antisperm antibodies, studies of men attending a clinic for sexually transmitted diseases showed the same level as in normal, fertile men, making it unlikely that venereal disease will trigger antisperm antibody production[62].

In more than 50% of men, vasectomy leads to the production of auto-antibodies. The autoimmune response to sperm following vasectomy is triggered by the phagocytosis of sperm in the epididymis. In the humoral immune response, sperm agglutinating, sperm immobilizing and antibodies to sperm nuclear protamines occur as early as 3–4 days after vasectomy. The incidence reaches 60–70% within 1 year and remains almost the same even after 20 years[63]. Circulating immune complexes (CICs) are also produced.

However, there appear to be great interspecies differences between the time and degree of the immune response to vasectomy, which makes extrapolation to man of a lot of the rather alarming reports, for instance, of increased incidence of vascular disease in monkeys after the operation[64], more difficult.

For example, in men the progressive disappearance of CICs from the third month after vasectomy with the simultaneous increase in antisperm antibody percentage and titer suggests that CICs could be a temporary feature in vasectomized men and do not lead to chronic disease[65]. For this reason, although there is a great deal of concerning information from animal studies, it appears most relevant to concentrate mainly on the evidence from research in men.

Whatever the mechanism, there is considerable evidence that vasectomy produces significant damage to the human testis. For example, a study to determine whether or not there is an association between testicular histological changes and antisperm antibodies showed significant increases in seminiferous tubule wall thickness ($p < 0.001$), focal interstitial fibrosis ($p < 0.001$) and percentage composition of the interstitium ($p < 0.01$) in vasectomized men, compared with control subjects. Serum antisperm activity was present in 74% of the vasectomized men, but none of the control subjects ($p < 0.001$). There was no association between testicular histological changes and immune status. It was concluded that vasectomized men exhibit significant testicular histological changes and increased autoimmune activity as compared with fertile control subjects. These histological changes are not directly associated with antisperm antibody status, suggesting that some other pathophysiological process must be responsible[66].

Evidence about impaired endocrine function of the testis following vasectomy is unclear. In one of the biggest studies[67], testosterone, LH, FSH and prolactin were measured in 298 normal healthy males aged 30–73 years from rural areas of China, and in 505 similar men vasectomized between 1 and 25 years previously. Age-related increases in LH and FSH but not in testosterone or prolactin were noted in normal men. No adverse effects of vasectomy were observed, apart from a 16% increase in mean LH levels in the vasectomized compared with nonvasectomized men of similar ages.

Similarly, most of the early studies, although relatively short-term, were reassuring, and some even showed raised postoperative testosterone levels, albeit accompanied by raised gonadotropin levels, suggesting at least some endocrine effects. However, in most studies, the control groups were age-matched nonvasectomized men, who might be expected to have lower initial indices of androgen function than those in the more fertile and sexually active operated subjects.

Typical of these studies was that of Smith and colleagues, in which, beginning at 6 months after vasectomy, mean plasma testosterone levels demonstrated a statistically significant elevation, mean plasma estradiol levels were lower, mean plasma LH levels were elevated and mean plasma FSH levels were unchanged. By 2 years after vasectomy, a slight plasma FSH elevation had occurred, plasma estradiol levels had returned to baseline and plasma testosterone and LH levels remained elevated. These changes, although significant statistically, did not exceed the normal ranges found in normal adult males in their laboratory, and were of unclear physiological significance. Thus, it can be concluded from this study of 56 men studied for 2 years, 148 men studied for 1 year and 182 men studied for 6 months after vasectomy that no adverse hormonal effects of vasectomy were demonstrated[68].

Later studies, especially those using dynamic androgen stimulation tests, showed more marked endocrine effects of vasectomy, and links with its immunological consequences. Fisch and colleagues[69] measured the serum gonadotropin response to GnRH in 25 men who underwent vasectomy 2–64 months before the study. Ten age-matched fertile men were used as controls.

Baseline serum FSH, LH and testosterone levels were not significantly different between vasectomized men and controls. However, mean serum FSH and LH responses to an intravenous bolus injection of 100 μg GnRH were significantly greater in the vasectomy group ($p = 0.008$ and

$p = 0.003$, respectively). There was no correlation between these responses and the interval after vasectomy.

Serum antisperm antibodies were present in 13 vasectomized men (52%) using enzyme-linked immunosorbent assay and microagglutination techniques. A significant correlation ($p = 0.003$) was found between the presence of serum antisperm antibodies and a normal FSH response to GnRH stimulation. Of 13 patients with demonstrable antisperm antibody titers, nine (69%) had normal FSH responses, compared with only one of 12 (8%) without identifiable antisperm antibody titers. Their data were taken to suggest that certain men following vasectomy have abnormalities in seminiferous tubule and Leydig cell functions of the testes. These abnormalities are unrelated to the interval after vasectomy and are not identifiable with routine static hormonal measurements.

In another study which indicated an effect of the operation on androgen production, prevasectomy levels of plasma LH, FSH, testosterone (T), estradiol (E_2) and 20α-dihydroprogesterone (20α-DHP), as well as semen analyses including semen volume, sperm count and sperm motility, from 260 healthy men were evaluated for annual changes. A statistically significant ($p \leq 0.015$) high-amplitude seasonal variation with the peak in April–May was detected in semen volume, sperm count and sperm motility. A statistically significant ($p \leq 0.04$) annual change of moderate T to large FSH amplitude was detected in each of the five plasma endocrine variables as well. Plasma LH, T and E_2 peaked in autumn, while FSH and 20α-DHP peaked in summer.

Analysis of postvasectomy LH, FSH, E_2, 20α-DHP and T blood levels for the 3 years following vasectomy revealed loss of seasonal rhythmicity as a group phenomenon in LH, E_2 and T. The amplitude of the seasonal variation in FSH was decreased, and that in 20α-DHP was unchanged compared with before-vasectomy baselines. For those annual rhythms which persisted following vasectomy, the peak time was unchanged. Compared with the prevasectomy group annual mean, that for each of the endocrine values was unchanged, except for that of LH and total T, which was slightly, yet statistically significantly, elevated[70].

The sperm- and T-producing cells work together, literally side by side, on the common mission of producing and launching these 'egg-seeking missiles'. Recent research has shown just how closely these functions are linked in many ways, including their own hormonal communications, the so-called paracrine actions.

After the operation, there may be a variety of complications, which can be divided into short- and long-term.

Short-term   There is often mild to moderate discomfort which may cause the patient to be off work for anything from an hour to a week, depending on his pain threshold, motivation and how many of the fine nerve endings that run alongside the vas get caught up in the operation.

Hematoma, epididymitis or wound infection occurred in up to 10% of cases in one carefully reported Canadian study[71], especially where there was little experience of the technique, which is often delegated to junior staff. This series of 1224 men documented complications in 124 cases (10.1%) and included 46 minor infections (3.8%), two serious infections (0.16%), 23 instances of epididymitis (1.9%), 16 cases of sperm granuloma (1.3%) and four minor hemorrhages (0.33%). In some studies infection rates up to 32.9% have been reported[72]. Such immediate complication rates, even in expert hands, means that this common operation must be causing a large amount of morbidity worldwide, especially as antibiotic resistant postoperative infections increase.

Fortunately quite infrequently, a variety of other changes can occur which cause a persistent and disabling 'postvasectomy pain syndrome'. One UK study of chronic testicular pain following vasectomy, for example, involved a survey by postal questionnaire and telephone interview of 172 patients 4 years after the operation. Chronic testicular discomfort was present in 56 patients (33%), considered by 26 (15%) to be troublesome but not by the other 30 (17%). Testicular discomfort related to sexual intercourse occurred in nine cases (5%). Of the nine patients who had sought further medical help, only two had had further surgery (one an epididymectomy and one excision of a hydrocele). Only three patients regretted having had the vasectomy because of chronic pain. On ultrasound examination, epididymal cysts were a common finding on both asymptomatic and symptomatic patients following vasectomy. It was concluded that prior to vasectomy, all patients should be counseled with regard to the risk of chronic testicular pain[73]. However, this is still seldom done.

Similar complication rates were reported in two UK populations studied 1 and 10 years after vasectomy. Wound infection occurred in 8 and 13%, and persistent scrotal pain in 17% (6% severe) and 14% (4% severe) in the two groups respectively[74].

Granulomas have been estimated to occur in between 3 and 75% of cases, averaging about 60%[74], but are usually small and pain-free. They may, however, increase the chances of antibodies against the patient's own sperm. Also there may be scarring of the testis from the bruising, and damming-back of the sperm and other products of the testis, which now have nowhere to go, into small 'blowout' cysts of the vas.

Long-term   Long-term complications of vasectomy may be much more common and diverse than is generally recognized. Of the limited amount of research which has been done, some is reassuring and some less so.

Andropause   Whether vasectomy does in fact predispose men to andropause later in life is an important but arguable point. As listed above, there are a range of theoretical reasons why it might do so. Clinically, however, that a common operation performed 10–20 years earlier was responsible for androgen deficiency arising in mainly 50–60-year-old men is hard to prove. Most of the research on vasectomy and testicular endocrine function is relatively short-term, usually 3–5 years, and research funds are hard to come by in such a controversial field, particularly with potential financial and medicolegal consequences for the vast vasectomy industry.

In the UK Andropause Study (UKAS), the incidence of vasectomy was 24% (360 of 1500: see Appendix 3), which is considerably higher than the average frequency of the operation in the general UK population of that age. The age distribution of the vasectomy group was slightly, but significantly, lower (53.4 versus 54.3, $p = 0.009$); the severity of symptoms, in terms of total andropause score at the first visit, was greater (27.8 versus 24.5, $p = 0.000$) sexual activity in terms of total orgasms per month was lower (5.5 versus 6.5, $p = 0.032$); and LH was lower (3.42 versus 3.82, $p = 0.009$). Other endocrine variables (total testosterone, FAI, calculated FT, FSH, E_2, and PSA and its subfractions) showed no significant differences between the vasectomy and nonvasectomy andropausal subjects.

The most common time for the symptoms to appear is 10–15 years after the vasectomy. This time scale was confirmed independently by another group in London, who also showed a fall in testosterone levels at this time. Other studies from Denmark have shown that the amount of testosterone and one of its active fractions, DHT, in the ejaculate are reduced by 23% and 40%, respectively, by vasectomy[75].

Vascular disease Whether or not vasectomy is one of the etiological factors in vascular disease, especially coronary heart disease, is typical of the important debates which have been raging about this method of contraception since it became common over 30 years ago. Studies of this and other possibly related illnesses are subject to confounding variables such as cultural and religious bias in reporting the operation. Roman Catholics, for example, are likely to under-report the operation. Also, subjects choosing vasectomy may differ socially, psychologically or in their health habits from those using other methods of contraception. The effect of hormonal changes may vary with differences in the baseline androgen levels in different races at different ages.

The debate began in the 1970s with the work of Nancy Alexander, who was among the first to point out that vasectomy in both man and a variety of experimental animals, including two varieties of monkeys, caused the production of CICs, which she considered to be linked to increased atherosclerosis. The group's early work also showed a mild change in arteriolar vessels in a small study of vasectomized men, and found a mild but insignificant increase in systolic blood pressure in vasectomized men over time compared with an age-matched group[76].

Later work showed that the rise in CICs in men was more transitory than in monkeys[77], and, although in some studies the increase was greater in men with coronary heart disease[78], the National Institutes of Health in America[79] and a large record-linkage study in Oxford[80] appeared to refute any association.

Prostate cancer   Another condition which has been linked to vasectomy in some studies, but not in others, is cancer of the prostate. Evidence is particularly conflicting here, but again, if it is proven, the link could be explained by long-term hormonal disturbances. Reduced semen flow through the prostate has been suggested as another possible link, but seems unlikely, as vasectomy reduces semen volume only by 5%, and this form of cancer is not particularly common in men leading a celibate life, such as monks.

Evidence is divided, to say the least; examples of studies showing a positive association range from small-scale case–control studies[81] to larger, prospective, epidemiological studies[82].

Conflicting results denying a link were found in other, equally large and well-executed studies, as well as emphasizing the importance of confounding variables such as social class, health-care patterns, lifestyle factors, such as smoking and diet, and geographical location. A large-scale study in Colorado found that vasectomy and an increased length of time since vasectomy are not associated with a higher risk of prostate cancer[83]. More recent research in Denmark also strongly added to the evidence that there is no excess prostate cancer risk after vasectomy[84].

The state of the debate is probably best currently represented by a meta-analysis carried out recently by an American group[85], who conducted a quantitative review of prostate cancer studies, pooling relative risk (RR) estimates of the association between prostate cancer and vasectomy. Random-effects models were examined along with a linear model for time since vasectomy. The pooled RR estimate was 1.37 (95% confidence interval (CI) 1.15–1.62), based on five cohort studies and 17 case–control studies. The RR estimate varied by study design, with the lowest risk for population-based case–control studies. No difference was seen in risk by age at vasectomy. A linear trend based on the 16 studies reporting time since vasectomy suggested a 10% increase for each additional 10 years or a RR of 1.32 (95% CI 1.17–1.50) for 30 years since vasectomy. When null effects were assumed for the six studies not reporting information, the linear RR for the 22 studies were 1.07 (1.03–1.11) and 1.23 (1.11–1.37) for 10 and 30 years since vasectomy, respectively. These results suggest that vasectomized men may be at an increased risk of prostate cancer; however, the increase may not be causal, since potential bias cannot be discounted and could explain the overall small association.

Testicular cancer   The surge in LH and total T[70] could also explain why there have been several reports of an increased number of cases of testicular cancer within the first 4 years after vasectomy[86,87], reaching a maximum after 2, although there are other studies which contradict this[88,89]. The tumor, which is increasing at a rate of about 2% per annum, particularly in young men, is most common when the testicles fail to descend, which is a condition also associated with raised FSH levels. It has recently been linked to environmental estrogens, which may have a similar effect in contributing to testicular failure and high FSH levels. An alternative theory is that there is no causal relationship between vasectomy and testicular cancer, but that it might precipitate the development of testicular cancer from preinvasive carcinoma *in situ* (CIS)[90].

In summary, it is reassuring that, in 1992, a large-scale, retrospective, record-linkage study in Oxford showed no evidence of a link between vasectomy, coronary heart disease, prostate and testicular cancer, or any other of the wide range of diseases surveyed[80]. However, the question arises whether any new contraceptive drug or device with the full range of proven and potential side effects of vasectomy would be allowed on the market in the present safety-conscious medical climate.

Target organs

As well as being affected by many of the above drugs, AR in many of the target organs, and the intracellular concentrations of both testosterone and DHT, decrease with age to a variable degree. Scrotal skin, for example, maintains the same levels of testosterone and DHT throughout life, whereas pubic skin levels of both are halved over the age of 60[31]. The same is thought to happen in the cavernosal AR regulating NOS activity, which together could account for the loss in penile sensitivity and morning erections, which together with erectile dysfunction occur as part of the andropausal picture, and need testosterone treatment to reverse.

In some men, the inherited lengthening of the CAG or GGN repeat sectors of the AR reduces the sensitivity of the receptor later in life, as described above.

Cardiac and skeletal muscles both have lower concentrations of AR than the accessory sex organs, and reduced levels of testosterone with age. Maintaining levels of cardiovascular and musculoskeletal fitness can reduce or even reverse this age-related decline, and, together with testosterone supplementation where needed, can help to maintain the condition and mass of both types of muscle, as well as prevent osteoporosis.

The shift of cellular metabolism from aerobic to anaerobic, caused by changes such as reduced tissue oxygenation resulting from aging processes, such as impaired perfusion and impaired carbohydrate metabolism, particularly in diabetics, leads to anoxia in both the cardiac and skeletal muscle, which can be reversed in many cases by testosterone treatment[91].

Drugs such as the aromatase inhibitors, and α_1- and α_2-adrenoreceptor blocking agents, can increase tissue resistance to androgen action.

KEY MESSAGES

Every level of the regulation, synthesis and action of androgens should be considered when assessing, diagnosing and treating the andropause. Rather than just throwing testosterone at the problem and hoping it will go away, depending on the history, a complete program of treatment may need to include, where possible, lifestyle changes such as stress management, relationship counseling, an exercise program, weight and alcohol reduction, and change in drug regime to one with fewer side-effects.

This understanding leads to a broad approach to managing this increasingly common disorder, and one that can be well suited to the basic skills of the personal physician armed with the supplementary specialist knowledge contained in this book.

References

1. Carruthers M. The diagnosis of androgen deficiency. *Aging Male* 2002;4:254

2. Schwanzel-Fukuda M, Jorgenson KL, Bergen HT, Weesner GD, Pfaff DW. Biology of normal luteinizing hormone-releasing hormone neurons during and after their migration from olfactory placode. *Endocr Rev* 1992;13: 623–34

3. Weinbauer GF, Gromoll J, Simoni M, Nieschlag E. Physiology of testicular function. In Nieschlag E, Behre H, eds. *Andrology: Male Reproductive Health and Dysfunction*. Berlin: Springer, 1997: 25–57

4. Jockenhovel F, Fingscheidt U, Khan SA, Behre HM, Nieschlag E. Bio- and immuno-activity of FSH in serum after intramuscular injection of highly purified urinary human FSH in normal men. *Clin Endocrinol (Oxf)* 1990;33:573–84

5. Rommerts FFG. Testosterone: an overview of biosynthesis, transport, metabolism and non-genomic actions. In Nieschlag E, Behre HM, eds. *Testosterone: Action, Deficiency, Substitution*. Cambridge: Cambridge University Press, 2004:1–37

6. Shanbhag VP, Sodergard R. The temperature dependence of the binding of 5α-dihydrotestosterone, testosterone and estradiol to the sex hormone binding globulin (SHBG) of human plasma. *J Steroid Biochem* 1986;24:549–55

7. Pardridge WM. Transport of protein-bound hormones into tissues *in vivo*. *Endocr Rev* 1981;2: 103–23

8. Rosner W, Hryb DJ, Khan MS, Nakhla AM, Romas NA. Sex hormone-binding globulin mediates steroid hormone signal transduction at the plasma membrane. *J Steroid Biochem Mol Biol* 1999;69:481–5

9. Kahn SM, Hryb DJ, Nakhla AM, Romas NA, Rosner W. Sex hormone-binding globulin is synthesized in target cells. *J Endocrinol* 2002;175:113–20

10. Fortunati N. Sex hormone-binding globulin: not only a transport protein. What news is around the corner? *J Endocrinol Invest* 1999;22:223–34

11. Rosner W, Hryb DJ, Khan MS, Nakhla AM, Romas NA. Androgen and estrogen signaling at the cell membrane via G-proteins and

cyclic adenosine monophosphate. *Steroids* 1999;64:100–6

12. Fortunati N, Becchis M, Catalano MG, *et al.* Sex hormone-binding globulin, its membrane receptor, and breast cancer: a new approach to the modulation of estradiol action in neoplastic cells. *J Steroid Biochem Mol Biol* 1999;69:473–9

13. Damassa DA, Cates JM. Sex hormone-binding globulin and male sexual development. *Neurosci Biobehav Rev* 1995;19:165–75

14. Vermeulen A. Declining androgens with age: an overview. In Oddens B, Vermeulen A, eds. *Androgens and The Aging Male.* New York: The Parthenon Publishing Group, 1996:3–14

15. Farnsworth WE. Roles of estrogen and SHBG in prostate physiology. *Prostate* 1996;28:17–23

16. Botwood N, Hamilton-Fairley D, Kiddy D, Robinson S, Franks S. Sex hormone-binding globulin and female reproductive function. *J Steroid Biochem Mol Biol* 1995;53:529–31

17. Quigley CA. The androgen receptor: physiology and pathophysiology. In Nieschlag E, Behre HM, eds. *Testosterone: Action, Deficiency, Substitution.* Heidelberg: Springer, 1998:33–106

18. Zitzmann M, Nieschlag E. The CAG repeat polymorphism within the androgen receptor gene and maleness. *Int J Androl* 2003;26:76–83

19. Lundin KB, Giwercman A, Ruhayel J, Giwercman YL. Functional difference between the two most common alleles of the androgen receptor GGN repeat in Swedish infertile men. Proceedings of the 3rd International Symposium on *Testosterone: Action, Deficiency, Substitution,* 2003

20. Aschim EL, Nordenskjold A, Giw-ercman A, Haugen TB, Grotmol T, Giwercman YL. Genotyping of the androgen receptor CAG and GGN repeats in boys with hypospadias. Proceedings of the 3rd International Symposium on *Testosterone: Action, Deficiency, Substitution,* 2003

21. Krithivas K, Yurgalevitch SM, Mohr BA, *et al.* Evidence that the CAG repeat in the androgen receptor gene is associated with the age-related decline in serum androgen levels in men. *J Endocrinol* 1999;162:137–42

22. Vermeulen A, Kaufman JM. Diagnosis of hypogonadism in the aging male. *Aging Male* 2002;5:170–6

23. Hogervorst E, Williams J, Budge M, Barnetson L, Combrinck M, Smith AD. Serum total testosterone is lower in men with Alzheimer's disease. *Neuroendocrinol Lett* 2001;22:163–8

24. Elwan O, Abdallah M, Issa I, Taher Y, el Tamawy M. Hormonal changes in cerebral infarction in the young and elderly. *J Neurol Sci* 1990;98:235–43

25. Okun MS, McDonald WM, DeLong MR. Refractory nonmotor symptoms in male patients with Parkinson disease due to testosterone deficiency: a common unrecognized comorbidity. *Arch Neurol* 2002;59:807–11

26. Dong Q, Hawker F, McWilliam D, Bangah M, Burger H, Handelsman DJ. Circulating immunoreactive inhibin and testosterone levels in men with critical illness. *Clin Endocrinol* 1992;36:399–404

27. Fox CA, Ismail AA, Love DN, Kirkham KE, Loraine JA. Studies on the relationship between plasma testosterone levels and human sexual activity. *J Endocrinol* 1996; 52:51–8

28. Bancroft J. *Human Sexuality and Its Problems.* Edinburgh: Churchill Livingstone, 1989

29. Barnes TRE, Harvey CA. Psychiatric drugs and sexuality. In Riley AJ, Peet M, Wilson C, eds. *Sexual Pharmacology*. Oxford: Oxford University Press, 1993:176–96

30. Meikle AW, Bishop DT, Stringham JD, West DW. Quantitating genetic and non-genetic factors to determine plasma sex steroid variation in normal male twins. *Metabolism* 1987;35:1090–5

31. Vermeulen A. Androgens and male senescence. In Nieschlag E, Behre HM, eds. *Testosterone: Action, Deficiency, Substitution*. Heidelberg: Springer, 1990:261–76

32. Sarkola T, Fukunaga T, Makisalo H, Peter Eriksson CJ. Acute effect of alcohol on androgens in premenopausal women. *Alcohol Alcohol* 2000;35:84–90

33. Sarkola T, Eriksson CJ. Testosterone increases in men after a low dose of alcohol. *Alcohol Clin Exp Res* 2003;27:682–5

34. Sparrow D, Bosse R, Rowe JW. The influence of age, alcohol consumption, and body build on gonadal function in men. *J Clin Endocrinol Metab* 1980;51:508–12

35. Badr FM, Bartke A, Dalterio S, Bulger W. Suppression of testosterone production by ethyl alcohol. Possible mode of action. *Steroids* 1977;30:647–55

36. Rettori V, McCann SM. Role of nitric oxide and alcohol on gonadotropin release *in vitro* and *in vivo*. *Ann N Y Acad Sci* 1998;840:185–93

37. Wright J. Endocrine effects of alcohol. *Clin Endocrinol Metab* 1978;7:351–67

38. Heikkonen E, Ylikahri R, Roine R, Valimaki M, Harkonen M, Salaspuro M. The combined effect of alcohol and physical exercise on serum testosterone, luteinizing hormone, and cortisol in males. *Alcohol Clin Exp Res* 1996;20:711–16

39. Sudha S, Balasubramanian K, Arunakaran J, Govindarajulu P. Preliminary study of androgen, thyroid and adrenal status in alcoholic men during deaddiction. *Indian J Med Res* 1995;101:268–72

40. Zumoff B, Kream J, Strain GW, Levin J. Elevated 24-hour mean plasma concentration of FSH in men with cirrhosis of the liver. *J Reprod Med* 1984;29:123–5

41. Adams ML, Forman JB, Kalicki JM, Meyer ER, Sewing B, Cicero TJ. Antagonism of alcohol-induced suppression of rat testosterone secretion by an inhibitor of nitric oxide synthase. *Alcohol Clin Exp Res* 1993;17:660–4

42. Adams ML, Meyer ER, Sewing BN, Cicero TJ. Effects of nitric oxide-related agents on alcohol narcosis. *Alcohol Clin Exp Res* 1994;18:969–75

43. Sun H, Mayhan WG. Superoxide dismutase ameliorates impaired nitric oxide synthase-dependent dilatation of the basilar artery during chronic alcohol consumption. *Brain Res* 2001;891:116–22

44. Carruthers ME, Chen CN, Crisp AH, *et al*. Early morning migraine: nocturnal levels of catecholamines, tryptophan, glucose and free fatty acids and sleep encephalographs. *Lancet* 1976;1:445–7

45. Sun H, Patel KP, Mayhan WG. Impairment of neuronal nitric oxide synthase-dependent dilation of cerebral arterioles during chronic alcohol consumption. *Alcohol Clin Exp Res* 2002;26:663–70

46. Oshita M, Takei Y, Kawano S, Hijioka T, Fusamoto H, Kamada T. Alcohol and endogenous nitric oxide in hepatic microcirculation. *Alcohol Alcohol* 1994;29(Suppl 1):5–7

47. Parks DA, Booyse FM. Cardiovascular protection by alcohol and polyphenols: role of nitric oxide. *Ann N Y Acad Sci* 2002;957:115–21

48. English KM, Mandour O, Steeds RP, Diver MJ, Jones TH, Channer KS. Men with coronary artery disease have lower levels of androgens than men with normal coronary angiograms [see Comments]. *Eur Heart J* 2000;21:890–4

49. Swartz CM, Young MA. Low serum testosterone and myocardial infarction in geriatric male inpatients. *J Am Geriatr Soc* 1987;35:39–44

50. Hamalainen EK, Adlercreutz H, Puska P, Pietinen P. Decrease of serum total and free testosterone during a low-fat high-fibre diet. *J Steroid Biochem* 1983;18:369–70

51. Smith KW, Feldman HA, McKinlay JB. Construction and field validation of a self-administered screener for testosterone deficiency (hypogonadism) in ageing men. *Clin Endocrinol (Oxf)* 2000;53:703–11

52. Longcope C, Feldman HA, McKinlay JB, Araujo AB. Diet and sex hormone-binding globulin. *J Clin Endocrinol Metab* 2000;85:293–6

53. Vermeulen A, Kaufman JM, Giagulli VA. Influence of some biological indexes on sex hormone-binding globulin and androgen levels in aging or obese males. *J Clin Endocrinol Metab* 1996;81:1821–6

54. Longcope C, Goldfield SR, Brambilla DJ, McKinlay JB. Androgens, estrogens, and sex hormone-binding globulin in middle-aged men. *J Clin Endocrinol Metab* 1990;71:1442–6

55. Carruthers M. More effective testosterone treatment: combination with sildenafil and danazol. *Aging Male* 2000;3:16

56. Bujan L, Daudin M, Charlet JP, Thonneau P, Mieusset R. Increase in scrotal temperature in car drivers. *Hum Reprod* 2000;15:1355–7

57. Carruthers M. *Male Menopause: Restoring Vitality and Virility.* London: HarperCollins, 1996

58. Chehval MJ, Martin SA, Alexander NJ, Winkelmann T. The effect of unilateral injury to the vas deferens on the contralateral testis in immature and adult rats. *J Urol* 1995; 153:1313–15

59. Fisch H, Laor E, Reid RE, Tolia BM, Freed SZ. Gonadal dysfunction after testicular torsion: luteinizing hormone and follicle-stimulating hormone response to gonadotropin releasing hormone. *J Urol* 1988;139:961–4

60. Isidori A, Dondero F, Lenzi A. Immunobiology of male infertility. *Hum Reprod* 1988;3:75–7

61. Bohring C, Krause W. Differences in the antigen pattern recognized by antisperm antibodies in patients with infertility and vasectomy. *J Urol* 2001;166:1178–80

62. Hargreave TB, Harvey J, Elton RA, McMillan A. Serum agglutinating and immobilising sperm antibodies in men attending a sexually transmitted diseases clinic. *Andrologia* 1984;16:111–15

63. Shahani SK, Hattikudur NS. Immunological consequences of vasectomy. *Arch Androl* 1981;7: 193–9

64. Clarkson TB, Lombardi DM, Alexander NJ, Lewis JC. Diet and vasectomy: effects on atherogenesis in cynomolgus macaques. *Exp Mol Pathol* 1986;44:29–49

65. Lenzi A, Valesini G, Dondero F. Vasectomy: study of circulating immune-complexes and its correlation with antisperm immunity in man, with a twelve-month follow-up study. *Andrologia* 1985;17: 158–65

66. Jarow JP, Goluboff ET, Chang TS, Marshall FF. Relationship between antisperm antibodies and testicular

histologic changes in humans after vasectomy. *Urology* 1994;43:521-4

67. Peng XS, Li FD, Miao ZR, *et al.* Plasma reproductive hormones in normal and vasectomized Chinese males. *Int J Androl* 1987;10:471-9

68. Smith KD, Tcholakian RK, Chowdhury M, Steinberger E. An investigation of plasma hormone levels before and after vasectomy. *Fertil Steril* 1976;27:144-51

69. Fisch H, Laor E, BarChama N, Witkin SS, Tolia BM, Reid RE. Detection of testicular endocrine abnormalities and their correlation with serum antisperm antibodies in men following vasectomy. *J Urol* 1989;141:1129-32

70. Reinberg A, Smolensky MH, Hallek M, Smith KD, Steinberger E. Annual variation in semen characteristics and plasma hormone levels in men undergoing vasectomy. *Fertil Steril* 1988;49:309-15

71. Alderman PM. Complications in a series of 1224 vasectomies [see Comments]. *J Fam Pract* 1991;33:579-84

72. Randall PE, Ganguli L, Marcuson RW. Wound infection following vasectomy. *Br J Urol* 1983;55:564-7

73. McMahon AJ, Buckley J, Taylor A, Lloyd SN, Deane RF, Kirk D. Chronic testicular pain following vasectomy. *Br J Urol* 1992;69:188-91

74. McDonald SW. Vasectomy review: sequelae in the human epididymis and ductus deferens. *Clin Anat* 1996;9:337-42

75. Ying W, Hedman M, Diczfalusy E, *et al.* Effect of vasectomy on the steroid profile of human seminal plasma. *Int J Androl* 1983;6:116-24

76. Alexander NJ. Possible mechanisms of vasectomy-exacerbated atherosclerosis. *Aust J Biol Sci* 1982;35:469-79

77. Witkin SS, Alexander NJ, Frick J. Circulating immune complexes and sperm antibodies following vasectomy in Austrian men. *J Clin Lab Immunol* 1984;14:69-72

78. Alexander NJ, Fulgham DL, Plunkett ER, Witkin SS. Antisperm antibodies and circulating immune complexes of vasectomized men with and without coronary events. *Am J Reprod Immunol Microbiol* 1986;12:38-44

79. National Institutes of Health. Long-term vasectomy shows no association with coronary heart disease. *J Am Med Assoc* 1984;252:1005

80. Nienhuis H, Goldacre M, Seagroatt V, Gill L, Vessey M. Incidence of disease after vasectomy: a record linkage retrospective cohort study *Br Med J* 1992:304:743-6

81. Rosenberg L, Palmer JR, Zauber AG, Warshauer ME, Stolley PD, Shapiro S. Vasectomy and the risk of prostate cancer. *Am J Epidemiol* 1990;132:1051-5

82. Giovannucci E, Ascherio A, Rimm EB, Colditz GA, Stampfer MJ, Willett WC. A prospective cohort study of vasectomy and prostate cancer in US men. *J Am Med Assoc* 1993;269:873-7

83. DeAntoni EP, Goktas S, Stenner J, O'Donnell C, Crawford ED. A cross-sectional study of vasectomy, time since vasectomy and prostate cancer. *Prostate Cancer Prostatic Dis* 1997;1:73-8

84. Lynge E. Prostate cancer is not increased in men with vasectomy in Denmark. *J Urol* 2002;168:488-90

85. Dennis LK, Dawson DV, Resnick MI. Vasectomy and the risk of prostate cancer: a meta-analysis examining vasectomy status, age at vasectomy, and time since vasectomy. *Prostate Cancer Prostatic Dis* 2002;5:193-203

86. Cale AR, Farouk M, Prescott RJ,

Wallace IW. Does vasectomy accelerate testicular tumour? Importance of testicular examinations before and after vasectomy [see Comments]. *Br Med J* 1990;300: 370

87. Thornhill JA, Conroy RM, Kelly DG, Walsh A, Fennelly JJ, Fitzpatrick JM. An evaluation of predisposing factors for testis cancer in Ireland. *Eur Urol* 1988;14:429–33

88. Moller H, Knudsen LB, Lynge E. Risk of testicular cancer after vasectomy: cohort study of over 73 000 men. *Br Med J* 1994;309:295–9

89. Hewitt G, Logan CJ, Curry RC. Does vasectomy cause testicular cancer? *Br J Urol* 1993;71:607–8

90. Jorgensen N, Giwercman A, Hansen SW, Skakkebaek NE. Testicular cancer after vasectomy: origin from carcinoma *in situ* of the testis. *Eur J Cancer* 1993;29A: 1062–4

91. Moller J, Einfeldt H. *Testosterone Treatment of Cardiovascular Diseases*. Berlin: Springer-Verlag, 1984.

4 The diagnosis of androgen deficiency

INTRODUCTION

One of the greatest obstacles to the diagnosis of androgen deficiency in the adult male is the problem of achieving a suitable definition. If we return to the definition given in the preceding chapter,

> 'an absolute or relative insufficiency of testosterone or its metabolites in relation to the needs of that individual at that time in his life'[1],

the question centers on who is going to judge whether a patient is androgen deficient, the physician or the laboratory, or both working together?

Laboratory-based doctors, particularly endocrinologists, tend to put far more emphasis on endocrine tests, but often do not take into account the severe problems discussed below in obtaining a representative blood sample, analyzing it accurately and then interpreting it in the light of that patient's symptoms and clinical condition. They are used to seeing younger patients with clear-cut developmental or genetic abnormalities, and labeling them as having primary or secondary hypogonadism.

These labels do not fit the average andropausal male in his 50s too well, so the doctors resort to complex terms such as 'hypergonadotropic hypogonadism'. These terms are unsatisfactory for the general clinician, who is unclear what precisely they mean or imply in terms of causation. The patient does not like such labels much either, because he cannot understand them except that they seem to imply that his testicles are malfunctioning in some way. More important, because the largely laboratory-based doctor will have strict definitions of hypogonadism based on a particular level of testosterone, except for the rare cases fulfilling such criteria, treatment will be denied.

Because of these considerations it is suggested that the diagnosis of androgen deficiency should rest on a combination of a full history, physical examination and specific andropause rating scales, as well as laboratory tests. For reasons explained later in this chapter, it is suggested that where there is still doubt, and it is safe to give it, a therapeutic trial of testosterone treatment may be needed to confirm or deny the diagnosis.

DEFINITION OF ANDROPAUSE

Probably the best current definition of the term 'andropause' is that proposed by Tremblay and Morales:

> *when men exhibit several of the symptoms and/or clinical features of reduced testosterone availability to various systems or organ functions*[2].

This characteristic 'identikit' pattern of andropause symptoms is the same as that seen in androgen-deficient adult males generally, whether caused by testicular damage, suppression of testosterone by a prolactinoma, antiandrogens or increases in sex hormone-binding globulin (SHBG) caused by thyrotoxicosis or anticonvulsant drugs.

TAKING A HISTORY

A history of the *presenting problems* usually elicits many of the symptoms which will later be covered in detail in the screening questionnaire used, whether it is the Andropause Check List (ACL), or the Aging Males' Symptoms (AMS) version (see below for detailed description of both, and the Andropause Clinic form in Appendix 2B). It also focuses on the patient's priorities and those symptoms that distress him most. The duration of the symptoms often gives a clue as to the likely cause.

The *other problems* reported may also indicate other reasons why the man is androgen deficient, as indicated in the chapter on causation. A wide range of chronic illnesses such as diabetes or hypertension and psychological stress can also have an androgen-lowering effect.

Conversely, there are many iatrogenic causes of both androgen deficiency and erectile dysfunction, particularly those induced by medications for hypertension and cardiovascular disease, and by psychotropic drugs. Treatment for rheumatoid or osteoarthritis and asthma may involve the use of corticosteroids, which can antagonize androgen actions. A history of loss of height can also suggest osteoporosis, whether or not accompanied by kyphosis or scoliosis.

Previous urinary tract infections and sexually transmitted diseases, especially nonspecific urethritis, can suggest possible causes for androgen deficiency, as well as indicating a high level of androgen action earlier in the man's life. It may also, like hepatitis B, be a marker of predisposition to human immunodeficiency virus (HIV) infection, which is known to be associated with reduced androgen levels.

A history of epilepsy should lead to inquiry about exposure to anticonvulsants, many of which can cause raised SHBG levels. Previous anxiety and depression can indicate that stress may be playing a large part in the individual's condition, or that the symptoms may be more due to a recurrence of his depressive state than to androgen deficiency. Conversely, if it is the first time in the man's life that he has become anxious or depressed, and there is no obvious external cause, a diagnosis of andropause becomes more likely.

Testicular problems may include a history of nondescent which was treated medically or surgically, and mumps any time after the age of 10, particularly if accompanied by orchitis. There is some evidence that any severe viral infection such as glandular fever (infectious mononucleosis) may cause damage, especially when the testis is developing its immunological defense system during a phase of rapid expansion at puberty.

Unilateral orchidectomy for any reason will obviously reduce the ability to produce androgens, and although there may be enough to complete normal puberty and for full fertility, the chances of developing andropause at an earlier age, and susceptibility to other contributory factors, are likely to be increased.

Traumatic episodes, such as blows with cricket balls or baseballs, especially if causing prolonged pain or bruising, can also cause mechanical or immunological damage. Similarly, torsion of the testis, even though only unilateral, can cause bilateral atrophy through sympathetic innervation or immune mechanisms.

Hydroceles and varicoceles are well-established factors in contributing to infertility and possibly reducing androgen production or metabolism, because of their water-jacketing effect in raising testicular temperature, but surgery to correct them may also further impair its function. Any operation on the testis or epididymis should generally be suspected as a possible cause of impaired function, and although controversial, for reasons discussed in the chapter on causation, it is suggested that vasectomy should be included among these. Hernia operations can occasionally damage structures passing through the inguinal canal, but this is usually evident shortly after the operation, and may present with local pain or testicular atrophy.

The patient should also be asked about exposure to toxic drugs such as agrochemicals or petrochemicals, which may have xenoestrogenic or anti-androgenic actions. Farmers particularly may have inhaled or absorbed through the skin the hormonally active compounds used to increase meat production, or pesticides and insecticides, such as dichlorodiphenyl-trichloroethane (DDT). Some fumes from welding and other industrial processes may also have hormonally disrupting actions.

Anabolic steroid abuse, either at present or any time in the past, can also cause testicular atrophy and suppression of the hypophyseal–gonadal axis of unknown duration. Similarly, abuse of a wide range of addictive drugs, especially opiates, and even possibly cannabis, can affect androgen production or action.

Current and previous medication, specifically tranquilizers, hypnotics, beta-blockers, other cardioactive drugs, alpha-blockers, aromatase inhibitors, antihypertensives, anti-inflammatory agents and antifungals, should all be assessed. Even hormonally active agents applied to the scalp such as finasteride, spasmolytic inhalations and nasal decongestants have all been reported as contributory factors in erectile dysfunction.

As well as inquiry about a history of urinary tract infections, urological operations and catheterizations may all indicate renal, bladder or most commonly prostatic pathology needing further investigation by an expert urologist before androgen treatment can be started. An evaluation of lower urinary tract symptoms also gives a pretreatment baseline to monitor any possible side-effects of androgens.

However, it must be emphasized that while current or previous prostatic cancer must be generally regarded as an absolute contraindication to androgen treatment, all except the most severe degrees of benign prostatic hyperplasia are not. Indeed, some of the symptoms of irritable bladder syndrome, and recurrent cystitis, may improve on androgen replacement therapy (ART), as the condition of the bladder epithelium and muscle improves under the action of testosterone. This is equivalent to the improvement in bladder function and resistance to infection seen in women on hormone replacement therapy (HRT).

Lifestyle factors such as smoking habits, present and previous alcohol consumption, and exercise should also be assessed, as they can all affect androgen production and action, as well as overall health and the progress of treatment.

The family history, as well as indicating a predisposition to hereditary disorders such as diabetes and cardiovascular disease, can also indicate genetic links to neoplastic and psychological conditions such as depression. In particular, the physician should inquire about a history of benign or malignant prostate disorders in close male relatives such as grandparents, father, uncles and brothers. A history of one such relative with prostate cancer doubles the risk, while with two the incidence goes up four times.

A history of marriages or other long-term relationships can indicate the lifetime sexual activity and orientation of the patient, as well as predisposition to sexually transmitted diseases. The number and age of children give a good indication of whether and when the patient was fertile, which may have important implications for his previous and, to a lesser extent, his present androgen production.

Before proceeding to the detailed assessment of symptoms related to androgen insufficiency, a general *psychosocial history* is taken to establish whether the patient is in a supportive and satisfactory relationship, or whether there is conflict such as in a divorce or separation situation, which is contributing to, or even causing his problems. The extremes of excessive stress and understimulation, as when unemployed, leading to either 'burnout' or 'rust-out', can both affect androgen production and erectile function. In general, anything which results in a loss of status or self-esteem and 'puts a man down' puts down his testosterone levels, and raises resistance to their action.

PHYSICAL EXAMINATION

As a broad approach to the diagnosis and treatment of androgen-related disorders is essential, a general medical examination is required in all cases.

This should include measurement of the height, weight and blood pressure, and some measure of adiposity, whether it is body mass index (BMI), waist/hip ratio or one of the more detailed measurements of body fat provided by skin-fold thickness measurements at several sites, or one of the electronic devices used for the purpose. Abdominal obesity particularly is linked with cardiovascular disease, and can also indicate syndrome X, both of which are associated with lowered androgen levels.

Gynecomastia may be a feature of excess body fat generally, or located within the breast tissue, when it is more likely to be a useful marker of endocrine imbalance. This can be linked with the hyperestrogenism caused by the aromatase activity in excess body fat, resulting from xenoestrogens in beer or agrochemicals, from the side-effects of a range of drugs mentioned in the chapter on causation and even from anabolic steroid abuse. Gynecomastia is recognized in gymnasia as 'witches' tits', a term of insult in body-building circles.

Less informative generally, although it is taken as one of the classical signs of androgen deficiency in boys with delayed puberty and other congenital hormonal disorders such as Klinefelter's syndrome, is reduced body hair. A patient can have severe balding, and abundant hair on the chest, abdomen, axillae and arms, and still be severely androgen deficient in the present day – an inactive testosterone volcano. Failure to allow for this results in many cases of andropause being missed.

Only infrequently, and usually as a natural feature of aging along with sprouting nasal, ear and eyebrow hair, is there reduction in either the density, or distribution upwards towards the umbilicus, of pubic hair. Reduction in frequency of shaving is also rarely noticed except in extreme cases. Overall, hair growth is a very unreliable guide to androgen production. It must be remembered that hair can continue to grow on a dead body.

The dryness, wrinkling and inelasticity of the skin, especially when accompanied by thinning, together with liability to injuries which heal poorly especially on the shins and feet, is a more useful indicator. The state of nutrition of the feet, the presence of hair on the dorsum and the state of the peripheral pulses can also be useful markers of androgen status in older patients.

Penile atrophy is rarely marked, but patients may complain that it appears to be shrinking recently. A few cases of true micropenis or partial hypospadias, which may be accompanied by a poorly developed scrotum, can have been missed by medical examiners from childhood onwards, and present even late in adulthood. This lifelong androgen deficiency can have blighted a man's social and sexual development, and the heightened assertiveness and libido which androgen treatment can produce in such cases comes as something of a shock.

Unless there is marked atrophy, or a difference between the two sides, testicular size is rarely informative, although some clinicians use orchiometers routinely. The consistency of the testis can also give some information on its condition, as well as excluding testicular tumors. The scrotum should be examined initially with the patient standing to exclude variccoele and hydrocele, which are more easily detected in this position. The cremasteric reflex is best elicited with the patient lying on his back, and scrotal cysts are also easier to find in this position.

Last, but not least, a digital rectal examination (DRE) should be performed to rate the commonly encountered benign enlargement of the prostate, and aid the exclusion of prostatic carcinoma. When in doubt, and particularly in patients over 50 with a high-normal or elevated prostate-specific antigen (PSA) level, a transrectal ultrasound examination should be performed by an expert in the procedure, and if necessary any suspicious areas biopsied. In this way a number of early carcinomas will be detected as part of routine prescreening with DRE and PSA, and the serious clinical error of treating such a case with androgens avoided.

INCIDENCE OF ANDROPAUSE

Although originally described as a rare condition[3], there is evidence that the incidence of andropause is increasing.

Based on screening questionnaires, estimates vary according to the sampling technique. Heinemann and colleagues[4], using a new AMS rating scale in a sample of 959 German males aged 40–69 years selected for random telephone interviews, judged 27% to have moderate to severe scores. In the same study in a group of 116 male patients in a similar age range from general practice clinics in Berlin, 44% were considered to have moderate or severe andropause symptoms.

Again, estimates using laboratory data alone tend to be lower than those based on prevalence of symptoms, and depend on the androgens selected and the lower cutoff reference points. The work of Vermeulen shows that, using free testosterone (FT) as a preferable marker to total testosterone (TT), 10% of males aged 40–60, and 30% of men aged 60–80, could be considered androgen deficient[5]. He also observed that some tissues might have decreased androgen sensitivity in elderly men. This includes androgen receptors (AR) in the corpora cavernosa and the pubic skin, and suggests that such factors could explain why elderly males may need higher testosterone levels than younger males for adequate sexual activity.

The most recent study by Leifke and colleagues[6] in a group of 575 healthy, nonobese men aged 20–80 showed a mean lifetime fall of 51% for TT, 64% for FT and 70% for bioavailable testosterone (BT). These changes started in the third decade, and of the 60–80 age group, 25%, 40% and 60%, respectively, could be considered androgen deficient by comparison with the lowest levels seen in the 20–29 age group.

Similarly, Smith, Feldman and McKinlay reported an incidence of 'testosterone deficiency', defined by a consensus of 53 experts from the Endocrine Society as a TT level below 12.1 nmol/l (350 ng/dl), of 20.4% in 1660 subjects aged 40–60 in the Massachusetts Male Aging Study, and 42.1% in a similarly aged sample of 304 men from a primary health-care clinic[7]. This coincides with the latest data from the Massachusetts Male Aging Study[8], which shows 30-year falls in TT in individuals averaging 48%, and in FT of 85%.

Do nearly 60% of even apparently healthy men over the age of 60 have a significant androgen deficit, as the work of Leifke and colleagues would suggest[6], or is it 0.01% as defined by Huhtaniemi and his colleagues[9]? If nearer the former estimate, every physician dealing with the adult male should have an interest. If close to the latter, then this is a rare condition with little impact on clinical medicine or pharmacology.

How can estimates of the frequency of a medical condition in similar populations differ by 6000%? Mainly it seems to be a question of definition and criteria, combined with acceptance or rejection of the concept.

Also, it raises issues of whether you take into account its incidence in sick people or in the whole population; its incidence in which country and in which races and at what ages. There is general acceptance that androgens decrease with age, especially the crucial free and bioavailable fractions of testosterone. The reductions start to occur usually in the 30s, and there is on average a steady decrease for the rest of a man's life, which can be accelerated by the wide range of factors indicated in the previous chapter.

In comparison with women, the work of Burger has shown that a fall of 50% in estrogen levels at the menopause is sufficient to precipitate the classical symptoms[10], which 'makes FSH [follicle-stimulating hormone] and estradiol unreliable markers of menopausal status'. As Gooren argues, why should the halving of a man's testosterone from a youthful 35 nmol/l (1000 ng/dl) to 17.5 nmol/l (500 ng/dl) be regarded as insufficient to bring on andropausal symptoms[11]?

In the following sections the reasons for this steadily increasing frequency of diagnosis of andropause, and the higher incidence according to questionnaire studies than in those based on androgen levels alone, are explored. As will become apparent, this is the crux of the andropause problem: should we be relying predominantly on the patient's symptoms or the laboratory for the diagnosis?

SYMPTOM RATING SCALES

Development of rating scales

Because symptom rating is by definition the most important factor in establishing the diagnosis of the andropause and monitoring the effectiveness of the treatment, it is important to follow the evolution of the rating scales, and to form a view on which may be the best currently available for screening purposes, and for detailed clinical assessment. The contribution and experience of each of the clinicians with experience in the field will be considered in turn. Since the syndrome of the 'male climacteric' was first described by Dr August Werner in 1939[12], recognition of the diagnostic pattern of andropausal symptoms, which depended on a skilled and experienced clinical observer, has been replaced with more objective and widely applicable rating scales.

There is remarkable consistency in the clinical experience recorded by various observers, with diverse backgrounds, working in different countries and populations over more than 60 years, and arriving at the same conclusions (Table 1)[13].

Rating scale design

There are a number of features that should be built into the design of a rating scale, according to its applicability to clinical practice, research or preferably both. The aim generally is to produce a simple instrument that can be used in clinical practice to classify patients, and measure the effects of intervention. This is an ongoing process of validating any questionnaire, in which the following requirements have to be assessed:

(1) Both good sensitivity (among subjects who have the condition, the proportion who test positive) and specificity (among subjects who have the condition, test negative). These are usually conflicting elements, and decision limits, or cutoff points, have to be derived from ROC (receiver operating characteristic) curves. The significance of the false- positive and false-negative rates depends on the costs of misclassification, and the prevalence of the condition in the population being examined. This form of analysis has been claimed to be 'a comprehensive test of pure accuracy, i.e. discriminating ability over the entire range of the test'[18], and is used extensively in this chapter.

(2) Discrimination, which is the power of each question to differentiate between cases and noncases, as judged above, is the criterion for assessing whether each question is worth including in any scale. Questions with poor discrimination dilute the power of the rest of the scale.

(3) Reliability, which represents the accuracy with which measurements can be made. This includes:

   (a) Internal consistency, which is how much the different items in the questionnaire correlate with each other, and with the total score.

Table 1 Comparison of the incidence of symptoms (% or frequency) attributed to the andropause in various studies[13]

				Year study started			
Author	1939[3] Werner	1953[14] Reiter	1989[15] Carruthers	1996[16] Carruthers	1998[2] Tremblay	1999[4] Heinemann	1999[17] Morley
Scale title	Male Climacteric	IDUT	ACL	web ACL	CAS	AMS	ADAM
Responses	yes/no	0–12	0, 1, 2, 3, 4	0, 1, 2, 3, 4	yes/no	1, 2, 3, 4, 5	yes/no
Subjects (n)	273	100	1500	1533	300	992	316
Symptoms							
Erectile dysfunction	90	++	84	83	++	88	+++
Libido/sex drive/desire	81	++	82	87	++	84	+++
Fatigue/energy reduced	80	+	78	94	+	80	++
Depression	77	++	62	88	+	75	+
Anxiety/nervousness	91	++	++	85	+	69	
Memory/concentration	76	+	42	90	+		+
Irritability/anger	80	+	57	85	+	72	+
Aches/pains joints	33		57	83		77	
Sweating especially at night	18		50	63	+	66	
Vasomotor/flushes	46		27		+		
Aging/older than years			43	55		59	
Dry skin/thinning	30		40	63			

IDUT, Impotence, Depression, Urinary disturbance, Thyroidism; ACL, Andropause Check List; CAS, Canadian Andropause Society; AMS, Aging Male Symptoms; ADAM, Androgen Deficiency in Aging Males

(b) Test–retest reliability, which is the stability of scores across time. With andropause rating scales, the time intervals for this measurement need to be short, e.g. 1–2 weeks, as symptoms can fluctuate rapidly in severity even in the absence of treatment. This is a compromise between variability in the subject's state, and his ability to recall the answers he gave previously.

(c) Interrater reliability, which can occur even with self-reported scales, according to the level of education, training and expectations of the rater. This should be as high as possible, and ideally the scale should be made simple and unambiguous enough to enable it to be self-reported or applied by either experienced or inexperienced raters.

(d) Bias of the subject or rater, which can be either unconscious, or deliberately faking-good, or faking-bad, according to the desire of the subject to be or not to be a case, and of the rater to include or exclude a case.

(e) Between-language and between-culture reliability, to enable it to be widely applied and interpreted.

(4) Scalability, which varies with the number of responses possible for each item, and the number of items. The design of individual questions and analysis of the responses are discussed in relation to 'the detection of psychiatric illness by questionnaire' using the General Health Questionnaire (GHQ) by Goldberg[19].

(5) Brevity, like the soul of wit, is essential in all but research studies. This can severely limit the applicability of a rating scale either in a busy clinical setting or as a general screener.

The recent developments in andropause rating scales are now reviewed with these attributes in mind.

Andropause Check List (ACL; Carruthers 1998[14]) (for full scale see Appendix 2B)

When the UK Andropause Study (UKAS) began in 1989, a symptom check list was drawn up, based on the male climacteric symptoms first described by Dr August Werner in 1939[12]. These had been repeatedly confirmed by Dr Werner in his subsequent papers[3,20–23], other American clinicians[24,25] and Dr Tiberius Reiter in the UK[14,26,27].

That the symptoms were in fact due to testosterone deficiency was shown by Werner's report that, of the 177 men treated with 25 mg intramuscular injections of testosterone propionate three times a week, 173 showed benefit[3]. While identifying the same symptoms, in a single-blind treatment study of 20 patients, with the diagnosis supported by bioassay of urinary gonadotropins, Heller and Myers[24] reported a positive response in all their patients.

However, it was considered necessary to extend the list of symptoms used by previous authors to take various other factors into account:

(1) Duration of symptoms: usually the symptoms come on gradually over a number of years, and the pattern and time of onset can sometimes give useful information on the cause of the condition, e.g. stressful life events, interruptions in relationships, viral illnesses, etc.

(2) Severity of symptoms: the degree to which the subject experiences the symptoms both before and after various periods of treatment is an invaluable guide to progress. It provides a systematic and objective assessment of how he perceives the intensity of each complaint at the initial and follow-up visits.

(3) Detailed assessment of the degree and impact of erectile dysfunction: this overlaps to a considerable extent with the assessment provided by the 1997 International Index of Erectile Function (IIEF)[28]. However, the ACL tries to avoid apparent overlap of the items studied, which appears inherent in that scale.

The ACL also rates changes in the frequency of morning erections. This is often both the first warning of impending problems with erections in the andropause, and the first sign of improvement on treatment. Being more physiological than psychological, it is also largely independent of relationship issues and performance anxiety.

Like the IIEF, it rates the frequency of intercourse in terms of penetrative sex per month, and also includes daily rates. Furthermore it provides estimates of frequency of masturbation on both a monthly and a daily basis, which both allows for the unavailability or unwillingness of partners, and is less homophobic than other questionnaires.

Unlike the IIEF, it inquires about both premature and delayed ejaculation, which can be major problems even when penetrative sex is possible. The libido (which is taken to be equivalent in most patients' vocabulary to sex drive) of both the subject and his partner needs to be taken into account. Similarly, the satisfaction of both partners with whatever form of sexual activity is undertaken is a useful index of the outcome of treatment.

Finally, whether the subject has a partner, and if so the quality of the relationship between them, is often affected by the andropause, and improved at many levels by treatment.

When applied to the 1500 patients in the UKAS study, the ACL (Appendix 2B) gave the following results:

(1) The ACL scores and symptom subscales were normally distributed. Approximately 95% of the total scores were between 10 and 45, the mean being 25.8.

(2) The mean duration of the symptoms varied between 3 and 5 years (Table 2).

Table 2 Duration, severity and incidence of symptoms in UK Andropause Study (UKAS)

Symptom	Years	Severity	%
Fatigue/energy reduction	4.3	1.70	78.1
Depression	4.1	1.09	61.9
Irritability	3.7	1.09	56.6
Memory/concentration	4.9	0.73	42.4
Impaired relationship with partner	4.1	1.11	50.9
Dry/thinning skin	4.6	0.64	40.2
Sweating/night sweats	3.5	1.02	50.3
Vasomotor/flushing	3.4	0.49	27.3
Aches/pains/stiffness	3.8	1.03	56.9
Aging/older than years	3.2	0.70	42.8
Reduced libido/self	4.1	2.07	82.3
Reduced libido /partner	5.1	0.58	31.2
Erectile dysfunction/initiation	4.1	1.87	83.1
Erectile dysfunction /maintaining	4.1	2.16	83.7
Erectile dysfunction/morning	3.9	2.10	79.3
Ejaculation/ premature	4.6	0.50	25.7
Ejaculation/delayed	3.6	0.49	21.5
Orgasm of partner impaired	3.8	2.08	68.5
Sexual satisfaction/ self	3.1	2.41	93.8
Sexual satisfaction/partner	3.3	1.97	81.3

3. The internal consistency of the constituent items of the ACL was shown by their correlations with the total ACL score, and with each other. Also there were significant correlations between the items in the various domains, especially 'sexual', which unlike the items in the other domains were all strongly negatively correlated with total sexual activity per month, except for delayed ejaculation.

4. The ROC curves showed each item to be sensitive and specific in relation to the total ACL score (Figure 1), with a significance less than 0.05, except for partner's libido and premature ejaculation.

ACL summary

Advantages The ACL is based on a wide range of symptoms recognized for over 60 years as being characteristic of the andropause. It has been found over a period of 15 years to be clinically useful in the diagnosis and treatment of the andropause, and is related to the large amount of clinical and endocrine evidence in the UKAS. It goes into more detail than other andropause questionnaires on the erectile dysfunction aspects of the andropause, and the consequences in terms of reduced sexual satisfaction and sexual activity in both the patient and his partner. It fulfills most of the requirements of questionnaire design, particularly good sensitivity and specificity of the individual items, and internal consistency between each

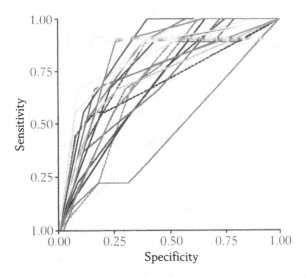

Figure 1   Receiver operating characteristic (ROC) curves for initial Andropause Check List symptoms in relation to total score; diagonal segments are produced by ties

other, particularly in their respective domains, and with the total score and sexual activity.

Disadvantages   Other than the majority of key items which overlap with the AMS scale, the ACL has not been translated into other languages, and undergone cultural and linguistic validation in each. Also, studies have not been carried out in randomly selected men of different ages. Like the majority of questions in the psychological domain likely to have weaker predictive power because of the high prevalence of true primary psychological disturbances in the general population, the ACL does not have items on anxiety, nervousness, or sleep. Other than the evidence presented in this book, it has not been previously published or validated.

Aging Males' Symptoms rating scale (AMS; Heinemann and colleagues, 1999[4]) (for full scale see Appendix 2A)

Although relatively recent, the AMS is the best validated in terms of the constituent items, and has been translated from German into English[29], and 14 other languages, including Bulgarian, Dutch, Finnish, Flemish, French, Indonesian, Japanese, Korean, Polish, Portuguese, Russian, Spanish, Swedish and Thai[30], which make it by far the most widely applicable questionnaire currently available. These versions of the AMS scale are generously made freely available for download on the internet at http://www.hqlo.com.

There are many similarities to the ACL. Like the ACL, the AMS is based on symptoms originally described by Dr Werner, combined with the observations of a clinician with many years' practical clinical experience in the field of aging males, Dr Alex Vermeulen, the coauthor who originally proposed most of the items in the check list. The domains of psychological, somatic and sexual symptoms overlap with those in the ACL, and the wording of many of the questions is identical.

Interestingly, the intensity of each symptom is also rated on a five-point scale: 'no' 1, 'mild' 2, 'moderate' 3, 'severe' 4, 'very severe' 5. The difference here is that each point in the scale awards one more point than the ACL scale, which starts at zero, awarding no points for each symptom that is absent, and making a total score of nil possible for the entirely symptom-free. This compares with a minimum score of 17 on the 17-item AMS questionnaire, which seems a less logical baseline for perfect health.

Like the ACL, however, the AMS was developed 'to compare severity of symptoms over time, and to measure changes pre and post treatment. It was not intended to design a screening instrument for androgen deficiency in aging males'[29]. This, as we shall see later in a more detailed comparison of symptomatology as assessed by the ACL rating system and androgen levels, is in any case an unsuitable and unobtainable goal.

In spite of these declared aims, however, the original construction of the AMS scale was from a check list of symptoms 'considered by physicians in medical practice in Germany to document complaints of men with hormonal deficiency'[4]. This implied relationship, although denied in the later article[29], was also shown by inclusion of the rare complaint of 'decrease in beard growth', which was 'listed as an exception to the 0.5 (factor weight) rule because it is a symptom in severe hormone deficiency'.

A comparison of the three main domains on the ACL and AMS scales shows more similarities than differences, providing that factors relating to partners' responses are omitted (Table 3):

(1) Psychological symptoms: the key components of fatigue (burnout), depression and irritability are identical on the two scales. Nervousness and anxiety are closely related and often overlapping symptoms, which were originally reported by Werner[12] and again by Reiter[27], who, because of the frequent association with sweating and palpitations, considered them related to 'thyroidism'. Although originally included in the ACL score, they were replaced by an overlapping question about reduced memory/concentration, which was also influenced by the psychological stress and tension described in the related AMS question. This is often a source of impaired performance and loss of 'competitive edge' at work, and noticeably improves on testosterone treatment, together with the other psychological symptoms.

(2) Somatic symptoms: these are in addition to a general feeling of premature aging more rapidly than friends and contemporaries, which is both physical and psychological, and made worse by aching, which is most

Table 3 Correlation table for individual items in the Andropause Check List (ACL) (1500 patients) with Aging Males' Symptoms (AMS) factor weights derived from factor analysis of a patient group (n = 116)[4]

	ACL		AMS	
	Item no.	Factor weight	Item no.	Factor weight
Psychological symptoms				
Fatigue	1	0.83	13	0.80
Depression	2	0.85	11	0.75
Irritability	3	0.85	6	0.72
Memory/concentration	4	0.70	7	0.59
Anxiety			8	0.69
Somatic symptoms				
Skin dry/thin	5	0.79		
Sweating	6	0.81	3	0.66
Vasomotor	7	0.72	3	0.66
Aches	8	0.83	2	0.77
Aging	9	0.77	1	0.56
Sleep problems			4	0.56
Increased sleep			5	0.64
Sexual symptoms				
Libido, self	10	0.71	17	0.84
Libido, partner	11	0.47		
Erection, initial	12	0.66	15	0.88
Erection, sustained	13	0.69	15	0.88
Erection, morning	14	0.77	16	0.86
Ejaculation, premature	15	0.43		
Ejaculation, delayed	16	0.70		
Orgasm, partner	17	0.74		
Sexual satisfaction, self	18	0.83	12	0.59
Sexual satisfaction, partner	19	0.76		
General relationship with partner	20	0.69		
Beard growth			14	0.20
Total score	0–80		17–85	

commonly experienced in the ankles and feet, especially in the morning. Joint symptoms, often associated with pain and stiffness in the calf muscles, lower back and shoulders, are closely similar to those experienced by menopausal women, and similarly relieved by hormonal treatment. The reasons for this will be discussed in Chapter 5 on the physical results of treatment.

(3) Sexual symptoms: these are the most frequent symptoms in all studies, and in both the ACL and AMS have the greatest weight in the factor analysis. Both have an item on reduction in morning erections, which can be one of the earliest signs of erectile dysfunction, particularly as it is partner-independent. The ACL covers erectile dysfunction in greater detail, as with the IIEF discussed later. This includes both initiating and

sustaining an erection, adequate for penetration and bringing the partner to orgasm where possible. This leads to consideration of problems with premature and delayed ejaculation, which are not dealt with specifically in the AMS questionnaire. Also, the patients' resulting sexual satisfaction is not referred to unless it is covered by the AMS question on 'having passed your peak', which is highly ambiguous in the English translation of the original German questionnaire.

The overall severity of complaints derived from the total AMS scores was: none: 17–26; little: 27–36; moderate: 37–49; severe: ≥ 50.

Cross-validation with the ACL

Because of the wide availability and excellent validation of the AMS questionnaire, a correlation study with the ACL was carried out in a group of 42 patients attending the London Andropause Clinic for their initial assessment visit. The ACL questionnaire was applied by the physician, and the AMS rating scale was self-administered.

The results showed that on the AMS total score, 17 were rated as having severe symptoms, 18 as moderate, five as mild and only two as having none. Since the majority of the questions are similar, if not identical, on the two scales, as would be expected, there were highly significant correlations between not only the total questionnaire scores (0.664), but also the subscales for psychological (0.709), somatic (0.705) and sexual (0.407) symptoms.

The correlations between the total scores and sexual scores for the two questionnaires could be further improved, to 0.731 and 0.549, respectively, by removing the items in the ACL relating to ejaculation problems and to the partner, which are not covered in the AMS.

AMS summary

Advantages   The scale has been carefully designed, has undergone cultural and linguistic validation in several published papers, and is available in 16 languages[30]. It is scalable and well suited to both diagnosis of the andropause and monitoring its treatment and has been shown to be highly effective in this latter context[31]. It is highly correlated both in total and in its subscales with the ACL questionnaire. It is being used increasingly in many clinical studies worldwide, and is rapidly becoming one of the standard outcome measures in the field of testosterone treatment.

Disadvantages   There are little data currently available concerning the relationship, if any, of the total or individual symptom scores with androgen levels, though a study of this will shortly be reported. There is overlap of some items, such as anxiety and nervousness, and in the two questions relating to sleep. There is limited information on erectile dysfunction, disturbances of orgasm, frequency of penetrative sex and masturbation, and the effect of these variables on the partner and the patient's relationship with them, though a new scale on quality of sexual functioning is in preparation (Heinemann LA, personal communication). The question about 'Feeling you have passed your peak' is ambiguous in English, but has a specific meaning of failing sexual performance in the original German version. The minimum score is not zero, which makes interpretation of initial and follow-up scores less clear.

Androgen Deficiency in Aging Males questionnaire (ADAM; Morley and Perry, 1999[17])

Based on his clinical experience in a geriatric medical unit at St Louis University, Morley identified 10 symptoms which he took to be commonly observed in older males with low bioavailable testosterone (BT) levels, and devised the questionnaire to detect this. The questions were arbitrarily selected without any apparent preliminary study of sensitivity or specificity of individual items, factor weighting or other criteria of questionnaire design discussed above. The questions were not scalable, being of yes/no format, as given in Table 4.

The following aspects of this questionnaire can be regarded as making it unsatisfactory, compared with the previous two questionnaires, for either routine screening for the andropause or monitoring its treatment, as seen in relation to each question in the list in Table 4:

(1) Decreases in libido are the norm with aging, stress and most disease processes, and a solitary yes/no response is likely to be a poor indicator of andropause.

(2) Do we not all have some degree of energy loss as we grow older? Is this mental or physical energy?

(3) Is this not the norm with age?

Table 4 Androgen Deficiency in Aging Males (ADAM) questionnaire[17]

(1) Do you have a decrease in libido (sex drive)?
(2) Do you have a lack of energy?
(3) Do you have a decrease in strength and/or endurance?
(4) Have you lost height?
(5) Have you noticed a decreased 'enjoyment of life'?
(6) Are you sad and/or grumpy?
(7) Are your erections less strong?
(8) Have you noticed a recent deterioration in your ability to participate in sports?
(9) Are you falling asleep after dinner?
(10) Has there been a recent deterioration in your work performance?

A positive questionnaire result is defined as a 'yes' answer to questions (1) or (7) or any three other questions

(4) This is a rare feature of andropause, especially in men below the age of 60, and indicates severe osteoporosis. Although the osteoporosis may be helped by testosterone treatment, the loss of height may be halted, but is not reversed. It cannot therefore be used to monitor the effects of treatment.

(5) A decreased enjoyment of life may be caused by loss of a relationship or a job, occurrence of which increase with age.

(6) The incidence of depression increases with age in men, and has been shown along with the other psychological domain questions which make up four of the ten items in the ADAM questionnaire to be a weak predictor of andropause, and it is a common cause of false positives.

(7) Although one of the commonest symptoms of andropause, erectile dysfunction, albeit sufficient in this questionnaire to give a positive response on its own, is generally considered to be rarely due to androgen deficiency, and may be another marker of age.

(8) The majority of men do not participate in sports after the age of 40, or else give up soon after, even with perfectly normal BTs for their age, and without andropausal symptoms.

(9) Stress, post-work fatigue or loss of social or sexual stimulation are more common causes in men of all ages than andropause.

(10) Being another question in the psychological domain, deterioration in work performance is more likely to be due to age, loss of employment or retirement than a marker of andropause or low BT.

In a further paper[33], Morley and his coworkers claimed to have validated the questionnaire by a study in 316 Canadian physicians aged between 40 and 82 years (52.8 ± 0.5, mean $\pm$ SEM), where positive results were compared with total testosterone (TT), BT and luteinizing hormone (LH).

Weak negative correlations were found between the incidence of positive responses to the questionnaire and the level of BT, but not TT or LH. However, age was not controlled for in this study. As the incidence of symptoms listed in the questionnaire is likely to increase with age, and testosterone has been proved, and indeed is shown in the study, to decrease with age, so finding a weak inverse correlation between the two is likely to have little bearing on whether the patient is andropausal, or be a better predictor of low BT than age alone.

In the same paper, 34 patients in a sexual dysfunction clinic, with a positive ADAM questionnaire, were found to include 13 with normal BT, a false-positive rate of 38%. Reductions in ADAM scores in 18 of the 21 low-BT subgroup were then taken to indicate that it was a 'useful tool for evaluating the therapeutic response to testosterone therapy'. It is difficult to agree with this conclusion, or, in view of the large amount of clinical work in previously cited studies over more than half a century, with the authors' assertion that: 'This study defines for the first time a symptom complex associated with declining testosterone levels in middle-aged and old males.'

ADAM summary

Advantages   It is short.

Disadvantages   It uses yes/no responses to a limited range of andropause symptoms, many of which are in the high false-positive psychological domain. The design and validation are poor, particularly in relation to sensitivity and specificity, and it appears highly age-dependent. It is insufficiently scalable and comprehensive to be used in monitoring testosterone treatment.

LABORATORY DIAGNOSIS OF ANDROGEN DEFICIENCY

Laboratory diagnosis of the andropause is an area fraught with difficulty and controversy. Often, laboratory data, because of their poor correlation with symptoms and widely varying 'normal' or 'reference' ranges, have been used in attempts to disprove the concept of the andropause and the need for treatment. Certainly in the eyes of many endocrinologists, treatment of symptoms, in the absence of laboratory data which are within their chosen 'reference' ranges, is regarded as 'unscientific', even if the symptoms are characteristic of androgen deficiency and relieved by giving androgens.

Samples available for routine clinical diagnosis are blood and saliva, with tissue biopsies and urine being generally confined to the fields of research and investigation of steroid abuse, both beyond the scope of this text.

VALIDITY OF ANDROGEN ASSAYS

As with other hormone estimations[34], there are many potential sources of error which can throw doubt on the validity of androgen levels as measured in blood for the clinical diagnosis of andropause, and the requirements for that individual to maintain high levels of androgens, especially in the 'high-testosterone male'. Apart from problems inherent in interpreting the results obtained, which are considered in detail later in this section, there are many sources of possible error in the assessment of androgen levels. Each of these is considered in turn.

Sampling problems

Circadian variation

Although the normal diurnal variation of androgens is well recognized, and has been described by most authors[35,36], the practical implications of this in routine clinical medicine are seldom considered.

Levels of testosterone increase by up to 35% overnight in younger men[37] with the pulsatile increase in LH which occurs during sleep, although this response may be blunted in older men[38]. It has also been known for many years that decreases of up to 14% in plasma proteins and molecules such as cholesterol occur with the hemodilution of recumbency[39]. During sleep, whose anabolic effect was described by Shakespeare as that which 'knits up the ravell'd sleave of care', the zenith of the first effect coincides with the nadir of the second. Because testosterone is bound strongly to SHBG and weakly to albumin, the combination of increased testosterone and a decrease in its binding proteins can cause marked differences in both BT and FT between high levels at night, and values up to 40% lower within a couple of hours of rising. This may explain why the disappearance of androgen-dependent nocturnal erections may be one of the earliest signs of the andropause.

These diurnal variations, and the effect of age, were clearly shown by Plymate, Tenover and Bremner[36], who took hourly blood samples throughout 24-h periods for TT, SHBG, BT and total protein levels in ten young normal men (mean age 27.3 years) and ten elderly men (mean age 70.7 years).

As well as having higher androgen levels both during the day and at night, the younger men had greater variability, particularly in BT, than did the older men (Figure 2). In both groups, having fallen to the daily minimum by 9 a.m., the BT remained at its lowest ebb until 3 p.m., while the TT was much more variable.

The drop in BT from nighttime to daytime levels was most marked between 7 and 9 a.m., when people are waking, which shifts the balance from parasympathetic dominated androgen secretion to the sympathetic-dominated stress of getting dressed and going to work. The effects were probably minimized in this experiment, because sleeping in hospital beds with indwelling catheters is not designed to give optimal conditions of rest, especially in the elderly, and therefore TT levels were likely to have been lower. Also, in this group the SHBG levels were less than in the younger men, whereas usually they might be expected to be significantly greater. This would minimize the drop in BT caused by hemoconcentration on rising.

These considerations are important in routine clinical practice. In most outpatient clinics, patients will arrive and have their blood samples taken at 9–10 a.m. at the earliest, by which time they will have been awake and subject to various degrees of physical activity and stress in traveling. The recommendation to have the sample taken in the morning covers a period of time during which an individual's testosterone levels may decrease by 20% and BT levels by 40%.

Jet-lag in patients attending from abroad may further confuse the timing of samples, as melatonin-based rhythms, such as those thought partially to regulate the increased testosterone secretion at night, may be out of phase for up to a week after long intercontinental flights[40], and the season may be different in the country of origin.

This may also explain why research studies such as the Massachusetts

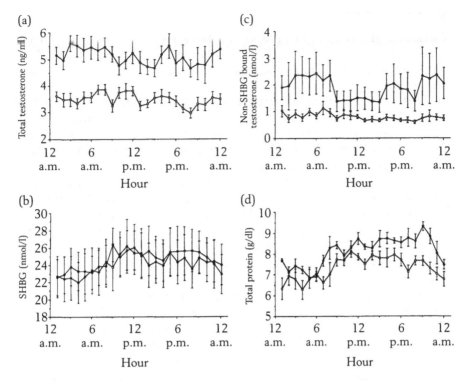

Figure 2 Serum total testosterone (a), sex hormone-binding globulin (SHBG) (b), non-SHBG-bound testosterone (c) and total protein (d) measurements in normal young (filled circles) and elderly (open circles) men measured hourly for a 24-h period. Reproduced with permission from reference 36

Male Aging Study (MMAS)[8,41], in which two blood samples, 30 min apart, were taken in the patient's home under resting conditions 'within 2 hours of waking', found small and inconsistent annual reductions in TT and FT with age. It also means that the researchers found few elderly men with testosterone levels below 12.13 nmol/l (350 ng/ml), who they would accept as truly hypogonadal[7]. However, because of the steepness of the decline in BT during this period, it is unlikely fully to 'control for diurnal variation in hormone levels' as claimed[7]. It may, however, partially explain the lower incidence of hypogonadism found in MMAS participants (20.4%) than in clinic patients (42.1%).

In view of the wide age range of the subjects in both home and clinic groups, 39–79 years (mean 58), it seems difficult to justify using any particular cutoff point for androgen deficiency. Also, many of the yes/no questions in the screener were age-related, which, as with the ADAM questionnaire above, is likely to make any correlation with testosterone levels largely artifactual.

Seasonal variations

Circannual variations in TT of up to 25% have been described by Smals and colleagues, who took 3-monthly blood samples in 15 healthy men. Peak levels were found in summer and early autumn and a nadir in the winter and early spring[42].

Dabbs[43] measured serum testosterone concentrations in 4462 military veterans, aged 32–44, to study the effects of age and seasonal variation. Testosterone concentrations were assayed from a single serum sample from each subject. All samples were drawn before breakfast, at about 8 a.m., from subjects recruited over a 16-month study period. Mean levels declined with age ($p < 0.001$), from 30.1 nmol/l (864 ng/dl) at age 32 to 26.9 nmol/l (773 ng/dl) at age 44. Mean levels also varied with month of testing ($p < 0.01$), with a seasonal peak in December (the seasonal peak was in November for men in their early 30s). The age effect was greater than the seasonal effect. He concluded that both effects may bear upon behavior and should be treated as possible sources of error in studies of testosterone.

In a comparable occupational group of 100 younger recruits to the Greek army, TT levels were measured between 9 and 11 a.m. on their first day in the army. Unlike Dabbs' veterans, these raw recruits, aged 18–22, who were unlikely to have slept well the night before, and were probably stressed by joining up, had a mean TT of 34.0 nmol/l (977 ng/dl). This level, allowing for decline with age, correlates well with the Dabbs figures, and suggests a lifetime peak around the age of 20 of about 35 nmol/l (1000 ng/dl) for young, fit, sexually and physically active men.

Dietary factors

The long-term effects of diet on androgen levels are discussed in detail in the chapter on causes of the andropause. The most important effects appear to be mainly on SHBG, which is decreased by high-protein, high-fat diets, and increased by vegetarian and high-fiber diets. These changes may be mainly via insulin levels, which tend to be lower in vegetarians, and are inversely related to SHBG.

There is little information on the acute effect of fasting overnight, but fasting male college wrestlers had a decrease in salivary testosterone while nonfasting subjects had an increase[44]. When prolonged for over 48 h fasting has been found to reduce gonadotropic testicular drive[45]. High levels of free fatty acids interfere with the binding of sex steroids to SHBG, which might theoretically affect the measurement of FT[37].

Alcohol

Alcohol in low doses has been shown to raise testosterone levels in both men[46] and women[47]. Conversely, acute alcohol intoxication, especially if accompanied by strenuous exercise, can reduce testosterone levels temporarily by up to 25%[48].

As indicated in the chapter on causation, long-term excess alcohol can damage the testes and lower testosterone levels, and by contributing to obesity, also lower SHBG levels. Gordon and colleagues showed that[49] chronic alcohol use decreases the function of the enzyme which controls an important rate-limiting step in the metabolism of testosterone in the liver, and that this effect may be due primarily to alcohol. The acute effects of alcohol in men on testosterone levels are not known, but in women they can certainly cause a rapid increase.

Physical activity

As well as influencing blood androgen estimations by causing hemoconcentration, as discussed above, depending on the fitness of the individual, various intensities of exercise can cause wide variations in androgen levels.

Long term, by increasing muscle mass and decreasing fat mass, exercise of moderate intensity can increase TT, and decrease SHBG, with double benefit to the free androgen index (FAI), calculated free testosterone (CFT) and BT derived from them.

Short term, depending on its intensity, exercise may either increase or decrease androgen levels, either directly or through its effects on other hormones. To examine the adaptations of the endocrine system to heavy-resistance training in younger versus older men, Kraemer and colleagues[50] studied two groups of men (30 and 62 years old) who participated in a 10-week strength–power training program.

Squat strength and thigh muscle cross-sectional area increased for both groups. The younger group demonstrated higher TT and FT and insulin-like growth factor-I (IGF-I) than the older men, and training-induced increases in FT at rest and with exercise. The older group demonstrated a significant increase in TT in response to exercise stress along with significant decreases in resting cortisol. These data indicate that older men respond with an enhanced hormonal profile in the early phase of a resistance-training program, but the response is different from that of younger men

Hemoconcentration and decreased metabolic clearance have been suggested as mechanisms to explain exercise-associated testosterone increase. Such nonspecific mechanisms should apply to other steroid hormones as well as to testosterone. To investigate whether the exercise-induced changes in other steroid hormones were similar to that of testosterone, Cumming and associates[51] measured serum levels of testosterone, androstenedione, dehydroepiandrosterone and cortisol, as well as gonadotropins, LH and FSH, and prolactin at 5–15-min intervals throughout progressive maximal intensity exercise on a cycle ergometer.

Significant increases were observed for all hormones with exercise. The increase in serum testosterone began prior to exercise, peaked at 20 min after the beginning of exercise and fell to baseline within 10 min. The serum LH increase was synchronous with that of testosterone, suggesting that gonadotropin stimulation was not responsible for the testosterone increment. The increases in serum cortisol, androstenedione, dehydroepiandrosterone and prolactin levels were simultaneous but began 25–30 min after that of testosterone in all subjects. These findings, therefore, suggest that, contrary to previous evidence, the exercise-associated increase in serum testosterone results predominantly from a specific mechanism, presumably involving increased testicular production without gonadotropin stimulation.

The same group[52] measured serum testosterone levels before and after a maximal-intensity swimming test in ten elite male and ten elite female swimmers. Levels of circulating testosterone fell in 19 of 20 swimmers in contrast to previous reports of exercise in the vertical position. In women, mean testosterone levels declined by 39.4% from baseline values and in males, fell by 19.0%. Since the incremental protocol was similar in design to maximal-intensity tests conducted on a treadmill or bicycle ergometer, these data suggest that the differing physical circumstances of swimming lead to a qualitatively different testosterone response to exercise.

The responses of plasma TT, SHBG binding capacity, androstenedione (A) and LH to 21 km of marching exercise and to sleep deprivation stress were studied by Zmuda and colleagues[53] in army recruits. The effect of physical fitness on the exercise responses was evaluated, cross-sectionally, by comparing the stress responses in 11 fit and 11 less fit subjects, and, longitudinally, in 11 subjects after 4 months of physical training.

The submaximal marching exercise did not significantly alter the plasma hormone levels compared with the control day levels. The fit subjects had a tendency towards smaller decreases in the mean plasma TT and testosterone/SHBG ratio during both control and exercise days than the less fit subjects[54].

After 4 months of training, the mean plasma TT and testosterone/SHBG ratio tended to decrease less during both control and exercise days, and this was more evident in the well-conditioned subjects. The exercise caused a decrease in mean plasma LH, especially in the less fit subjects. This confirmed the general picture that 'training' and submaximal exercise cause increases in testosterone levels, while 'straining', with maximum exercise, decreases it.

In addition, it has been found that after exercise, there is a reduction 15–60 min later, which can last for up to 3 days. This tends to be longer with more intense forms of exercise and lesser degrees of fitness[55].

After sleep deprivation stress, the morning levels of plasma TT, A and LH were significantly depressed, as a result of which the normal diurnal variation of the hormones disappeared.

Type of sample and storage

Unlike plasma catecholamines[34], where samples have to be separated and stored frozen immediately, androgens are reported as being quite stable for up to 4 days at room temperature and up to a week at 4 °C. When frozen at 20 °C, they are stable for up to 3 months, and over 6 months at −70 °C. In some epidemiological studies, these limits have been carried to extremes, samples being reanalyzed after periods of up to 10 years[8]. Certainly, it is inadvisable to thaw and freeze samples repeatedly, as proteins such as SHBG are likely to denature, giving different results for these assays and for CFT.

Also, plasma and serum samples are assumed to be equivalent (UK Supraregional Assay Service Regional Handbook), although original proof of these assumptions has not been found. To the contrary, considerable variations have been reported if plasma rather than serum is used[37]. Values obtained with heparin plasma are reported as 3–6% lower, with ethylenediaminetetraacetic acid (EDTA) plasma 17.5% lower and with citrate plasma 34.8% lower.

Sodium azide is often added to either serum or plasma quality-control samples as a preservative. In some methods it has been found to cause elevation of testosterone levels by around 8% or more, especially at low levels, and even up to 16% at hypogonadal levels. If this compound was present in calibration sera, it would lower analytical values by similar amounts. With male estrogens, where precision is notoriously poor anyway, the effect may be even worse, and could rise to over 40%.

Medical problems

Illness

Serious physical illnesses, ranging from life-threatening trauma[56], coronary heart disease[57] and liver disease[58] to leprosy[59], have also been related to reduced testosterone levels, although it is always difficult to establish which came first. The MMAS showed that as a group the 18% apparently healthy men in their follow-up study had TT levels 15% above the rest of the 1156 men remaining out of the original group of 1709[8]. These health-related factors are again dealt with in the chapter on causation.

Stress

As is detailed in the chapters on causation, and androgens and the brain, stress can profoundly affect the entire hypothalamic–pituitary–gonadal axis. In both the short and the long term, stress generally causes a fall in TT.

There is a wealth of evidence from both primate and human research that a male's testosterone level changes when his status changes, rising when he achieves or defends a dominant position, and falling when he is dominated. Mazur and Lamb reported three experiments confirming this in men[60].

In the first experiment, subjects played in doubles tennis matches in which winners received $100 apiece. Most winners of the matches who had decisive victories showed subsequent rises in testosterone relative to the losers of these matches; however, the winners of one very close match, in which there was no clear-cut triumph, did not show testosterone rises.

In the second experiment, subjects won $100 prizes, or not, depending on the random draw of a lottery. Winners in this situation, where their fortune came without any effort of their own, did not show subsequent testosterone rises compared with the losers.

The third experiment used the natural setting of a medical school graduation. Rises in testosterone were observed among new recipients of the M.D. degree, 1 and 2 days after the ceremony. In these experiments, changes in testosterone showed some relationship to subjects' moods. These results suggest that when a man achieves a rise in status through his own efforts, and he has an elation of mood over the achievement, then he is likely to have a rise in testosterone.

However, even fans supporting winning teams of basketball or football players can have a rise in testosterone, while supporters of losing teams showed a fall[61].

Both excessive and unpleasant physical and mental stress can activate the hypothalamic–pituitary–adrenal axis and reduce either the amount or the activity of androgens. A review by Christiansen in 1998[62] of the effects of various types of stress included a variety of mental and physical stressors. Extreme endurance training in military cadets, involving psychic stress and deprivation of food and sleep, resulted in a marked drop in testosterone levels, as have intensive on-duty periods in resident physicians.

Less acute psychological stress, such as financial problems, serious quarrels and loss of close friends or relatives, have also been shown to lower androgen levels.

Sexual activity

In general, the effects of sexual activity on testosterone appear to be greater than the reverse. This was well demonstrated in a research study by Dabbs and Mohammed[63] in which salivary testosterone concentrations were measured in male and female members of four heterosexual couples on a total of 11 evenings before and after sexual intercourse and 11 evenings on which there was no intercourse. Testosterone increased across the evening when there was intercourse, and decreased when there was none. The pattern was the same for males and females. The early-evening measure did not differ on the two kinds of days, suggesting that sexual activity affects testosterone more than initial testosterone affects sexual activity.

Knussmann and Christiansen[64] studied a sample of 33 healthy young men, from whom six blood samples were obtained in the course of 2 weeks, and testosterone, dihydrotestosterone (DHT) and estradiol levels were determined. The amount of FT in the saliva was also ascertained for 23 of the subjects. All participants kept a daily record of their sexual activity during the investigation period.

They concluded that the comparison of hormone levels to sexual behavior, prior to and after individual sampling, revealed significant positive correlations between serum testosterone and the extent of FT on the one hand and both the preceding and subsequent frequency of orgasms on the other. The estradiol levels showed a significant negative correlation with both the preceding and the subsequent frequencies of sexual activity without orgasm.

However, Mantzoros and Georgiadis, in their study of young Greek army recruits, suggested that in young adults, DHT levels are 'the most important, and perhaps only important androgen in determining male sexual behavior as reflected in the frequency of orgasms'[65]. Masturbation has also been found to raise TT levels[66].

As with physical exercise, to which sexual intercourse may be a close comparison, it seems that at least in young, fit men there is a rise in TT and DHT before and after sexual stimulation and orgasm. However, they often desire sex within the hour, or at least the same day, whereas, with certain notable exceptions, men over 50 rarely have sex two or more times a day on a regular basis. Also, little research has been done on androgen levels immediately after sexual intercourse in older men, particularly those with hypogonadism.

Certainly, the experience of exhaustion after sex, which could be called the 'post-coitum triste' syndrome, appears common in andropausal patients. This may last hours, days, or in a few cases weeks, and can cause the patient to dread intercourse because of the exhaustion that follows. Andrologists often insist on several days' abstention from intercourse before taking a semen sample for infertility investigations. Should they do the same before taking a blood sample for androgen estimations?

Smoking

Smokers have been found to have both TT and FT levels 5–15% higher than those of nonsmokers[67]. Increases in both testosterone (9%) and SHBG (8%) were found by Field and colleagues[68], while DHT increased by 14%. The greater increase in the last suggests that this, combined with some of the pleasurable aspects of nicotine-stimulated nor-epinephrine secretion[69], might explain some of the link between smoking and sexual activity. The immediate effects of smoking do not appear to have been studied, and so it is unclear what the effect of smoking in the morning before the test might be.

Analytical problems

Methodology

There are often between five and ten different methods being used in measuring each steroid in any one country at any time. Each has its individual bias in relation to the true assay value as measured by a reference method, usually gas chromatography and mass spectrometry. For routine clinical purposes, extraction radioimmunoassay methods have been phased out, and replaced by fully automated, nonextraction, competitive protein-binding immunoassay methods. These are much quicker, and less expensive, but may be more prone to interfering substances such as azide in control sera, high levels of SHBG, and agents used to strip testosterone from its binding proteins, particularly danazol. Because less expert laboratory staff are needed for the fully automated methods, there may be a tendency to be less critical of the results the analyzers turn out.

Quality control

Nonanalytical errors (blunders or flyers) were found in an average of nearly 2% of the over 300 laboratories in the UK, NEQAS (National External Quality Assessment Schemes) Birmingham quality-control schemes reported in the year 2000[70]. These are usually due to either faulty sampling or inaccurate reporting of results.

A bias of plus or minus 15% is generally considered acceptable, and often only when it goes consistently outside these limits is any action taken. This is usually in the case of about 6% of laboratories each year in the UK, and then the method is often 'recalibrated' by the manufacturers of the machines and kits that go with them. The overall interlaboratory coefficient of variation is generally below 15%, and the within-laboratory variation below 10%.

Similar figures were reported for the EQUAS scheme of the German Society of Clinical Chemistry for the year 2000[71]. For TT, although a normal distribution was assumed, there was a negative bias from the true mean of 25% over the whole range of 5–30 nmol/l. The author concludes that 'reference values must be established locally, based on the technology used at each site. Extrapolation from data in the literature may be disadvantageous for the patient.' However, this proposal may be impractical for the majority of laboratories, who will not have large sources of reference sera, and are likely to use the questionable reference values of the reagent manufacturers.

As a result of this policy, variations in TT estimations of up to 50%, especially below 10 nmol/l, are being accepted in Germany as within allowable limits. The variation is even greater, up to 46% positive bias, worldwide in levels measured in the normal female range of below 3 nmol/l[72]. A similar situation in relation to the estimation of estrogens in men exists because the automated methods are established to measure testosterone within the male range, and estrogens within the range for premenopausal females. Satisfactory accuracy and precision levels are unlikely to be reached until sex-specific methods are established for both these vital sex-steroid measurements.

With SHBG, interlaboratory variation was 9–12% between 30 and 50 nmol/l, rising to 15% at levels of 60 nmol/l. Similar figures were reported for the UK NEQAS. It must be remembered that when calculating the FAI and CFT, errors in the testosterone and SHBG methods are compounded, especially if they are in opposite directions.

Interpretation problems

Log-normal distribution of hormones

Early in the search for a definition of a normal range in scientific measurements, it was pointed out by Galton in 1879 that what was called the 'normal law of errors' predicted negative observations[73]. The example given was that the existence of men of more than double the average weight implies the existence of men with negative weight. He also observed that when logarithmic transformation of the measurements is carried out, this difficulty does not arise.

This fundamental truth about the log-normal distribution of the large majority of biological variables was reiterated as a general principle by Gaddum in 1945[74]. He gave as examples some of the effects of drugs on enzymes, and of oxygen on hemoglobin, which can be explained by the theory that molecules of a protein in a solution show continuous variations among themselves, and that certain of their properties are log-normally distributed[75].

When it became possible to make accurate quantitative measurements of biochemical constituents of blood, urine and other body fluids, it was necessary to establish laboratory 'normal ranges' to aid diagnosis of individual cases. Observations in 'normal subjects' showed again that the majority of variables proved to be log-normally distributed[76], usually revealed by the fact that the distribution covers more than a two-fold range, as in the case of most hormones, including androgens. In spite of this, 'improper statistics'[77] continued to be used to characterize the normal range of biochemical and endocrine measurements, and, especially in the interpretation of both clinical and research data on androgens, this has important implications. Neglect of this basic biological principle, as Henry pointed out in 1960, 'has led to frequent, grossly misleading implications, and in some instances, to absurdities'.

Effect of log transformation of androgen values

As part of a retrospective audit of the findings in 1500 men of mean age 54 (range 31–88) presenting with symptoms of androgen deficiency at a private andrology clinic in London over a 15-year period (UK Andropause Study, Appendix 3), endocrine, biochemical and hematological profiling was carried out using fasting blood samples taken between 9 and 10 a.m. at their initial pretreatment visit, and the results of the androgen assays are shown in Figure 3.

At first glance it can be seen that the actual distribution of the values for each hormone plotted in a linear mode is a poor fit to the superimposed 'normal distribution curve'. It also has illogicalities such as extending the two standard deviation (2 SD) lower limits well below what is observed clinically, in some cases suggesting that it should include negative values. There also appears to be an excess of values beyond the upper 2 SD limits. The mathematical fit and clinical relevance are both greatly improved by log to the base 10 transformations of the variables for each set of results.

Similar log-normal distributions were also evident in this patient population for DHT, LH, FSH, estradiol (E_2), prostate-specific antigen (PSA), prolactin, cortisol and TSH, but not free T_4.

The log transformation of the androgen-related values in the UK Andropause Study had a marked effect on their distribution, changing both the mean and mathematical expression of the variance in terms of standard deviations from the mean. This is shown in Table 5. Using the log distribution curves shifts the means downward and the upper and lower (± 2 SD) limits significantly upward, and this has a crucial effect on the interpretation of clinical results.

It also affects the results of all the statistical tests applied to such figures, such as those used in the analysis of variance, because parametric tests are being applied to nonparametric data. These figures are much more in accordance with both the observed values and the clinical pictures seen.

Application of log transformation to 'reference ranges' On average, the logarithmic-transformed means are 10% lower than the arithmetic means, and the lower reference limits raised by 25% of the arithmetic means, with the upper limits increased by 30% of the arithmetic means. There may be more exact mathematical treatments possible, but these figures give a working basis for transforming results from the linear to the log scale. Although it needs to be confirmed by reanalysis of the original investigators' data, assuming that the degree of skew of androgen results is similar in the values obtained in the study of 'normal' populations, it may be possible to estimate more appropriate 'reference ranges' from the figures given in the existing literature.

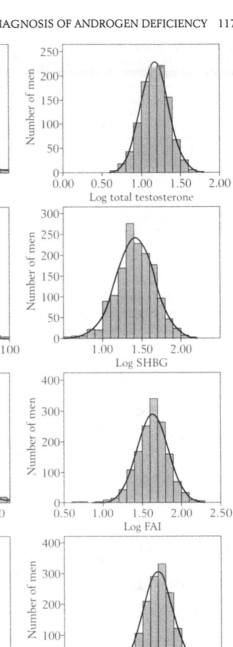

Figure 3 Normal and log-normal histograms for pre-treatment androgen-related variables of 1500 men in the UK Andropause Study (UKAS). SHBG, sex hormone-binding globulin; FAI, free androgen index; CFT, calculated free testosterone

Table 5 Changes in means and upper and lower limits of androgen-related variables (± 2 SD) in first-visit UK Andropause Study (UKAS) data on going from arithmetic (Arith.) to logarithmic (Log) distributions

Hormone	Arith. mean	Arith. lower limit	Arith. upper limit	Log mean	Log lower limit	Log upper limit	Change mean %	Change lower limit %	Change upper limit %
TT (nmol/l)	16.3	2.2	30.3	14.9	6.5	34.8	−9.4	+24.2	+31.3
SHBG (nmol/l)	38.1	3.1	73.1	35.0	14.2	84.1	−9.8	+26.4	+30.8
FAI (%)	47.8	1.1	94.5	43.0	16.8	109.7	−11.3	+29.5	+35.7
CFT (pmol/l)	310	38	582	283	119	675	−9.5	+26.5	+31.0

TT, total testosterone; SHBG, sex hormone-binding globulin; FAI, free androgen index; CFT, calculated free testosterone

Applying these results to the ranges of TT in different age groups given by Vermeulen[78] gives the results seen in Figure 4.

When establishing reference ranges for androgens, and doing statistical tests for variance between groups, it is important first to carry out log trans-

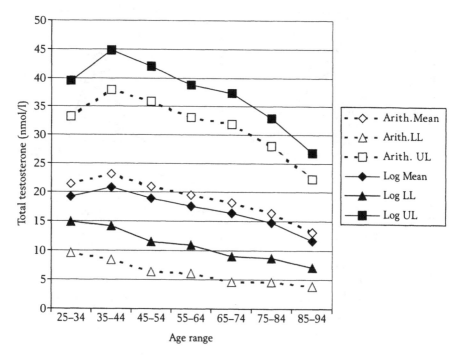

Figure 4 Changes in means and 2 SD 'reference ranges' for total testosterone levels at different ages according to the figures of Vermeuleun[78] for 249 healthy men, comparing figures calculated from arithmetic and logarithmic distributions

formation of the data. A totally different picture of conditions associated with androgen deficiency in the adult male is likely to result from this simple but important analytical change. When in doubt, transform.

Age-related effects

Definition of a 'normal range' for androgens is central to arguments for and against the existence of the andropause. The clinically compelling similarity with the menopause in women was denied on the basis of the absence of any sudden drop in testosterone level to values considered clinically subnormal in the majority of cases[79].

Although later measurements of urine testosterone showed a marked decline with age, the reduction in average plasma TT values appeared to be slight. Kaufman and Vermeulen have emphasized the importance of defining the 'normality' of the subjects to be included in establishing the variation of androgen levels in different body compartments with age, and have carried out the most detailed studies of these[80].

These considerations may explain why a review of reported studies on plasma TT levels in male senescence by Vermeulen in 1990 listed five out of a total of 16 as showing no decrease in TT levels with age[81]. However, the same article pointed out the 'virtual unanimity' in the view that free, biologically active testosterone levels do decrease with age, mainly due to an increase in SHBG[82,83]. However, as far as can be ascertained, none of these studies allowed for the log-normal distribution of the measurements, and so cannot be used without logarithmic transformation to establish biologically significant 'normal ranges'.

Although designed as the definitive study on androgens and aging, the Massachusetts Male Aging Study (MMAS) threw up several interesting questions relevant to any large-scale epidemiological investigation of this type[8,84]. From the outset in 1987, it appeared to be a biased, self-selected sample, mainly made up of white, more educated, heavy-drinking, unhealthy men, half of whom had some degree of erectile dysfunction.

Between the two reports in 1991 and 2002, it was apparent that there were key differences in hormone assay methods that resulted in significantly different results, 11 of the 13 methodologies listed having changed. Crucially, by the new methods, correcting for age- and health-related effects as described in the two papers, the baseline TT figures had increased by 85%, the FT by 87%, the CFT by 92% and the albumin-bound testosterone by 89%.

So what do these MMAS figures tell us about the rate of annual decline? The original cross-sectional figures showed annual drops of TT of 0.3% (FT −1.0%), and the follow-up figures for TT of 0.8% (FT −1.7%). The change data for individuals reported in the second study showed even larger falls of 1.6% in TT and 2.8% for FT. Taken over a 30-year period, this would give decreases of 48% in TT and 85% in FT.

This raises the question of how much reliance should be put on a study of androgen changes, as measured in a self-selected group of largely unhealthy men observed at two intervals 7–10 years apart, using androgen assays giving results with an average variation of 88%. Also, does an in-depth analysis of these figures from MMAS justify abandoning the concept of the andropause, together with 60 years of worldwide clinical experience that men with andropausal symptoms can benefit from androgen treatment?

High-testosterone males

We have many past and present examples of how testosterone, the 'hormone of kings – king of hormones'[16], can bring about the rise and fall of presidents and potentates, princes and politicians.

To some extent testosterone can be regarded as the 'success hormone'. A National Institutes of Health (NIH) study comparing testosterone levels with personality type in over 1700 men[85] found that, typically, the male with high levels, the 'high-testosterone man', who in primate studies would probably be called the 'alpha male', 'attempts to influence and control other people ... expresses his opinion forcibly and his anger freely, and ... dominates social interactions'. Having innate and persistent high levels of testosterone seems to make these men hard-driving, competitive and sometimes more successful.

Similarly, studies by Professor James Dabbs at Georgia State University[86] have shown that both men and women in more extrovert, domineering professions, such as lawyers, had higher levels of testosterone than non-competitive, more laid-back individuals. Such factors will be discussed further in Chapter 6 under the heading 'Testosterone and behavior'.

These considerations led to the idea that each man may have his own 'reference range' for several endocrine variables, including testosterone. Genetic[87] and behavioral patterns can play a major role in deciding at what level an individual feels he is functioning best in terms of general and sexual drive, energy, enthusiasm and physical activity. Certainly, 15 years' clinical experience with a range of captains of industry, tycoons, politicians and men who are sometimes called 'movers and shakers' shows that they need higher doses of testosterone to restore their competitive edge than the less ambitious.

Ethnic differences

There is emerging evidence that different races have significantly different distributions of androgen levels in their male populations. Recently, multi-center clinical trials to determine male contraceptive efficacy showed that testosterone-induced suppression of spermatogenesis to azoospermia occurred in about 90% of Asian but only 60–70% of white men. Compared with white men, Asian men respond earlier and with more marked suppression of pulsatile LH secretion to graded doses of testosterone[88]. Other studies have shown that smaller testes coupled with reduced Sertoli cell number and function and reduced daily sperm production could predispose Asian men to have a heightened negative response of testes to steroidal contraceptives, as compared with Caucasian men[89]. These observations have been taken to be due to polymorphism of the genomes controlling androgen regulation and action. While 9–37 CAG repeats can be regarded as being within the normal range, the mean number varies between ethnic groups, with Africans having 18–20, Caucasians 21–22, and East Asians 22–23[90].

In support of this is a report comparing three ethnic groups living in Manchester, UK, who were sampled randomly from population registers, being of white European ($n = 55$), Pakistani ($n = 50$) and Afro–Caribbean (AfC) origin ($n = 75$). It was found that TT levels were lower in Pakistani men (mean 14.6 nmol/l, 95% confidence interval 12.6–16.6 nmol/l) than in Europeans (18.7, 16.8–20.6 nmol/l) or AfCs (18.0, 16.4–19.6 nmol/l) ($F = 4.8$, $p = 0.009$). Despite SHBG levels also being lower in Pakistani men (22.9, 19.4–26.5 nmol/l) compared with Europeans (28.7, 25.7–31.8 nmol/l) and AfCs (26.9, 23.9–30.0 nmol/l) ($F = 3.0$, $p < 0.05$), circulating FT was significantly lower in the Pakistani group (367, 326–408 pmol/l) than in Europeans (455, 416–494 pmol/l) or AfCs (458, 424–492 pmol/l) ($F = 6.8$, $p = 0.001$). Pakistani men were on average 4 cm shorter than men in other groups. However, the lower FT persisted even when adjusted for height or waist/hip ratio.

The lower SHBG in the Pakistani men was paralleled by a lower insulin sensitivity (0.40, 0.25–0.56) compared with Europeans (0.77, 0.61–0.93) and AfCs (0.80, 0.66–0.93) ($F = 8.2$, $p < 0.0001$). SHBG correlated positively with insulin sensitivity ($\rho = 0.28$, $p < 0.001$) and strongly with TT ($\rho = 0.54$, $p < 0.001$). There was no difference in insulin secretory capacity in Pakistani men compared with Europeans and AfCs. Multiple linear regression analysis showed that TT was independently and negatively related to the log of fasting insulin ($\beta = -0.28$, $p < 0.001$) and age ($\beta = -0.17$, $p = 0.02$) and positively to the log of SHBG ($\beta = 0.23$, $p < 0.001$) and height ($\beta = 0.22$, $p = 0.001$). There was no relationship with ethnicity or waist/hip ratio. The finding that both total bound and CFT were lower in Pakistani men, and that their SHBG levels were lower, was in keeping with their poorer insulin sensitivity.

As well as giving useful baseline data on these groups, the authors make the case that further work is necessary to establish ethnic-specific ranges for the interpretation of total circulating and FT levels in men[91].

Androgen receptors (AR)

Steroid-abusing athletes are well aware that AR can be uprated or down-regulated by different patterns of testosterone usage over a period of time. For example, low levels of testosterone may upregulate the activity of 5α-reductase, and sustained high levels can do the reverse. This is seen clinically in the initial reduction in andropausal symptoms for the first week or two on oral androgens, the honeymoon period, which then fades in a few patients. Fortunately, by slightly increasing the dose, the benefits can usually be restored and maintained indefinitely.

The reverse response can be seen in aging men, where although TT and FT are declining, the dihydrotestosterone levels are usually maintained[8].

Recently there has been increasing awareness that the activity of the AR is modulated by a polymorphic CAG trinucleotide repeat in the AR gene, which is thought to be one of the most polymorphic genes in the human body. A study of andropausal symptoms, hormone levels and AR CAG triplets in 213 41–70-year-old men[92] showed that the proportion of men with serum LH in the uppermost quartile ($> 6.0\,IU/l$) with normal serum testosterone ($> 9.8\,nmol/l$, above the lowest 10%) increased significantly with age ($p = 0.01$). There were fewer men with this hormonal condition among those with CAG repeat number in the uppermost quartile (≥ 23 repeats) ($p = 0.03$). These men also reported less decreased potency ($p < 0.05$). The repeat number was positively correlated with depression, as expressed by the wish to be dead ($r = 0.45$, $p < 0.0001$), depressed mood ($r = 0.23$, p = 0.003), anxiety ($r = 0.15$, p < 0.05) and deterioration of general well-being ($r = 0.22$, $p = 0.004$), as well as decreased beard growth ($r = 0.49$, $p < 0.0001$).

It was concluded that only certain types of age-related changes in aging men were associated with the length of the AR gene CAG repeat, suggesting that this parameter may play a role in setting different thresholds for the array of androgen actions in the male.

The MMAS gave further evidence that a shorter polymorphic CAG repeat length in exon 1 of the AR gene is associated with higher transcription activation by the AR[93]. In this study they determined the number of CAG repeats for 882 men aged between 40 and 70 years. The CAG repeat length was significantly associated with testosterone ($p = 0.041$), albumin-bound testosterone ($p = 0.025$) and FT ($p = 0.003$) when controlled for age, baseline hormone levels and anthropometrics. Follow-up levels of testosterone decreased by 0.74% ± 0.36% per CAG repeat decrement. Likewise, the percentages of FT and albumin-bound testosterone decreased by 0.93% ± 0.31 and 0.71% ± 0.32% per CAG repeat decrement, respectively. It was concluded that these results suggested that androgen levels may be modulated by AR genotype.

Research has also shown that a low number of CAG repeats were independently associated with protective parameters in relation to the 'metabolic syndrome' or 'syndrome X' (low body fat mass and plasma insulin) as well as with adverse parameters (low high-density lipoprotein cholesterol concentrations). This suggests that the pivotal role of this polymorphism in modulating androgen effects on cardiovascular risk factors is of a complex nature, and implies that its clinical impact, similar to that of androgens, is dependent on exogenous cofactors[94].

It has also been found that a high number of CAG repeats within the AR gene attenuate testosterone effects on bone density and bone metabolism, and that this seems to be associated with accelerated age-dependent bone loss[95].

Even predisposition to benign or malignant enlargement of the prostate has been linked to CAG repeat links[93]. CAG repeat length in exon 1 of the AR gene correlates inversely with transcriptional transactivation activity of the AR. Men with shorter AR CAG repeat lengths are at higher risk of prostate cancer. Because benign prostatic hyperplasia (BPH) is an androgen-dependent condition, Giovannucci and his coworkers[96] examined the hypothesis that a shorter AR gene CAG repeat length increases the risk of developing of BPH. They found that among 14 916 men of the Physicians' Health Study, in the 310 men who had surgery for BPH during up to 7.5 years of follow-up, compared with 1041 controls, the risk of surgery increased linearly with decreasing AR CAG repeat length (p (trend) = 0.03). Relative to men with a CAG repeat length ≥ 25, men with a repeat length ≤ 19 had an odds ratio of BPH surgery of 1.76 (95% confidence interval 1.16–2.65).

Obviously, these small modifications in the AR can have a profound effect on the action of testosterone and its metabolites[90], which can further confound the clinical interpretation of laboratory androgen estimations.

Choice of androgen measures in the diagnosis of andropause

As can be seen from the above discussion, there is no perfect measure of androgen activity, although some appear more useful than others.

Total testosterone (TT)   Although unfortunately it is the most commonly measured and quoted, TT is a poor indicator of clinical androgen activity, falling least with age, and bearing the weakest relationship with most clinical states and their response to testosterone treatment.

We can only agree with the view expressed by Atkinson and colleagues[97] that 'Because of the variability in serum testosterone concentration in the normal male during the day, from person to person, and among assays, there is no accepted testosterone value used as a cutoff to define testosterone deficiency. Symptoms, etiology, clinical impression, and a very low or low-normal testosterone aid the diagnosis of hypogonadism.'

Free androgen index (FAI)   This has the merit of being easy to calculate, and makes some allowance for the important effect of SHBG. It has, however, been attacked on theoretical grounds by Kapoor and colleagues[98] when used in men, on the basis that the binding capacity of SHBG needs to exceed greatly the concentration of its ligand testosterone for the equation to be valid.

However, they produce evidence from only 20 female and 19 male subjects, aged between 20 and 78 years, which was far from conclusive. It also lacked any directly measured FT estimations, or the calculated FT which they recommended in place of the FAI. More detailed work in which all these measurements were made on the same sample[99] showed a good correlation between FAI and FT measured by equilibrium dialysis, especially in the clinically more important situations where the FAI is below 50%, and the FT below 400 pmol/l.

The question also arises of the interpretation of the meaning of FAIs of over 100%. Being an indirect ratio, it also compounds the errors of both TT and SHBG estimations.

Despite these theoretical objections, FAI has remained a useful guide in diagnosis and treatment of the andropause, and especially with logarithmic transformation of the values, correlates well with the CFT, as seen from the pretreatment UKAS data (Figure 3).

Bioavailable testosterone (BT) Also known as 'free and weakly bound' testosterone, this has the advantage that with the ammonium sulfate precipitation method it can be measured cheaply and directly, and has been recommended for screening for the andropause[100].

Although often used in America and Canada, BT is seldom measured in Europe, as it obscures the information gained by measuring SHBG. This is often of major clinical importance in finding the origin of andropausal symptoms in individual patients, and in treating them, especially with SHBG-lowering agents such as danazol.

There is also the question of whether the testosterone bound weakly to albumin is actually free and biologically active in its short transit through the capillaries in all parts of the body. The albumin-bound fraction is also considerably greater, but less variable, than the free fraction, and variations in the former may mask smaller but potentially more important changes in the latter, which is usually only 5–10% of the BT.

Calculated free testosterone (CFT) As it has been shown that CFT and FT measured by equilibrium dialysis[99] exhibit a higher correlation than any of the other measures, it was concluded that 'calculated FT is a reliable index of FT, that calculated non-specifically bound T reflects non-SHBG-T, and that immunoassayable SHBG is a reliable measure of SHBG binding sites.' These key statements from this detailed study must be regarded as the definitive ideas at present in this complex field, and make CFT the laboratory measure of choice.

A nomogram for deriving CFT from the equation provided by Vermeulen and colleagues[101] is shown as the frontispiece to this book.

Lack of correlation between symptoms and androgen levels

It has been consistently found in studies from all over the world that there is little or no correlation between andropause symptoms and androgen levels. This is generally taken by endocrinologists to be conclusive proof of the unreliability of questionnaires, but in view of the issues raised above in

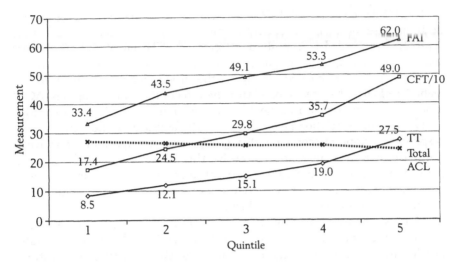

Figure 5 Lack of correlation of endocrine variables and total Andropause Check List (ACL) scores. UK Andropause Study data divided according to quintiles of total testosterone (total testosterone (TT) nmol/l, free androgen index (FAI)%, calculated free testosterone (CFT) pmol/l divided by 10)

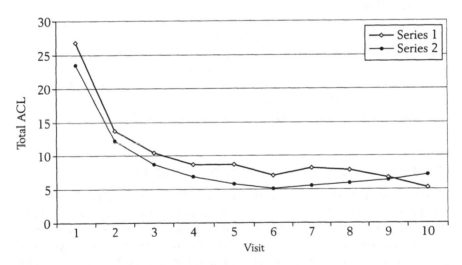

Figure 6 Comparison of the response to all forms of testosterone treatment of lowest total testosterone (TT) quintile (series 1) with highest TT quintile (series 2). ACL, Andropause Check List of symptoms

relation to the validity of androgen assays, the question could equally well be asked whether the patients' symptoms might represent a more accurate bioassay of the overall androgenic effect in that individual. Some light is shed on this question by the findings from the UKAS.

The UKAS consisted of 1500 men who were diagnosed as andropausal, both because of their characteristic initial symptoms, and because these symptoms responded to testosterone treatment. The initial androgen values were divided into quintiles of 300 patients, from the lowest to the highest TT groups, which corresponded closely to the groups with the lowest to the highest FAI and CFT. It was found that the total of the initial symptom (ACL) scores showed no trend across the full range of androgen variables (Figure 5).

The lack of correlation between any of the androgen values and the corresponding symptom scores for that group raises the question of which is the better diagnostic measure. To resolve this dilemma, the results of treating the lowest and highest androgen quintile groups with all three forms of treatment used – testosterone undecanoate, mesterolone and testosterone pellet implants – were examined (Figure 6).

This showed that the group with the highest androgen levels responded just as well to testosterone treatment as those with the lowest initial androgen levels, which further underlines the unsuitability of laboratory estimations as the major arbiter of testosterone treatment.

Further confirmation of this lack of correlation between symptoms and androgen levels was obtained by plotting the receiver operating characteristic (ROC) curves for all the endocrine variables in the UKAS patients at the first visit (Figure 7).

The curves in Figure 7 show that none of the endocrine variables are significantly different from the null hypothesis; i.e. they have no discriminating power in the diagnosis of andropause. This was confirmed by the area under the curves and significance calculations.

The conclusion drawn from the ROC curves is that not one of TT, FAI, CFT, estradiol or SHBG bear any statistical relationship to the andropausal symptoms, other than the last two having a weak, insignificant, negative correlation, as would be expected.

Androgen levels in the diagnosis of andropause

The androgen values at the initial visit for patients in the UKAS were used to try to establish what levels might be diagnostic of andropause, assuming the diagnosis was initially based on the presence of symptoms according to the ACL questionnaire (Appendix 2B). Figure 8 shows that if you take 8 nmol/l (230 ng/dl) TT as the cut-off point you miss 95% of andropause cases; if you take 12 nmol/l (350 ng/gl/) as the cut-off point you miss 75% of andropause cases; and if you take 14 nmol/l (400 ng/dl) as the cut-off point you miss 60% of andropause cases. The conclusion is that none of these cut-off points are appropriate for the diagnosis of andropause.

As with TT, the figures for FAI and CFT (Figures 9 and 10 respectively) suggest that there is no suitable cut-off point for the diagnosis of androgen deficiency, as the levels found in andropausal men extend right across the full range of measurements.

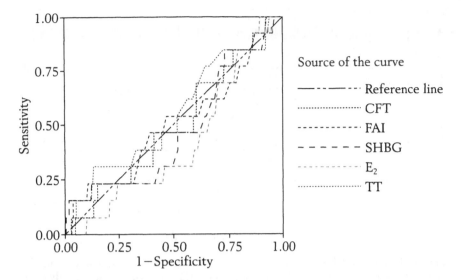

Figure 7   Receiver operating characteristic (ROC) curves for endocrine variables and the diagnosis of andropause in UKAS patients: diagonal segments are produced by ties. CFT, calculated free testosterone; FAI, free androgen index; SHBG, sex hormone-binding globulin; E_2, estradiol; TT, total testosterone

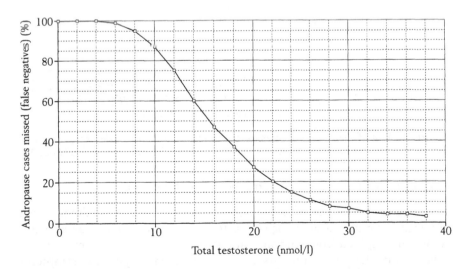

Figure 8   Plot of false-negative rates for the diagnosis of andropause using total testosterone levels alone as the diagnostic criterion (UK Andropause Study data)

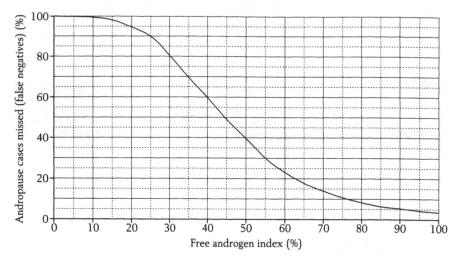

Figure 9 Plot of false-negative rates for the diagnosis of andropause using free androgen index levels alone as the diagnostic criterion (UK Andropause Study data)

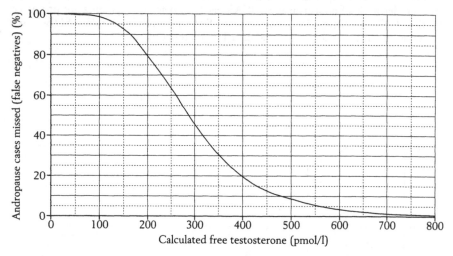

Figure 10 Plot of false-negative rates for the diagnosis of andropause using calculated free testosterone levels alone as the diagnostic criterion (UK Andropause Study data)

Androgen levels at which symptoms recur after treatment

Further evidence of the relatively high levels of the various androgens that are needed for men over the age of 50 to remain free of andropausal symptoms can be gained from studying patients whose testosterone implants are wearing off after 6 months. As can be seen from Figure 11, symptoms reappear at a wide range of TT, FAI and especially CFT values, spanning and extending beyond all known reference ranges.

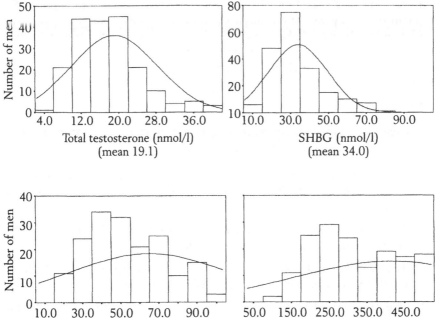

Figure 11   Androgen levels at which symptoms recur after testosterone pellet implant treatment; UK Andropause Study, $n = 489$, 6 months after pellet implant. SHBG, sex hormone-binding globulin

If results in studies of androgen levels in the diagnosis of androgen deficiency in adult males are being compared with those found in youth or early middle age, and the aim of treatment is to restore them to the same target levels, then a shift in the lower limit of the 'normal range' from, say, 8 to 14 nmol/l is highly significant.

In the case of the UK Andropause Study (UKAS), this would mean that under the criteria recently laid down by the Australian Endocrine Society[102], and used as mandatory prescribing guidelines for doctors in that country, only 5% would qualify for treatment. If a level of 14 nmol/l were considered more representative of the true limits of an appropriate reference range, then at least 40% would be eligible. Not until a level of 26 nmol/l are 90% of cases included.

However, the figures given by Vermeulen and Kaufman[78] indicate that the largest falloff in androgens with age is either the CFT, as confirmed by the work of Tremblay[100], or the FAI. If the lower limit of the latter is taken to be 50%, rather than the 20% quoted by most Australian laboratories, then 60% of the UKAS cases would be considered to have androgen deficiency, rather than 5%. Not until an FAI of 75 are 90% of cases included. Similarly, the often-quoted CFT of 200 pmol/l would miss 80%, and a cutoff point of around 500 is needed for the accurate classification of 90% of cases.

This analysis also suggests that the total level of ACL symptoms is independent of TT, FAI or CFT. This makes lower limit 'cutoff' points for laboratory androgens totally unsatisfactory as a means of diagnosing the andropause. Denying a therapeutic trial of testosterone treatment to men with characteristic androgen deficiency symptoms on the basis of androgen assays alone is a misuse of laboratory data.

CONCLUSIONS

Although laboratory tests can help to support a diagnosis of andropause, they should not be used to exclude it because we do not know:

(1) The exact sampling conditions in relation to circadian and seasonal variations, diet and alcohol, physical activity and posture, and sample preservation and storage;

(2) The medical problems of patients in relation to their state of health, stress, sexual activity and smoking habits;

(3) The accuracy and precision of the androgen analyses used, which are unreliable, and subject to wide interlaboratory variation;

(4) The true reference ranges: androgen values are log-normally distributed, and yet reference ranges are often derived from normal distribution curves, and applied to all age-groups;

(5) The levels needed in later life for optimal responses from different organs. Men may need the hormones of their youth to feel and function well, particularly if they are 'high-testosterone' men;

(6) What combination of testosterone and its metabolites is working against what combination of antagonists such as SHBG, estrogens, catecholamines, cortisol and antiandrogens;

(7) The cellular levels of androgens needed in various organs to maintain optimal function in relation to aging endocrine systems and varying AR status.

References

1. Carruthers M. The diagnosis of androgen deficiency. *Aging Male* 2002;4:254

2. Tremblay RR, Morales AJ. Canadian practice recommendations for screening, monitoring and treating men affected by andropause or partial androgen deficiency. *Aging Male* 1998;1:213–18

3. Werner AA. The male climacteric: report of two hundred and seventy-three cases. *J Am Med Assoc* 1946; 132:188–94

4. Heinemann LAJ, Zimmermann T, Vermeulen A, Thiel C, Hummel W. A new 'Aging Males' Symptoms' (AMS) rating scale. *Aging Male* 1999;2:105–14

5. Vermeulen A. The future of hormone replacement treatment in the aging male. *Aging Male* 2000;3:210–13

6. Leifke E, Gorenoi V, Wichers C, Von Zur MA, Von Buren E, Brabant G. Age-related changes of serum sex hormones, insulin-like growth factor-1 and sex-hormone binding globulin levels in men: cross-sectional data from a healthy male cohort. *Clin Endocrinol (Oxf)* 2000;53:689–95

7. Smith KW, Feldman HA, McKinlay JB. Construction and field validation of a self-administered screener for testosterone deficiency (hypogonadism) in ageing men. *Clin Endocrinol (Oxf)* 2000;53:703–11

8. Feldman HA, Longcope C, Derby CA, *et al.* Age trends in the level of serum testosterone and other hormones in middle-aged men: longitudinal results from the Massachusetts Male Aging Study. *J Clin Endocrinol Metab* 2002;87: 589–98

9. Makinen J, Pollanen P, Perheentupa A, *et al.* How few men are really suitable for androgen replacement therapy? In Carruthers M, ed. London: The Andropause Society, 2003: 3rd International Conference, London

10. Burger HG. The endocrinology of the menopause. *J Steroid Biochem Mol Biol* 1999;69:31–5

11. Gooren LG. Quality-of-life issues in the aging male. *Aging Male* 2000;3:185–9

12. Werner AA. The male climacteric. *J Am Med Assoc* 1939;112:1441–3

13. Carruthers M. A multifactorial approach to understanding andropause. *J Sex Reproductive Med* 2001;1:69–74

14. Reiter T. Testosterone implantation: a clinical study of 240 implantations in ageing males. *J Am Geriatr Soc* 1963;11:540–50

15. Carruthers M. HRT for the aging male: a clinical study in 1000 men. *Aging Male* 1998;1:34

16. Carruthers M. *Male Menopause: Restoring Vitality and Virility.* London: HarperCollins, 1996

17. Morley JE, Perry HM. Androgen deficiency in aging men. *Med Clin North Am* 1999;83:1279–89

18. Zweig MH, Campbell G. Receiver-operating characteristic (ROC) plots: a fundamental evaluation tool in clinical medicine. *Clin Chem* 1993;39:561–77

19. Goldberg DP. *The Detection of Psychiatric Illness by Questionnaire.* Oxford: Oxford University Press, 1972

20. Werner AA. *Research in Endocrinology.* St Louis, MO: Von Hoffman Press, 1952

21. Werner AA. The male climacteric. *Gen Practitioners' Digest* 1951;2:165

22. Werner AA. The male climacteric: report of fifty-four cases. *J Am Med Assoc* 1945;127:705–10

23. Werner AA. Male climacteric: additional observations of thirty-seven patients. *J Urol* 1943;49:872–82

24. Heller CG, Myers GB. The male climacteric: its symptomatology, diagnosis and treatment. *J Am Med Assoc* 1944;126:472–7

25. Sevringhaus EL. *The Management of the Climacteric.* Springfield, IL: CC Thomas, 1948

26. Reiter T, Horn H, Ben-Uzilio R, Finkelstein M. Plasma levels of testosterone in ageing male patients following implantation of testosterone. *J Am Geriatr Soc* 1964;12: 515–16

27. Reiter T. Treatment of male climacteric by combined implantation. *Practitioner* 1953;170:181

28. Rosen RC, Riley A, Wagner G, Osterloh IH, Kirkpatrick J, Mishra A. The International Index of Erectile Function (IIEF): a multidimensional

scale for assessment of erectile dysfunction. *Urology* 1997; 49:822–30

29. Heinemann LAJ, Saad F, Thiele K. The Aging Males' Symptoms rating scale: cultural and linguistic validation into English. *Aging Male* 2001; 4:14–22

30. Heinemann LA, Saad F, Zimmermann T, *et al*. The Aging Males' Symptoms (AMS) scale: update and compilation of international versions. *Health Qual Life Outcomes* 2003;1:77

31. Daig I, Heinemann LA, Kim S, *et al*. The Aging Males' Symptom (AMS) scale: review of it's methodological characteristics. *Health Qual Life Outcomes* 2003;1:77

32. Heinemann LA, Saad F, Heinemann K, Thai DM. Can results of the AMS scale predict those of screening scales for androgen deficiency? *Aging Male* 2004; in press

33. Morley JE, Charlton E, Patrick P, *et al*. Validation of a screening questionnaire for androgen deficiency in aging males. *Metabolism* 2000;49: 1239–42

34. Carruthers M, Conway N, Somerville W, Taggart P, Bates D. Validity of plasma-catecholamine estimations. *Lancet* 1970;1:62–7

35. Kaufman JM, T'Sjoen G, Vermeulen A. Androgens in male senescence. In Nieschlag E, Behre HM, eds. *Testosterone: Action, Deficiency, Substitution*. Cambridge University Press, 2004:497–541

36. Plymate SR, Tenover JS, Bremner WJ. Circadian variation in testosterone, sex hormone-binding globulin, and calculated non-sex hormone-binding globulin bound testosterone in healthy young and elderly men. *J Androl* 1989;10:366–71

37. Vermeulen A, Kaufman JM. Diagnosis of hypogonadism in the aging male. *Aging Male* 2002;5:170–6

38. Bremner WJ, Vitiello MV, Prinz PN. Loss of circadian rhythmicity in blood testosterone levels with aging in normal men. *J Clin Endocrinol Metab* 1983;56:1278–81

39. Stoker DJ, Wynn V, Robertson G. Effect of posture on the plasma cholesterol level. *Br Med J* 1966; 5483:336–8

40. Carruthers M, Arguelles AE, Mosovich A. Man in transit: biochemical and physiological changes during intercontinental flights. *Lancet* 1976;1:977–81

41. Gray A, Berlin JA, McKinlay JB, Longcope C. An examination of research design effects on the association of testosterone and male aging: results of a meta-analysis. *J Clin Epidemiol* 1991;44:671–84

42. Smals AG, Kloppenborg PW, Benraad TJ. Circannual cycle in plasma testosterone levels in man. *J Clin Endocrinol Metab* 1976;42: 979–82

43. Dabbs JM. Age and seasonal variation in serum testosterone concentration among men. *Chronobiol Int* 1990;7:245–9

44. Booth A, Mazur AC, Dabbs JM. Endogenous testosterone and competition: the effect of "fasting". *Steroids* 1993;58:348–50

45. Cameron JL, Weltzin TE, McConaha C, Helmreich DL, Kaye WH. Slowing of pulsatile luteinizing hormone secretion in men after forty-eight hours of fasting. *J Clin Endocrinol Metab* 1991;73:35–41

46. Sarkola T, Eriksson CJ. Testosterone increases in men after a low dose of alcohol. *Alcohol Clin Exp Res* 2003;27:682–5

47. Sarkola T, Fukunaga T, Makisalo H, Peter Eriksson CJ. Acute effect of alcohol on androgens in premenopausal women. *Alcohol Alcohol* 2000;35:84–90

48. Heikkonen E, Ylikahri R, Roine R,

Valimaki M, Harkonen M, Salaspuro M. The combined effect of alcohol and physical exercise on serum testosterone, luteinizing hormone, and cortisol in males. *Alcohol Clin Exp Res* 1996;20:711–16

49. Gordon GG, Vittek J, Ho R, Rosenthal WS, Southren AL, Lieber CS. Effect of chronic alcohol use on hepatic testosterone 5α-A-ring reductase in the baboon and in the human being. *Gastroenterology* 1979;77:110–14

50. Kraemer WJ, Hakkinen K, Newton RU, et al. Effects of heavy-resistance training on hormonal response patterns in younger vs. older men. *J Appl Physiol* 1999;87:982–92

51. Cumming DC, Brunsting LA, Strich G, Ries AL, Rebar RW. Reproductive hormone increases in response to acute exercise in men. *Med Sci Sports Exerc* 1986;18:369–73

52. Cumming DC, Wall SR, Quinney HA, Belcastro AN. Decrease in serum testosterone levels with maximal intensity swimming exercise in trained male and female swimmers. *Endocr Res* 1987;13:31–41

53. Zmuda JM, Thompson PD, Winters SJ. Exercise increases serum testosterone and sex hormone-binding globulin levels in older men. *Metabolism* 1996;45:935–9

54. Remes K, Kuoppasalmi K, Adlercreutz H. Effect of physical exercise and sleep deprivation on plasma androgen levels: modifying effect of physical fitness. *Int J Sports Med* 1985;6:131–5

55. Adlercreutz H, Harkonen M, Kuoppasalmi K, Kosunen K, Naveri H, Rehunen S. Physical activity and hormones. *Adv Cardiol* 1976;18:144–57

56. Spratt DI, Bigos ST, Beitins I, Cox P, Longcope C, Orav J. Both hyper- and hypogonadotropic hypogonadism occur transiently in acute illness: bio- and immunoactive gonadotropins. *J Clin Endocrinol Metab* 1992;75:1562–70

57. Swartz CM, Young MA. Low serum testosterone and myocardial infarction in geriatric male inpatients. *J Am Geriatr Soc* 1987;35:39–44

58. Handelsman DJ. Testicular dysfunction in systemic disease. *Endocrinol Metab Clin North Am* 1994;23:839–56

59. Morley JE, Distiller LA, Sagel J et al. Hormonal changes associated with testicular atrophy and gynaecomastia in patients with leprosy. *Clin Endocrinol (Oxf)* 1977;6:299–303

60. Mazur A, Lamb TA. Testosterone, status and mood in human males. *Horm Behav* 1980;14:236–46

61. Bernhardt PC, Dabbs JM, Fielden JA, Lutter CD. Testosterone changes during vicarious experiences of winning and losing among fans at sporting events. *Physiol Behav* 1998;65:59–62

62. Christiansen K. Behavioural correlates of testosterone. In Nieschlag E, Behre HM, eds. *Testosterone: Action, Deficiency, Substitution.* Berlin: Springer-Verlag, 1998:107–42

63. Dabbs JM, Mohammed S. Male and female salivary testosterone concentrations before and after sexual activity. *Physiol Behav* 1992;52:195–7

64. Knussmann R, Christiansen K, Couwenbergs C. Relations between sex hormone levels and sexual behavior in men. *Arch Sex Behav* 1986;15:429–45

65. Mantzoros CS, Georgiadis EI, Trichopoulos D. Contribution of dihydrotestosterone to male sexual

behaviour. *Br Med J* 1995;310: 1289–91

66. Brown WA, Monti PM, Corriveau DP. Serum testosterone and sexual activity and interest in men. *Arch Sex Behav* 1978;7:97–103

67. Vermeulen A, Kaufman JM, Giagulli VA. Influence of some biological indexes on sex hormone-binding globulin and androgen levels in aging or obese males. *J Clin Endocrinol Metab* 1996;81:1821–6

68. Field AE, Colditz GA, Willett WC, Longcope C, McKinlay JB. The relation of smoking, age, relative weight, and dietary intake to serum adrenal steroids, sex hormones, and sex hormone-binding globulin in middle-aged men. *J Clin Endocrinol Metab* 1994;79:1310–16

69. Carruthers M. Modification of the noradrenaline related effects of smoking by beta-blockade. *Psychol Med* 1976;6:251–6

70. Middle J. UK NEQAS for steroid hormones. 2000

71. Thijssen JH. Laboratory tests in the endocrine evaluation of aging males. In Lunenfeld B, Gooren L, eds. *Textbook of Men's Health.* London: Parthenon Publishing, 2002:44–50

72. Taieb J, Mathian B, Millot F, *et al.* Testosterone measured by 10 immunoassays and by isotope-dilution gas chromatography–mass spectrometry in sera from 116 men, women, and children. *Clin Chem* 2003;49:1381–95

73. Galton F. The geometric mean, in vital and social statistics. *Proc R Soc* 1879;29:365

74. Gaddum JH. Lognormal distributions. *Nature (London)* 1945;156: 463–6

75. Gaddum JH. *Proc R Soc* 1937; 121:598

76. Wootton ID, King EJ, Smith JM. The quantitative approach to hospital biochemistry: normal values and the use of biochemical determinations for diagnosis and prognosis. *Br Med Bull* 1951;7:307–11

77. Henry RJ. Improper statistics characterising the normal range. *Am J Clin Pathol* 1960;34:326–7

78. Vermeulen A. Declining androgens with age: an overview. In Oddens B, Vermeulen A, eds. *Androgens and the Aging Male.* New York: Parthenon Publishing, 1996:3–14

79. Burns-Cox N, Gingell C. The andropause: fact or fiction? *Postgrad Med J* 1997;73:553–6

80. Kaufman JM, Vermeulen A. Declining gonadal function in elderly men. *Baillieres Clin Endocrinol Metab* 1997;11:289–309

81. Vermeulen A. Androgens and male senescence. In Nieschlag E, Behre HM, eds. *Testosterone: Action, Deficiency, Substitution.* Heidelberg: Springer, 1990:261–76

82. Vermeulen A, Verdonck L. Some studies on the biological significance of free testosterone. *J Steroid Biochem* 1972;3:421–6

83. Tenover JS, Matsumoto AM, Plymate SR, Bremner WJ. The effects of aging in normal men on bioavailable testosterone and luteinizing hormone secretion: response to clomiphene citrate. *J Clin Endocrinol Metab* 1987;65: 1118–26

84. Gray A, Feldman HA, McKinlay JB, Longcope C. Age, disease, and changing sex hormone levels in middle-aged men: results of the Massachusetts Male Aging Study. *J Clin Endocrinol Metab* 1991;73: 1016–25

85. Gray A, Jackson DN, McKinlay JB. The relation between dominance, anger, and hormones in normally aging men: results from the Massachusetts Male Aging Study. *Psychosom Med* 1991;53:375–85

86. Dabbs JM, de La RD, Williams PM.

Testosterone and occupational choice: actors, ministers, and other men. *J Pers Soc Psychol* 1990;59: 1261-5

87. Meikle AW, Stringham J, Bishop D, West D. Quantitation of genetic and non-genetic factors influencing androgen production and clearance rates in men. *J Clin Endocrinol Metab* 1988;67:104-9

88. Wang C, Berman NG, Veldhuis JD et al. Graded testosterone infusions distinguish gonadotropin negative-feedback responsiveness in Asian and white men – a Clinical Research Center study. *J Clin Endocrinol Metab* 1998;83:870-6

89. Johnson L, Barnard JJ, Rodriguez L et al. Ethnic differences in testicular structure and spermatogenic potential may predispose testes of Asian men to a heightened sensitivity to steroidal contraceptives. *J Androl* 1998;19:348-57

90. Hiort O, Zitzmann M. Androgen receptor: pathophysiology. In Nieschlag E, Behre HM, eds. *Testosterone: Action, Deficiency, Substitution.* Cambridge University Press, 2004:93-124

91. Heald AH, Ivison F, Anderson SG, Cruickshank K, Laing I, Gibson JM. Significant ethnic variation in total and free testosterone concentration. *Clin Endocrinol (Oxf)* 2003; 58:262-6

92. Harkonen K, Huhtaniemi I, Makinen J, et al. The polymorphic androgen receptor gene CAG repeat, pituitary-testicular function and andropausal symptoms in ageing men. *Int J Androl* 2003;26:187-94

93. Krithivas K, Yurgalevitch SM, Mohr BA, et al. Evidence that the CAG repeat in the androgen receptor gene is associated with the age-related decline in serum androgen levels in men. *J Endocrinol* 1999; 162:137-42

94. Zitzmann M, Gromoll J, Von Eckardstein A, Nieschlag E. The CAG repeat polymorphism in the androgen receptor gene modulates body fat mass and serum concentrations of leptin and insulin in men. *Diabetologia* 2003;46:31-9

95. Zitzmann M, Brune M, Kornmann B, Gromoll J, Junker R, Nieschlag E. The CAG repeat polymorphism in the androgen receptor gene affects bone density and bone metabolism in healthy males. *Clin Endocrinol (Oxf)* 2001;55:649-57

96. Giovannucci E, Stampfer MJ, Chan A, et al. CAG repeat within the androgen receptor gene and incidence of surgery for benign prostatic hyperplasia in US physicians. *Prostate* 1999;39:130-4

97. Atkinson LE, Chang Y, Snyder PJ. Long-term experience with testosterone replacement through scrotal skin. In Nieschlag E, Behre HM, eds. *Testosterone: Action, Deficiency, Substitution.* Berlin: Springer-Verlag, 1998:365-88

98. Kapoor P, Luttrell BM, Williams D. The free androgen index is not valid for adult males. *J Steroid Biochem Mol Biol* 1993;45:325-6

99. Vermeulen A, Verdonck L, Kaufman JM. A critical evaluation of simple methods for the estimation of free testosterone in serum. *J Clin Endocrinol Metab* 1999;84: 3666-72

100. Tremblay RR. Practical consequences of the validation of a mathematical model in assessment of partial androgen deficiency in the aging male using bioavailable testosterone. *Aging Male* 2001;4:23-9

101. Vermeulen A, Verdonck L, Kaufman JM. A critical evaluation of simple methods for the estimation of free testosterone in serum. *J Clin Endocrinol Metab* 1999;84: 3666-72

102. Conway AJ, Handelsman DJ, Lording DW, Stuckey B, Zajac JD. Use, misuse and abuse of androgens. The Endocrine Society of Australia consensus guidelines for androgen prescribing. *Med J Aust* 2000;172:220–4.

5 Androgen replacement therapy

INTRODUCTION

The treatment principles and practice given here are the synthesis of two sets of recommendations published in the past 5 years, combined with 25 years of personal experience of testosterone treatment.

The first set of recommendations is that of Morales and Lunenfeld on 'Investigation, treatment and monitoring of late-onset hypogonadism in males'[1]. These 'Standards, Guidelines and Recommendations of the International Society for the Study of the Aging Male (ISSAM),' were developed from the 'Canadian practice recommendations for screening, monitoring and treating men affected by andropause or partial androgen deficiency'[2], coauthored by Tremblay and Morales of the Canadian Andropause Society. After a year's consultation with the members of ISSAM, the draft recommendations put forward in 2001[3] were adopted as the official ones in 2002, and will be referred to as the 'ISSAM recommendations'. (Given in full in Appendix 1A.)

The second set of recommendations was adopted by the First and Second Annual Andropause Consensus Meetings of the Endocrine Society in 2000[4] and 2001[5], and were independently reviewed and approved by the Society's Clinical Affairs Committee. They will be referred to as 'Endocrine Society Management Recommendations'. (Given in full in Appendix 1B.)

GENERAL PRINCIPLES

'First do no harm' is the guiding principle for safe and effective androgen treatment. Central to this is careful and complete evaluation of the patient's symptoms, history, physical examination and the results of a full endocrine, biochemical and hematological profile, followed by careful monitoring of the effects of treatment.

Fortunately, there is evidence that testosterone is one of the safest forms of pharmacotherapy. For example, a survey was carried out of adverse reactions to all forms of testosterone treatment as reported to the Medicines

Control Agency in the UK. This receives reports of suspected adverse drug reactions (ADRs) directly from doctors, dentists and coroners, and indirectly from pharmaceutical companies. These are placed on a specialized computer system, Adverse Drug Reactions On-line Information Tracking System (ADROIT). This has provided a complete list of all adverse reactions reported between 1963, when the yellow-card scheme for reporting adverse reactions was set up, and 2002, i.e. nearly 40 years of the clinical use of all forms of testosterone.

This extensive database gives the following reassuring information (Table 1). First, there were no reactions to testosterone reported until 1978, about 15 years from the start of the reporting system. From then a total of 214 reactions were reported in 185 patients by the end of the survey period, some patients having more than one reaction. Of these reactions, half were minor skin reactions, pain at injection sites or loss of pellet implants. The rest were widely scattered through the organ systems, with only three 'fatal outcomes', including one overdose, one suicide and one sarcoma of unknown site, i.e. less than one possibly unconnected fatality every 10 years. This is an amazing safety record, which totally contradicts the adverse medical and lay images of testosterone treatment, even allowing for a tendency for underreporting.

Table 1 Adverse reactions to testosterone 1963–2002 from UK Medicines Control Agency data (yellow card)

Cutaneous + local reaction, $n = 117$	implant + injection complications 90, rash 15
Psychiatric + general, $n = 27$	aggression 6, depression 3 (suicide 1)
Endocrine + metabolic + musculoskeletal, $n = 17$	muscle cramps 3, arthralgia 3, hirsutism 1, diabetes 1
Gastrointestinal + liver + respiratory, $n = 16$	diarrhea 7, nausea 3, abdominal pain 3, jaundice 2
Vascular, $n = 15$	cardiac 8, CVA 2, DVT 4, embolus 1
Neurological + eye, $n = 13$	paresthesia 6, headache 6 (OD–CVA 1)
Neoplasms + urological, $n = 9$	?prostate 2 (sarcoma 1), breast 1, priapism 2, testicular pain 2, renal failure 1

CVA, cerebrovascular accident; DVT, deep vein thrombosis; OD, overdose

Only one case of acute testosterone overdose following an injection has been reported in the literature. This was a cerebrovascular accident in a patient with a gross overdosage giving a plasma testosterone concentration of 395 nmol/l (11 380 ng/dl), over ten times the upper limit of normal.

Studies of the commonly perceived dangers of anabolic steroid abuse[6] in fact show a high margin of safety given the very large doses of a wide range of clinically unsuitable drugs used, and often total lack of medical supervision. As the above article states, especially in women, 'many of the effects reported could be labeled as un-cosmetic but clinically harmless'.

The second principle is that the testosterone therapy is only part of the broad medical approach to treating these cases, just as insulin or oral antidiabetic drugs are not the only measures used in the overall management of a diabetic. Stress, alcohol and weight reduction, as well as review of any current medication which might be interfering with the synthesis or action of testosterone, or contributing to erectile dysfunction, should also be routinely considered.

Third, the wishes and needs of the patient with regard to the form, dose and acceptability of different types of treatment should be taken into account. Some are quite happy to take tablets once or twice a day. Others prefer fortnightly injections, or even testosterone pellet implants once every 6 months. Also, the dose may need to be progressively increased to give androgen levels within the physiological range for that individual in his youth to achieve symptom relief, or to the supraphysiological levels required for specific indications such as the treatment of ischemic limb ulcers and possibly Alzheimer's disease.

This principle coincides with the view of the Workshop Conference on Androgen Therapy organized jointly by the World Health Organization (WHO), US National Institutes of Health (NIH), and US Food and Drug Administration (FDA) in 1990 on the best therapeutic guidelines:

> *The consensus view was that the major goal of therapy is to replace testosterone levels at as close to physiological concentrations as is possible[7].*

This recommendation might now need to be refined by including reference to normalization of androgen binding and receptor levels to as near youthful physiological levels as possible.

Finally, in considering the therapeutic effects and safety profiles of the different testosterone preparations, it is unjustified to generalize in terms of testosterone treatment does this, or testosterone treatment does that. The pharmacological effects of the different preparations vary widely, and too often the alleged side-effects of any one preparation as listed in the manufacturer's data sheet are a compendium of all of those attributed to every known testosterone preparation.

COMMENTARY ON THE ISSAM GUIDELINES, AND COMPARISON WITH THE MANAGEMENT RECOMMENDATIONS OF THE ENDOCRINE SOCIETY

The ISSAM Guidelines and the Endocrine Society Management Recommendations for androgen replacement are given in full in Appendix 1B.

ISSAM 1

> *Definition (of ADAM): A biochemical syndrome associated with advancing aging and characterized by a deficiency in serum androgen levels with or without a decreased genomic sensitivity to androgens. It*

may result in significant alterations in the quality of life and adversely affect the function of multiple organ systems.

This recommendation was absent in the first 'draft' guidelines, and appears to add little by its inclusion in the later 'official' ones. First, according to the *Oxford English Dictionary*, a syndrome is 'a concurrence of several symptoms in a disease', and while the characteristic symptoms of andropause may have a common endocrine origin, it seems imprecise to use the word 'biochemical' as an adjective in this context.

Also, the term 'advancing aging' places undue emphasis on age as a cause, and belies the fact that while symptoms of the andropause most commonly occur in men in their 50s, a few cases occur up to 20 years earlier. Most people in their 50s, and many in their 60s and even 70s, would deny being of 'advanced age'. It would also appear to make it less important to treat this syndrome, as it is just 'aging'.

In the ISSAM Guidelines this definition follows the diagnostic criteria of the condition in terms of screening, diagnostic and treatment monitoring questionnaires such as that produced by Heinemann and colleagues[8]. To characterize the condition then on the basis of laboratory criteria such as 'a deficiency in serum androgen levels' appears both tautological and inaccurate and to make the clinical diagnosis overdependent on inaccurate and arbitrary endocrine norms. Serum, as distinct from plasma, exists only in the laboratory, there may be resistance to even high levels of androgens, e.g. from raised sex hormone-binding globulin (SHBG), and it might be that tissue androgens are a crucial factor in some cases.

Finally, how is 'genomic sensitivity to androgens' to be assessed by the clinician, and, like the comments on the 'quality of life' and 'function of multiple organ systems', how does it help establish the diagnosis of androgen deficiency?

The relevant section of the Endocrine Society guidelines raises similar problems in its introduction when it lists many characteristic andropausal symptoms, and then states:

> *A definition of andropause (clinically significant androgen deficiency in the elderly male) should include some or all of these symptoms and signs plus a low serum testosterone (T).*

Similar objections to the word 'elderly' and need for a low serum testosterone apply

ISSAM 2

> *ADAM [androgen deficiency in the adult male], or the andropause is a syndrome characterized primarily by:*
>
> *(1) The easily recognized features of diminished sexual desire and erectile quality, particularly nocturnal erections;*

(2) Changes in mood with concomitant decreases in intellectual activity, spatial orientation ability, fatigue, depressed mood and irritability;

(3) Decrease in lean body mass with associated diminution in muscle volume and strength;

(4) Decrease in body hair and skin alterations;

(5) Decreased bone mineral density resulting in osteopenia and osteoporosis;

(6) Increase in visceral fat.

(These manifestations need not all be present to identify the syndrome. In addition, the severity of one or more of them does not necessarily match the severity of the others, nor do we yet understand the uneven appearance of these manifestations. Moreover, the clinical picture may or may not be associated with low testosterone. Therefore, the clinical diagnosis should be supported by biochemical tests confirming the presence of hypogonadism.)

Endocrine Society Recommendations list these symptoms, and add insulin resistance, and an increased risk of diabetes and cardiovascular disorders, to the possible health risks of testosterone deficiency.

ISSAM 3

In patients at risk or suspected of hypogonadism, the following biochemical investigations should be performed:

(1) Serum sample for testosterone determination between 08.00 and 11.00. The most reliable and widely acceptable parameter to establish the presence of hypogonadism is the measurement of bioavailable testosterone or, alternatively, calculated free testosterone.

(2) If testosterone levels are below, or at the lower limit of, the accepted normal values, it is prudent to confirm the result with a second determination together with assessment of follicle stimulating hormone (FSH), luteinizing hormone (LH) and prolactin.

Endocrine Society guidelines also emphasize the need for 'early morning samples, and where total testosterone levels are below 14 nmol/l (400 ng/dl), doing calculated free or bio-available T, with LH [luteinizing hormone] and prolactin if these are abnormal'.

ISSAM 4

It is recognized that significant alterations in other endocrine systems occur in association with ageing but the significance of these changes is not well understood. In general terms, determinations of DHEA, DHEA-S [dehydroepiandrosterone and its sulfate], melatonin, GH [growth hormone] and IGF-1 [insulin-like growth factor-1] are not indicated in the uncomplicated evaluation of ADAM. Under special circumstances, or for well-defined clinical research, assessment of those and other hormones might be warranted.

These other hormones are not mentioned in the Endocrine Society Recommendations.

ISSAM 5

A clear indication (a clinical picture together with biochemical support) should exist prior to initiation of androgen therapy.

Although three andropause symptom questionnaires are mentioned, the emphasis seems to be mainly on the laboratory tests in the Endocrine Society consensus statement.

ISSAM 6

In the absence of defined contraindications, age is not a limiting factor to initiate ART [androgen replacement therapy] in aged men with hypogonadism.

The Endocrine Society suggest starting screening at age 50 and repeating 5-yearly with no upper age limit, quoting the percentage of men with low testosterone levels up to age 80+.

ISSAM 7

Currently available preparations of testosterone (with the exception of the alkylated ones) are safe and effective. The treating physician should have sufficient knowledge and adequate understanding of the advantages and drawbacks of each preparation.

This chapter is designed to provide the physician with the information needed to formulate a treatment program according to each patient's needs.

ISSAM 8

The purpose of ART is to bring and maintain serum testosterone levels within the physiological range. Supraphysiological levels are to be avoided.

This guideline is more arguable, as many physicians would see the aim of ART as being to remove the patient's symptoms, and to offer preventive medical benefits. The Endocrine Society suggests that:

Treatment goals include: 1) restoring metabolic parameters to the eugo-nadal state; 2) increasing muscle mass, strength, and function; 3) main-taining BMD [bone mineral density] and reducing fracture risk; 4) improving neuropsychological function (cognition and mood); 5) improving psychosexual function; and 6) enhancing quality of life.

Except that some clinicians might reverse the order of importance of these goals, this seems a good summary of the aims of ART. However, both definitions raise the question of what is the 'physiological' or 'eugonadal state' for that individual at that age.

ISSAM 9

Liver function studies are advisable prior to onset of therapy, quarterly during the first year and on a yearly basis thereafter during treatment.

This is not essential with modern preparations, which are not hepatotoxic, and are not mentioned in the Endocrine Society Recommendations. They can, however, be used to monitor alcohol intake, which is an important factor in both causation and treatment of androgen deficiency.

ISSAM 10

A fasting lipid profile to initiation of treatment and at regular intervals (no longer than one year) during treatment is recommended.

Again, this is not essential, but is an important part of the clinical management on a general medical basis.

ISSAM 11

Digital rectal examination (DRE) and determination of serum prostate-specific antigen (PSA) are mandatory in men over the age of 40 years as baseline measurements of prostate health prior to therapy with andro-gens, at quarterly intervals for the first 12 months and yearly thereafter. Transrectal ultrasound-guided biopsies of the prostate are indicated only if the DRE or the PSA are abnormal.

This is a key recommendation which is also emphasized in the Endocrine Society statement:

Serum PSA and DRE of the prostate should be performed before treatment, and at 3 and 6 months after initiating treatment, and then annually.
    If an increase in PSA of ≥ 1.5 ng/ml/year is verified on repeat testing,

if there is an average annual increase of ≥ 0.75 ng/ml over a minimum of 2 years, or if the PSA is greater than 4.0 ng/ml, urological consultation should be obtained.

These unanimous guidelines ensure that at least men being considered for ART have basic screening to exclude prostate cancer, which in countries such as the UK is not yet routinely offered under the state system. Also, it has been suggested that by giving ART for 3 months, and then checking the PSA again, if there is an early or occult hormone-sensitive cancer, it would be revealed by a significant rise in the PSA according to the criteria of the Endocrine Society[9].

A slight rise in PSA occasionally occurs in the first months of ART, but is usually only restoring the PSA to a level in the range which would be normal for a man of that age. This has been reported in other series[10–12], although some low-dosage testosterone studies, e.g. with testosterone undecanoate, where neither estrogen nor dihydrotestosterone (DHT) is markedly raised, have even reported a decrease in prostate volume, PSA and lower-urinary tract symptoms (LUTS) on starting treatment[13]. No significant change in total or free PSA, or their ratio, was found in the UK Andropause Study (UKAS) (see Appendix 3), where PSA was measured before starting treatment, and at 3 months, and 6-monthly intervals afterwards.

ISSAM 12

Androgen administration is absolutely contraindicated in men suspected of carcinoma of the prostate or breast cancer.

This crucial contraindication is recognized by the Endocrine Society, and virtually all other advisory authorities.

ISSAM 13

Androgen supplementation is contraindicated in men with severe bladder outlet obstruction due to an enlarged, clinically benign prostate. Moderate obstruction represents a partial contraindication to ART. Once the urinary obstruction has been successfully treated, these men are candidates for androgen supplementation.

The Endocrine Society list only 'severe obstructive symptoms of BPH [benign prostatic hyperplasia]', confirming that mild and moderate degrees of benign hypertrophy are not contraindications, and this might otherwise exclude 50% of men over the age of 50.

ISSAM 14

ART normally results in improvements in mood and well-being. The development of negative behavioral patterns during treatment calls for dose modifications or discontinuation of therapy.

Hypersexuality and excessive aggressive impulses are seldom seen with ART[14], and are mainly confined to young men grossly overdosing on steroids. Generally, androgen deficient men are restored to their previous individual 'normal' levels of sexuality and drive, and do not overshoot. They often become markedly less irritable, as frequently commented upon by both themselves and their partners.

ISSAM 15

Polycythemia occasionally develops during ART. Periodic hematological assessment is indicated. Dose adjustments may be necessary.

Fortunately, this is usually only a significant problem with a few patients on high-dosage parenteral ART preparations such as injections and implants (see safety section in this chapter). It can be dealt with by reducing the dosage, moving to a weaker preparation or regular phlebotomy.

The Endocrine Society specify that a hematocrit $\geq 55\%$ is an absolute contraindication to treatment, and $\geq 52\%$ a relative one. They also include congestive heart failure as a relative contraindication to treatment.

ISSAM 16

There is insufficient evidence for a recommendation regarding safety of ART in men with sleep apnea. It is suggested, therefore, that good clinical judgment and caution be employed in this situation.

The Endocrine Society just list 'untreated sleep apnea' as a relative contraindication, and as one of the symptoms to be monitored during treatment.

ISSAM 17

Monitoring during ART is a shared responsibility. The physician must emphasize to the patient the need for periodic evaluations and the patient must agree to comply with these requirements. Since ART is normally for life, monitoring is also a lifetime mutual duty.

To summarize, it is reassuring that the ISSAM Guidelines are generally in close agreement with the Endocrine Society ART Management Recommendations, which give an excellent one-page summary of their 11 key points, and an investigation flow chart, at the end of the paper.

TESTOSTERONE TREATMENT

The different forms of testosterone treatment will be dealt with according to their different routes of administration.

Testosterone injections

Development

As soon as testosterone was first synthesized, injections of free testosterone were tried, but found to be impractical, as in this form it only has a half-life of 10 min. Through research in the late 1930s and early 1940s it was found that adding a fatty-acid side-chain made it more slowly absorbed, the duration of action being roughly proportional to the length of the side-chain,

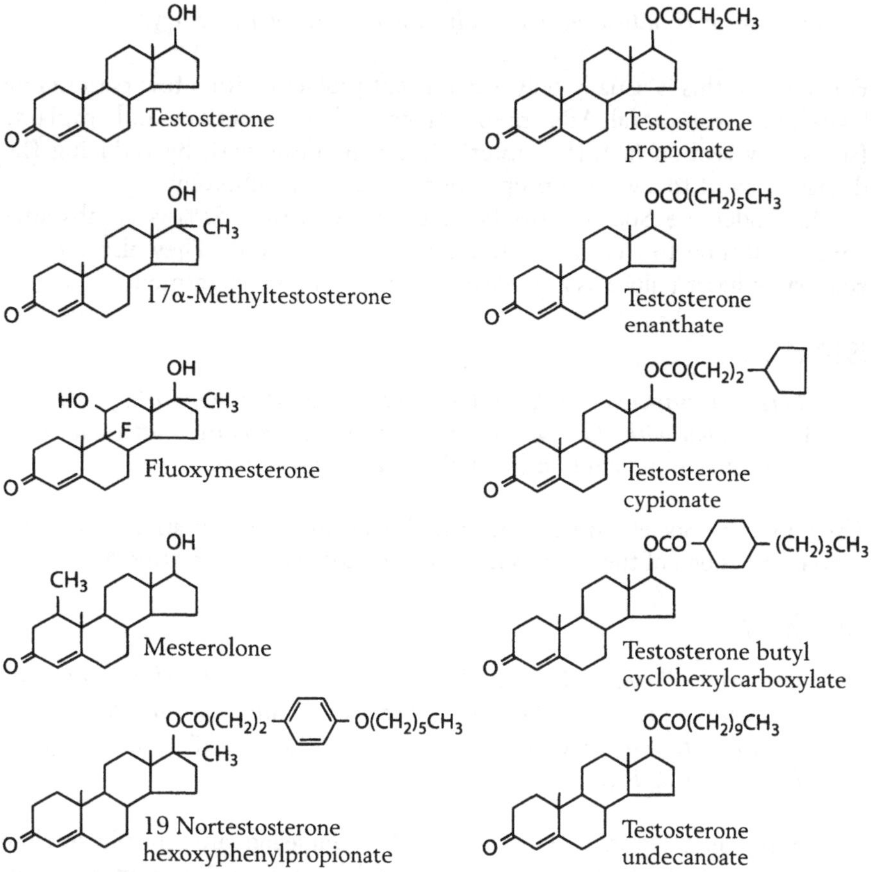

Figure 1 Molecular structure of testosterone and its derivatives. Reproduced with permission from reference 15

although certain further modifications could extend the half-life still further (Figure 1). Once absorbed, each of the esters is rapidly broken down to the unesterified testosterone, which has the same short half-life as the endogenous molecule.

The first of these esters to be synthesized in the late 1930s was testosterone propionate, which became the standard injectable alternative to either the toxic oral methyltestosterone, or pellet implants, until the 1960s. Although it was initially used with success by clinicians such as Dr Augustus Werner in treatment of the andropause[16,17], and enabled Heller and Myers to carry out placebo-controlled trials showing the efficacy of testosterone in this condition[18], it had to be given in 50-mg doses at least twice and preferably three times per week.

Also, it suffered the disadvantages common to all injectable testosterone preparations so far available to clinicians, of giving large fluctuations in hormone level, ranging from the initial supraphysiological surge, falling to low basal levels before the next dose. This put the patient on a roller-coaster ride, ranging from a hormonal high, in which he might feel hyperactive and almost manic the day after the injection, dropping to lethargy, impotence and depression at the end of the cycle.

These undesirable variations of energy and mood are still seen with the most commonly available injectable forms of testosterone used to this day. These are the enanthate, cypionate and cyclohexane carboxylate, which, although they have virtually the same pharmacokinetics, being generally given at 2–3-weekly intervals, are sometimes combined in preparations such as Sustenon®. This is popular in the UK, mainly on cost grounds, since it is less than half the price of the equivalent 250-mg dose of enanthate. However, as Behre and Nieschlag have pointed out, 'For treatment of male hypogonadism there is no advantage in combining short- and long-acting testosterone esters'[19]. Furthermore, not only is this preparation dissolved in arachis (peanut) oil, but also this cocktail of esters has nothing like the wealth of worldwide clinical experience of use and safety data of testosterone enanthate.

Because of the shortcomings of existing injectable preparations, in 1980 the WHO initiated a steroid synthesis program that resulted in the production of several formulations with extended durations of action. Of these, the buciclate ester, given in doses of 1000 mg, lasted 12–16 weeks, while testosterone enanthate bound to biodegradable latex microspheres lasted 8 weeks. However, though used in various research studies of hypogonadism and male hormonal contraception[15], none of these compounds have become available for routine clinical practice.

The first really long-acting injection to be become available to the clinician is a preparation of 1000 mg testosterone undecanoate in castor oil (Nebido™, Schering), which gives testosterone levels staying within the physiological normal range when given to hypogonadal men at 3-monthly intervals (Figure 2)[20]. Bodyweight, hemoglobin, serum lipids, PSA and

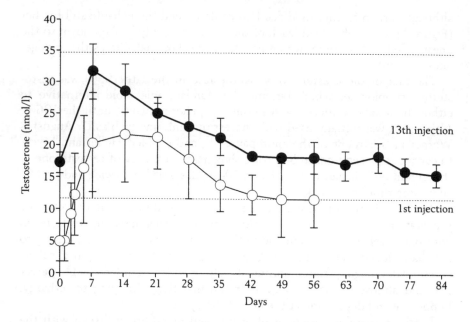

Figure 2 Serum testosterone (mean ± SD) after a single injection of 1000 mg testosterone undecanoate in castor oil in 14 untreated hypogonadal men (open circles) and after treatment with the same dose every 12 weeks for 102 weeks (closed circles). Broken lines indicate normal range of testosterone. Reproduced with permission from reference 20

prostate volume did not change significantly over 3.2 years, indicating that this is likely to be a safe and economical form of treatment. It also potentially can replace the need for testosterone pellet implantation, over which it has several advantages, including cost, convenience and being a more physiological form of treatment.

These views appear to be shared by the WHO and its panel of male contraceptive experts. They are summarized by Behre and co-workers[15], who suggest that 'As this preparation has been approved for clinical use in Europe, intramuscular testosterone undecanoate in castor oil will become a significantly improved testosterone preparation for treatment of male hypogonadism as well as for male contraception.'

However, the form of injectable testosterone that is most fully researched, has the largest amount of clinical evidence available on its safety, and is widely available throughout the world, is testosterone enanthate. The accumulated clinical experience with this long-established preparation is both impressive and reassuring.

Pharmacology

The pharmacokinetics of testosterone enanthate are given in detail because they are similar for all the intermediate acting esters available in routine clinical practice, including combined preparations such as Sustenon®.

The simulated pharmacokinetics of 250 mg of testosterone enanthate given in multiple intramuscular doses at intervals of 1–4 weeks are shown in Figure 3. These simulated 'sawtooth' curves coincide closely with blood levels measured in research studies[19], and with physicians' and patients' experiences in clinical use.

Clinical application

Intramuscular injections of 250 mg of testosterone enanthate every 2 weeks are the most commonly used dosage, keep the majority of patients within the physiological normal range, depending on how you define that (see previous chapter), and are usually sufficient to maintain the patient's symptomatic response.

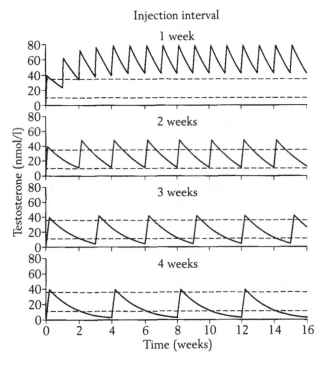

Figure 3 Testosterone levels with 250-mg injections of testosterone enanthate given at intervals of 1–4 weeks. Broken lines represent lower and upper limits of 'normal range' (10–35 nmol/l)

Only if supraphysiological levels of testosterone need to be maintained, as in the initial treatment of severe peripheral arterial disease cases, may weekly injections be required. The safety of these high dosages has been shown in the WHO multicenter trial of testosterone as a male contraceptive, in relation to lipids[21], hemostatic variables[22], prostate and testis[23], sexuality and mood[14].

Oral testosterone preparations

Methyltestosterone

Pure testosterone given orally has, since it was first synthesized in 1935, been known to be well absorbed, but is rapidly broken down in the liver, the first-pass effect. The search for an oral form rapidly resulted in the synthesis of the water-soluble methyltestosterone[24]. This was the main form of oral testosterone available through to the 1970s, but was recognized as being toxic to both the liver and heart.

The frequent and severe side-effects are due to the alkyl group in the 17α-position, and are shared by other steroids with this configuration, such as fluoxymesterone. Although methyltestosterone was taken off the market in most countries in the 1980s[25], it is still available in the USA for some reason, especially in combination with estrogens in the treatment of menopausal women. Even though the dosage is lower, reducing its hepatotoxicity, it still seems inadvisable to use it in either sex.

Mesterolone (Proviron® 25- and 50-mg tablets; Schering)

This relatively weak oral androgen was developed in the 1960s, and is protected from rapid breakdown in the liver by the addition of a methyl group in position 1 (Figure 1). It has a direct metabolic effect similar to DHT, and, unlike testosterone, cannot be aromatized to estrogen. This limits its clinical effectiveness, and means that it has only a partial androgenic action, as reported in the UK Andropause Study, producing no measurable effects on total testosterone, SHBG or estrogen levels.

While this makes it unlikely to cause complications such as gynecomastia, and produces little or no reduction in either LH or follicle stimulating hormone (FSH), the large increase in blood levels of either DHT, or the closely similar mesterolone molecule, may cause concern in relation to benign enlargement of the prostate or hair loss. 5α-Reductase blockers such as finasteride are used to reduce DHT levels in both these conditions. However, clinically, this is largely a theoretical objection, as neither appears to be significantly increased by using mesterolone over a period of up to 10 years.

Clinical application   While I am not going as far as to conclude that 'Altogether,   mesterolone   is   not   suited   for   the   substitution   of hypogonadism'[15], it is certainly only partially effective in cases where a weak effect, e.g. on libido, or facial hair growth, is required. Clinically it is sometimes of use where other oral agents such as testosterone undecanoate have failed, or are poorly tolerated.

An interesting report was of its use in depression[26], where its antidepressant effects were compared with those of amitriptyline in a double-blind, parallel-treatment design. The drugs were found to be equally effective in reducing depressive symptoms. Mesterolone produced significantly fewer adverse side-effects than amitriptyline.

Safety Early reports showed it to be safe[27-29], and although it raised DHT levels to a greater extent than other testosterone preparations, it had less effect on erythropoiesis[30]. However, in one study of severely hypogonadal patients, it was found to have a marked effect on lipid levels[31], raising total cholesterol, low-density lipoprotein (LDL), and triglycerides, and lowering high-density lipoprotein (HDL) cholesterol C. These latter findings were not confirmed by the UKAS.

The preparation comes in 25-mg tablets, and the dose used can be between 25 and 100 mg daily, given in two doses, preferably breakfast and lunchtime for the reasons to be discussed in relation to testosterone undecanoate.

Testosterone undecanoate (Andriol®, Restandol® and Testocaps®, 40-mg capsules)

Development Because testosterone itself, when given by mouth, is rapidly broken down in the liver, alternative strategies were investigated. Protecting the molecule from breakdown either made it hepatotoxic, as with methyl- or fluoxy- derivatives, or prevented aromatization, as with mesterolone.

In the mid-1970s, 40 years after testosterone was first synthesized, a preparation which largely solved this problem became available. By adding a long aliphatic side-chain in the form of undecanoic acid (Figure 1), absorption was switched from the portal vein to the lymphatic system draining into the thoracic duct[32,33]. It has the distinction of being the one form of testosterone treatment which has the 'male climacteric', now recognized as the andropause, as one of its licensed applications.

Early studies indicated that testosterone undecanoate in doses of 80–200 mg orally daily was an effective and safe compound for treating many cases of androgen deficiency. It appeared to be more suitable for older, andropausal men where there was only a mild to moderate reduction in basal androgen levels, which needed 'topping up', rather than severely deficient patients such as those with testicular nondescent, orchidectomy or prolactinoma.

The efficacy and safety of testosterone undecanoate have been studied in many countries since 1975 as Andriol® and Restandol®, but its use was severely limited by the fact that it was not available in America. It did, however, appear on the Canadian market in the late 1990s, and has been actively marketed there, mainly in relation to treatment of the andropause. Its use is likely to extend to the whole of the North American market within the next couple of years, particularly in the revised formulation of Testocaps®.

Pharmacology   Testosterone undecanoate is produced by Organon NV in 40-mg capsules, equivalent to 25 mg of testosterone. Absorption is almost entirely via the fat particles (chylomicra and very-low-density lipoprotein (VLDL)) formed by the enterocytes of the small intestine, draining into the lymphatic system through the thoracic duct[34]. This is why it is crucial that the capsules are taken with food, preferably containing some fat to improve solubilization and absorption[35].

The latest research preceding the introduction of Testocaps® confirmed the importance of fat in the food for absorption of this oral preparation, by giving a single dose of 80 mg of testosterone undecanoate (2 × 40-mg Testocaps®) to 16 healthy postmenopausal women who were either unfed, or given a normal breakfast. Figure 4 shows that in the unfed state there was virtually no absorption, while the fat content of the breakfast gave excellent absorption, levels reaching a peak 6 h later.

The earlier preparations of oral testosterone undecanoate were more temperature-labile than generally assumed, and many patients, acting on the instructions given in the package insert that they *must* store the capsules at room temperature (15–25 °C), frequently had a good initial clinical response, which faded after a month or two. The reason given for these storage instructions was that refrigeration would separate the oil and the testosterone and prevent transport into the lymphatic system, but that after 48 h at room temperature the two would recombine. In spite of this, the capsules were delivered to pharmacists in refrigerated containers, and they were advised to store them in the refrigerator 'to maintain long-term stability'.

Testocaps®, however, also contains 40 mg testosterone undecanoate, but dissolved in castor oil rather than oleic acid, together with a lipolytic surfactant (propylene glycol laurate). This formulation is claimed to have increased the shelf life at room temperature from 3 months to 3 years[36], which should be a great advance in maintaining a full clinical response. The manufacturers have only recently drawn attention to these important points, and now emphasize the need for the drug to be taken with food.

Recent clinical studies of the pharmacology of Testocaps® have also confirmed that absorption varies widely, in both amount and timing, from person to person[37]. Peak testosterone levels have been found to occur at any time 3–7 h after administration, with a mean of 6 h. It has been shown by studies in both men[36] and women[35] that there is a sharp exponential decay curve in testosterone, values falling to 50% of peak within about 2 h, with

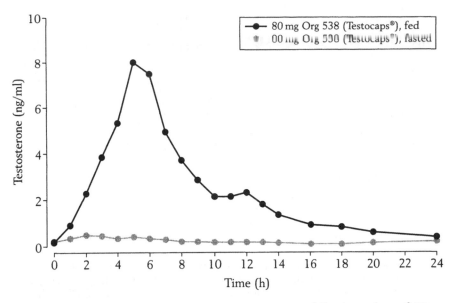

Figure 4 Testosterone mean concentration against time following a dose of 80 mg testosterone undecanoate, in either the fed or the unfed state. Reproduced with permission from reference 35

near baseline levels being regained 12–24 h after two doses 12 h apart (Figure 5).

The same research showed that testosterone undecanoate gave a relatively greater and more prolonged rise in DHT, levels being raised to 3–6 times the upper limit of normal at peak, and remaining raised for up to 12–24 h (Figure 5). However, there was no significant rise in estradiol, and these changes were similar to those seen in the larger population group of the UKAS (see Appendix 3).

What is rarely reported, however, is the important fact that testosterone undecanoate is the only commonly used form of testosterone treatment which consistently produces a fall in SHBG. In the UKAS, the sustained reduction was about 25%. This was confirmed by the studies of Skakkebaek and colleagues[38] in 1981, Davidson and associates[39] in 1987 and Conway and colleagues[40] in 1988. It therefore results in a proportionally greater rise in free testosterone than that with other preparations, which greatly enhances its therapeutic effect.

Clinical application   In the case of Andriol® or Restandol®, the precautions needed in relation to refrigeration of stock bottles by both the pharmacist and the patient must be emphasized. However, when the bottle of capsules is opened for use, it must be left in a cool place, at room temperature, to allow the testosterone undecanoate to become resuspended in the oleic

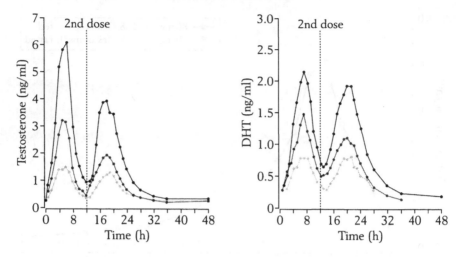

Figure 5 Mean concentration versus time curves of three different doses of testosterone undecanoate (2×20 mg, 2×40 mg and 2×80 mg) in 45 postmenopausal women, taking the medication at time zero and 12 h, with meals. DHT, dihydrotestosterone. Reproduced with permission from reference 36

acid. This precaution will not be needed for the new formulation of Testocaps®, which is stable at room temperature.

However, it must be emphasized, as the above research proved, that either preparation needs to be taken with a small amount of fat, to carry it into the lymphatic system draining the gut. A slice of buttered bread, or a pot of yogurt, particularly if combined with a cup of milky tea or coffee, is likely to be sufficient. Although the package insert suggests taking it after meals, it is unclear whether, for optimal absorption, during or even just before might be preferable. Small details of storage, and timing in relation to meals, can probably make a big difference to the success or failure of this form of androgen treatment.

Also, timing of the doses is critical. Practical experience has shown that it is best to try to mimic the normal diurnal variation of testosterone levels seen in a healthy young man. Rather than space the doses out to morning and evening, or spread them through the day, it is preferable to give the first, and often larger, dose with breakfast, and then the second dose with the midday meal, and none after that.

This timing has several advantages. First, it ensures that the major dose is taken before the patient starts his daily schedule, in which the second dose may be missed. This improves compliance, which can be a problem in men reluctant to take oral medication on a daily basis.

Second, it allows for the 3–7-h delay before peak absorption occurs, but maintains adequate levels for most of the waking hours. Testosterone seems to have an arousing, alerting effect, and some patients observe that if they have their second dose with their evening meal it can cause insomnia or dreaming.

Third, it causes less suppression of the early-morning surge in endogenous androgen synthesis arising from LH and FSH stimulation of the testes, because the lower night-time levels of testosterone result in reduced feedback inhibition of the pituitary gonadotropin-releasing hormones. It may also reduce any tendency towards downregulation of the androgen receptors, which may occur with the sustained high levels of testosterone produced by widely spaced doses.

The usual starting dose of testosterone undecanoate is two of the 40-mg capsules with breakfast and one with lunch. Usually there is a marked reduction in symptoms and improvement in well-being within 2 days to 2 weeks. Sometimes, the initial improvement fades after a week, the so-called 'honeymoon effect'. This may be due to reduction of endogenous synthesis, androgen receptor changes or even weakening of the initial placebo effect. The patient needs to be reassured if this occurs, and if full symptomatic improvement is not achieved at the lowest dose, at monthly intervals, if necessary, the dose is increased to 80 mg twice a day, and to a maximum of 120 mg twice daily, especially in high-body-weight patients.

The patient should then be reassessed at 3 months, with a morning blood sample taken at least 3 h after his usual morning dose of the capsules. Because the major goal of treatment is relief of symptoms, and the restoration and maintenance of the optimal quality of life which can be achieved, more attention should be paid to assessing these subjective factors than to overreliance on the laboratory data, which may miss the absorption peak and be disappointing.

However, the visit may indicate why the clinical response to treatment is impaired, if, for example, the SHBG remains too high, with a corresponding reduction in free testosterone, requiring a change to another modality of treatment, such as danazol or testosterone pellet implant. Also, the visit may show whether absorption of the oral testosterone undecanoate is inadequate, or causing the infrequent problems of gastric irritation or diarrhea.

It is also important at this 3-month visit to check whether the patient has managed to adopt any necessary lifestyle changes, such as stress, alcohol and weight reduction, needed to maximize and maintain the effects of treatment, and to monitor the PSA.

If these details of administration of testosterone undecanoate are carefully observed, the majority of andropausal men will be relieved of their symptoms and be maintained in good health for many years on two, three or four of the 40-mg capsules daily. Depending on whether the intention is relief of andropausal symptoms, or long-term prevention of disease, periodic withdrawal of the medication may be tried to see if symptoms recur. This may vary according to the lifestyle and circumstances mentioned above, with withdrawal symptoms usually appearing within a month, and disappearing a few weeks after restarting treatment.

Safety The safety of testosterone undecanoate has been shown both by the initial studies which reported very few side-effects other than in a few patients where it caused mild gastric irritation, and with the castor-oil-based Testocaps®, diarrhea, and by long-term research by Professor Louis Gooren[41]. In the latter 10-year safety study of 33 of 35 men originally included in the study, no alteration in the biochemical parameters of liver function could be detected. Upon annual measurements (7–9 h after ingestion of testosterone undecanoate), serum levels of testosterone ranged between 5.4 ± 1.9 and 6.5 ± 1.9 nmol/l (normal range 8–24) and of 5α-dihydrotestosterone between 3.2 ± 1.8 and 3.5 ± 1.7 nmol/l (normal range 0.8–2.5). These levels remained constant during the study period, indicating that there is no increased hepatic enzymatic breakdown of the androgen over time.

Eight men were older than 50 years at the start of the study. Over the 10-year period in two of them a mild reduction in urine flow was measured, whereas in the other six this could not be demonstrated. Digital examination of the prostate did not reveal signs of prostate tumors. The author concluded that testosterone undecanoate appears to be a safe oral androgen, and a yearly checkup of the patient on therapy with this androgen seems adequate.

Further evidence of safety in relation to the prostate was shown by Pechersky and colleagues[13], who measured testosterone and gondatropin levels, together with prostate volume, prostate-specific antigen (PSA) and lower-urinary tract symptom (International Prostate Symptoms Score, IPSS) score in 207 men, aged 40–83 years, presenting with clinical features of age-related androgen deficiency, who were treated for 6 months with oral testosterone undecanoate.

These men were divided into two groups, group 1 ($n = 92$, plasma testosterone levels > 13 nmol/l) were treated with 80 mg daily; group 2 ($n = 115$, plasma testosterone levels < 13 nmol/l) were treated with 120 mg daily.

Within 1 month of treatment, the elevated blood LH levels were markedly decreased in all men in group 1, as well as most men in group 2. Group 2 was subdivided into men whose LH levels were suppressed ($n = 95$, group 2a) and those whose LH levels were not suppressed ($n = 20$, group 2b). Men in groups 1 and 2a had marked decreases in prostate volume, PSA and lower urinary tract symptom (IPSS) scores, whereas no significant changes were observed in group 2b. Groups 1 and 2a also had more striking suppression of LH, FSH, DHT and estradiol, whereas group 2b had no significant increases in blood testosterone concentrations.

These findings suggested that exogenous testosterone in middle-aged and older men with some clinical features of age-related androgen deficiency can retard or reverse prostate growth, and confirmed that elevated plasma LH may be a useful index of severity of age-related androgen deficiency.

The safety of testosterone undecanoate in relation to the heart was recently demonstrated by Uyanik and coworkers[42]. In order to assess the effects of testosterone undecanoate (TU; 120 mg/day orally for 2 months) on serum lipid, lipoprotein and apolipoprotein levels in healthy elderly men, a placebo-controlled study was performed in 37 elderly men, aged between 53 and 80 years.

Blood samples taken after an overnight fast showed that in the placebo group, neither hormonal data nor lipid, lipoprotein and apolipoprotein levels showed significant changes. After TU supplementation, serum total cholesterol (TC), low-density lipoprotein cholesterol (LDL), and estradiol (E_2) levels decreased from 198 ± 30.7 mg/dl to 174 ± 41.9 mg/dl ($p < 0.05$), from 111 ± 18.14 mg/dl to 87.9 ± 29.4 mg/dl ($p < 0.01$) and from 86.2 ± 16.9 pmol/l to 70.5 ± 18 pmol/l ($p < 0.01$), respectively. Statistically significant differences were not observed in serum triglyceride (TG), high-density lipoprotein cholesterol (HDL), and apolipoprotein (apo) A-1 and apo B levels after TU treatment.

The mean ratios TC/HDL and LDL/HDL, considered to be coronary risk factors, decreased significantly in the TU group, but not in the placebo group. No obvious side-effect was observed in those who took TU except for gastric irritation in two of 17 elderly men.

The increased serum levels of total testosterone (TT) produced by administration of TU, 120 mg/day orally for 2 months, were taken to suppress levels of TC and LDL and E_2 but not significantly change levels of TC, HDL, apo A-1 and apo B. It was concluded that TU may be an effective drug for protecting against coronary heart disease in healthy elderly men with lowered TT and free testosterone levels.

These studies, when taken together with UKAS data on the use of testosterone undecanoate over a 10-year period in relation to the prostate, cardiovascular system, liver, metabolic and hematological values, and physiological measures, provide considerable reassurance of its safety.

Professor Eberhard Nieschlag, who conducted some of the earliest studies of this preparation in the mid-1970s, has concluded that, in spite of problems with absorption making it less than ideal, 'Along with injectable testosterone esters, oral testosterone undecanoate belongs to the standard repertoire for the treatment of hypogonadism'[15], and it is difficult to disagree with this view.

Testosterone pellet implants

Development

Pellet implants are one of the earliest forms of testosterone treatment, being developed within 2 years of the original synthesis of the hormone. It is remarkable that the same basic method of implantation is in use to this day, particularly for patients with primary hypogonadism who need lifelong treatment. It is a great tribute to the safety and efficacy of the treatment that some of these patients have been receiving supplementation by this route for up to 60 years. Because of the consistency of results over the

4–6-month period that each implant remains effective, without swings in energy, libido or mood, such patients usually choose to stay on this treatment in preference to injectable preparations.

The original preparation was in tablet form, manufactured by mixing testosterone crystals with a cholesterol excipient under high pressure[43,44]. These, although clinically effective, proved difficult to standardize, sterilize and insert, and they often fragmented or became pitted, giving variable absorption. The technique was improved in the 1940s by the introduction of a high-temperature molding of pure molten testosterone into narrow cylinders containing 100 or 200 mg of the steroid[45]. These were easier to insert through a trochar, caused less fibrotic reaction, and, as was clearly shown by weighing pellets extruded at different time intervals, gave smoothly declining absorption curves over a period of more than 6 months.

Testosterone pellet implantation became the method of choice for the long-term treatment of primary hypogonadism, and clinics were established in most major endocrinology centers having a special interest in these cases[46]. Although mentioned by Werner[17] as one of the treatment options for the 'male climacteric', it was used only sporadically in androgen-deficient older men, mainly in Europe.

Dr Tiberius Reiter in the UK wrote several articles on 'Testosterone implantation: the method of choice for treatment of testosterone deficiency'[47], and described in detail essentially the same methodology as is used today[48,49].

Two important points he emphasized were that the dose required to obtain optimum relief of symptoms was likely to be higher in men over the age of 50 than in younger men with primary hypogonadism seen in their 20s to 40s in the endocrinology clinics; that is, 6–10 of the 200-mg pellets were needed rather than 3–6, and for these bulkier doses the buttock provided a more convenient and less conspicuous implant site. The higher dosage appears to be logical if SHBG has doubled in older men, or if their receptors have been downregulated. This progression is usually seen in men with primary hypogonadism, needing higher doses as they age to remain symptom-free for 6 months. Such men, like other people receiving pellet implants, become very accurate observers of their clinical state in relation to their free testosterone levels.

That these higher doses are safe over long periods is shown by Dr Reiter's carefully observed clinical studies over 15 years, and by the UKAS over a similar period (see Appendix 3).

Pharmacokinetics of testosterone implants

For over 60 years the practical clinical requirements for testosterone implantation have been well known, and the fact that around 90% of the dose given was absorbed within 6 months had been determined by weighing

pellets extruded at various time intervals, but it is only recently that this
wealth of experience has been confirmed by detailed pharmacokinetic studies.

Handelsman and his colleagues[50] showed that both total and free testosterone levels rose to a peak within a month, and declined steadily, reaching
baseline levels at 4 months with either 3×200 mg or 6×100 mg, and
around 6 months with 6×200 mg, which is the minimum dose usually
required by the older andropausal male (Figure 6).

The rise in both total and free testosterone was shown to be rapid,
occurring within the first 2 weeks, once the implant area had become vascu-
larized (Figure 7). This coincides with most patients' experience of the
onset of effect of an implant.

The same group also showed that the suppression of gonadotropin levels
continued for the duration of the implants, and was virtually complete on

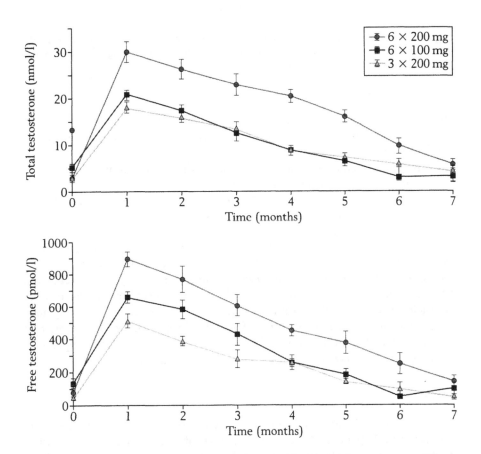

Figure 6 Total and free testosterone levels in 43 hypogonadal men on one of three
different regimes, with data given as mean and standard error of mean. Reproduced
with permission from reference 51

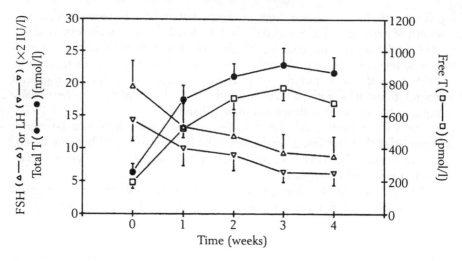

Figure 7 Total and free testosterone, and gonadotropin levels, in 15 hypogonadal men, measured for a month after the implantation of 6 × 100 mg of testosterone. Reproduced with permission from reference 52

the higher-dose implants (Figure 8), where both LH and FSH were generally below the lower limits of their normal range at the end of the 6-month implant period.

This suppression of gonadotropins, with corresponding temporary switching-off of endogenous testosterone production, accounts for the marked shrinkage of the testes noticed by many of the older men put on this form of treatment. Spermatogenesis is also suppressed to the point of azoospermia with higher doses of testosterone pellet implantation[53], as with high-dosage testosterone enanthate injections used for contraceptive purposes in the WHO trial[54]. Some patients with still-fertile partners regard this effect of the implant as a 'fringe benefit', especially when reassured that the reductions in testicular size and reduced sperm counts are restored to their previous levels within 3–6 months after stopping the implants, when their gonadotropins return[53]. They should be warned, however, that this method of contraception takes 1 or 2 months after the implant to become effective, nor is its time of wearing off predictable.

Clinical application

The practical details of performing testosterone pellet implant are described in Appendix 1C. Essentially, 6–10 of the small 200-mg cylinders of fused crystals of testosterone are implanted into the buttock under a local anesthetic with a trochar. The entire procedure takes 15–20 min, depending on the amount of preparation already done for the operator. The symptomatic improvements are usually experienced by the patient within 10–14 days, and the number of pellets adjusted at subsequent visits to a level where the patient is just becoming aware that the implant is wearing off a couple of weeks before the 6-monthly reimplantation visit.

Most patients appreciate the convenience of the implantation technique, and some prefer it to oral treatment because of the consistency and potency of the treatment, and problems with remembering to take twice daily medication. Consequently, continuation rates are high; in one series of 973 consecutive implantations studied prospectively in 221 men over 13 years, the rate was 93% overall, rising successively from 88% after the first implantation to 91% after the second, 95% after the third to the ninth and 99% after the tenth and subsequent procedures[55].

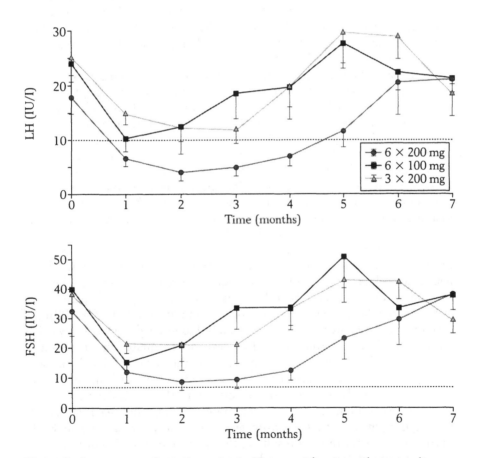

Figure 8 Suppression of gonadotropins in 22 men with primary hypogonadism on one of three different regimes, with data given as mean and standard error of mean. Reproduced with permission from reference 51

The same study listed an incidence of 11% of one or more adverse events following the procedure, which is about twice that experienced in over 1200 consecutive implants carried out in the UKAS.

Transdermal treatments

Development

Attempts at transdermal administration of testosterone began in the 1940s with the work of Dr Jayle, a French physician, who in 1942 prepared a cream containing testosterone which claimed some clinical success[56]. From the outset, this cream raised the problem faced by subsequent cream and gel preparations, that of transfer to female partners. Although this was infrequent, and usually only followed injudicious application to the lower abdomen by the patient immediately prior to intercourse, it was reported as occasionally being a cause of hirsutism of the face and thighs in the wives of men using medroxyprogesterone acetate and large amounts of testosterone cream, in research on male contraception[57].

This was followed, also in France, by a cream containing DHT, called Andractim®. However, although this was absorbed more rapidly, the somewhat impractical advice of showering a minimum of 10 min after application, prior to intercourse, was still recommended to prevent transfer. Another disadvantage was that it raised blood levels only of DHT, which, although theoretically a more potent androgen, in practice has a more limited range of clinical actions than testosterone, and cannot be aromatized to estrogen. It was shown to be less efficient than testosterone in preventing bone loss in androgen-deficient men, and the conclusion was that 'transdermal preparations of testosterone are more advisable than percutaneous DHT' for obtaining normal physiological levels of sex steroids[58].

As with all transdermal treatments, one of the chief limitations is the transport of steroids through the thick stratum corneum barrier. This is less of a problem in relation to estrogen treatment in women, where an amount an order of magnitude lower is sufficient to give adequate levels in the picomolar region. Here, one patch impregnated with 50–100 μg of estradiol is sufficient to maintain adequate blood levels for 3–4 days. The daily dose of testosterone needed to provide adequate supplementation with around 5 mg absorbed, however, is of the order of 10–25 mg as a patch, even with their special delivery systems, or 50–100 mg in a cream or gel. Interestingly, this corresponds closely to the 50–100 mg given daily as testosterone undecanoate (2–4 of the 40-mg capsules, each containing the equivalent of 25 mg testosterone). This low uptake through the dermis and the gut mucosa results in the wastage of 50–95% of the manufactured dose of testosterone, which makes it correspondingly expensive via either route, especially if an expensive delivery system is needed for each daily dose.

Testosterone creams have been produced for many years by compounding pharmacies throughout the world, but have never been extensively researched or taken up. This has partly been because of a low level of clinical interest, and corresponding investment by the major pharmaceutical companies, but also because of poor quality control by the small-scale producers. However, this seems set to change with a range of creams being produced by an Australian company, Lawley Pharmaceuticals in Perth. They have recently produced a range of creams including Andromen® Forte and Andromen® for men, containing 50 and 20 mg/g testosterone, respectively, and Andro-Feme® for women, containing 10 mg/g. This latter preparation has already undergone a clinical trial in the treatment of desire disorders, and proved to be well absorbed and tolerated, and highly effective in improving well-being, mood and sexual function in premenopausal women[59].

Clinical studies are being undertaken in several countries to explore the use of these testosterone creams via the scrotal and labial/vaginal routes (the female equivalent of the scrotum). These have already been shown by the extensive research[60] undertaken on scrotal patches (see below) to enhance uptake through the thinner stratum corneum and better blood supply of the skin in these areas, and to reduce the dosage and hence the cost of these forms of treatment. If these studies fulfill their early promise, the implications in terms of making low-cost androgen therapy available in an economical, physiological, safe and easy-to-administer form are extensive.

Scrotal patches (Testoderm®)

Attempts to improve absorption by using a patch applied to the thinner scrotal skin were encouraging, but never became more than an experimental method. A scrotal patch called Testoderm® was developed by Alza Research in the USA, and tested in Germany by Dals-Piatsch and colleagues[61] and in America[62]. The former group showed that over nearly 24 h, serum testosterone levels in normal men were moderately increased, with concentration curves almost parallel to basal levels. Seven hypogonadal patients also responded to this 'transdermal testosterone system (TTS)', and serum testosterone levels were in the normal range during a 12-week treatment period. There were no side-effects, and a low incidence of skin reactions.

Subsequent research[60] confirmed the safety and clinical efficacy of this preparation for periods of up to 8 years, and that there was much greater absorption of the testosterone through the scrotal skin than elsewhere in the body. Compared with other areas, scrotal skin has a thin stratum corneum and a rich superficial vascular supply. As shown in 12 healthy men, these features resulted in a 40 times greater absorption from this site than from chest skin, although this gradient was halved by the addition of permeation enhancers (Figure 9). Similar absorption of corticosteroids through the sponge-like scrotal skin had been reported by Feldmann and Maibach in 1967[63]. This absorption of

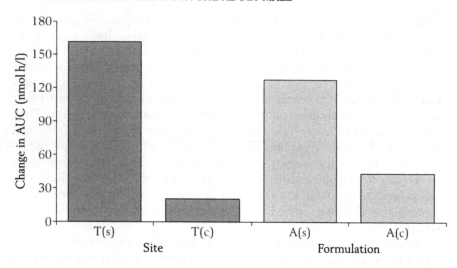

Figure 9   Skin site and formulation affect testosterone concentrations. Baseline-corrected mean area-under-the-curve (AUC) figures: T(s), Testoderm® applied to scrotal skin; T(c), Testoderm applied to chest; A(s), formulation A, containing skin permeation-enhancer, applied to scrotal skin; A(c), formulation A applied to chest. Reproduced with permission from reference 60

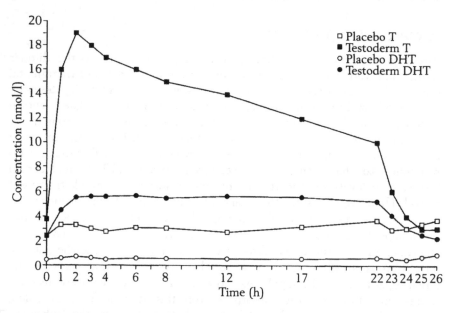

Figure 10   Effects of a Testoderm® scrotal patch, applied at time zero and removed at 22h, on total testosterone (T) and dihydrotestosterone (DHT), compared with placebo. Reproduced with permission from reference 64

over 50% of the applied dose of testosterone would appear to offer great scope for economy for all transdermal preparations if applied to scrotal skin.

Furthermore, this method of application appeared to give more rapid absorption, reaching a maximum after 2 h, than testosterone gels or creams, which are normally applied to the trunk or arms. This results in a more physiological pattern of diurnal variation, and potentially less suppression of nocturnal endogenous synthesis of testosterone (Figure 10).

The extensive clinical experience with the scrotal testosterone patch showed both a good safety profile and a wide range of clinical benefits. Compared with testosterone injections, it maintained total testosterone levels in the normal range, unlike the sawtooth effect of testosterone injections and consequent weekly fluctuations in emotional state already described (Figure 3). This was clearly demonstrated in a cross-over design study comparing the total testosterone levels in 11 hypogonadal men given 200 mg testosterone cypionate and the 6-mg Testoderm scrotal patch (Figure 11).

Apart from maintaining testosterone levels within the physiological range, the Testoderm system avoided the increases in estrogen levels seen with injections and implants, as well as the polycythemia which is a common problem when either of these routes is used. However, because of the high level of 5a-reductase in the scrotal skin, there is a 2–3 times increase in blood DHT levels with Testoderm (Figure 10). This did not appear to have any adverse effects, however on the prostate, skin or any other organ in this or other studies[60].

The clinical benefits associated with treatment with Testoderm were wide-ranging. It was shown to maintain bone mineral density in cortical

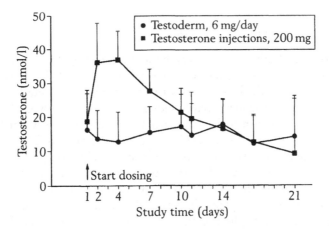

Figure 11 Comparison of total testosterone levels in 11 hypogonadal men treated with Testoderm® scrotal patch or testosterone injections. Reproduced with permission from reference 60

bone and increased it rapidly in vertebral bone. In men with low testosterone levels, an increase in lean body mass and decrease in abdominal fat, together with a slight increase in strength, was seen in the first 6 months of treatment, and did not improve further at a 1-year follow-up.

Skin patches

Another approach to the general safety principle in androgen therapy of mimicking the normal concentration of testosterone and its active metabolites[66] was the development of nonscrotal transdermal patches. These had the advantage that there was no need to shave the scrotal skin, but the disadvantages that they were conspicuous and often caused loss of hair and irritant reactions in the areas of the back, upper arm, abdomen and thigh where they were applied. Although these reactions could be reduced by pretreatment of the application site with corticosteroid cream, the systems never achieved wide acceptance, and have largely been abandoned. They did, however, provide a large amount of data on their clinical effectiveness in a wide range of conditions, as well as on the safety of long-term application[58,65,67]. Despite being provided in 2.5- and 5.0-mg dose systems, to achieve levels in the upper part of the physiological range, two or even three units might need to be applied, and again expense was a limiting factor.

Skin gels (AndroGel®, TestoGel® and Testim®)

These are the latest development in transdermal testosterone treatment, and again have undergone extensive research showing good physiological androgen replacement patterns, excellent safety and a wide range of clinical benefits.

Pharmacokinetics of testosterone gels

Testosterone and other steroids can be applied to the skin in alcoholic gels, which dry rapidly, leaving the hormone to be absorbed slowly through the stratum corneum, which serves as a reservoir. The very detailed studies of Swerdloff and colleagues[65] have shown that this reservoir in the skin releases testosterone into the circulation gradually over several hours. On single-dose application, peak levels are reached after 18–24 h, while with once-daily application steady-state levels are reached only 7–14 days later (Figure 12). Absorption was found to be 23% greater if the gel was applied at four sites rather than one. However, only 9–14% of the 50–100 mg testosterone applied as a daily dose was absorbed. The present formulation of the gel cannot be applied to the genitalia because the alcohol it contains causes pain in the delicate skin of these areas, and the amount absorbed from the scrotum would be excessive if applied in these relatively large amounts.

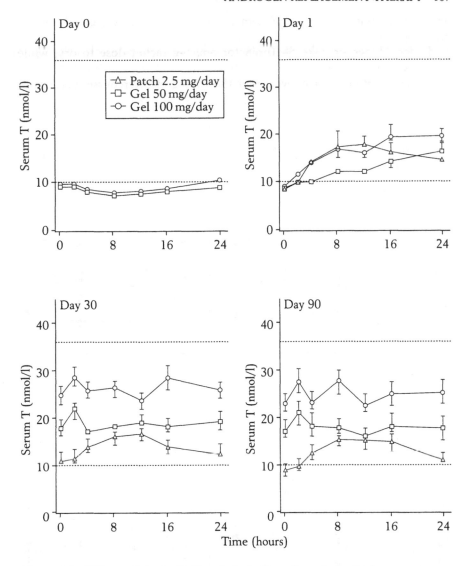

Figure 12 Effects of AndroGel® and AndroDerm® patch on 24-h serum testosterone (T) concentrations (mean ± SE) in 227 hypogonadal men (three groups with about 75 in each). Reproduced with permission from reference 65

Although the gel system of transdermal testosterone treatment is rapidly gaining acceptance in America and Europe, its pharmacokinetics raises certain problems in relation to its long-term use, which have to be weighed up against the benefits. The gel is highly acceptable to patients, as it is convenient and painless and promotes the macho image that it is not really a medication, but a natural supplement to be applied as part of regular morning toilet.

It does, however, take 5–10 min for one 5-g sachet dose to dry, while 10 g takes even longer. Also, it constrains the daily showering, bathing or swimming routine. It may even limit the timing of intercourse, because of

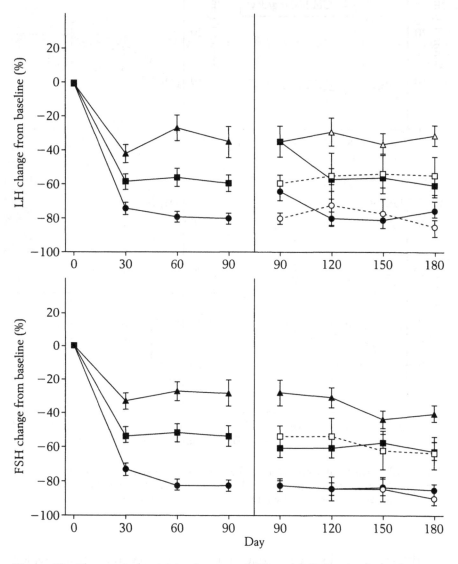

Figure 13   Changes in luteinizing hormone (LH) and follicle-stimulating hormone (FSH) in three groups of 75 men (total 227) given testosterone patch (triangle symbol), testosterone gel 5 g (square symbol) or testosterone gel 10 g (circle symbol). Open symbols represent intermediate doses of the gel. Reproduced with permission from reference 65

the possibilities of transfer to a female partner from the quite large areas of skin to which it needs to be applied, particularly in the higher dosage. Also, the cost of gels, which are often needed in 10-g doses daily, can be more than twice that given by injection, by implantation or orally.

The slow absorption pattern of the gel means that, although physiological levels can be maintained, there is abolition of the normal diurnal variation and hence a truly physiological pattern of androgen metabolism (Figure 12). This is also more likely to suppress the usual gonadotropin surge which occurs during sleep, and result in a greater decrease in endogenous synthesis compared with short-acting preparations such as testosterone undecanoate, those administered via the scrotum or even skin patches (Figure 13).

Similarly, because of the slower absorption of the gel, there are greater rises in estradiol and particularly DHT than with other preparations, including the patch (Figures 14 and 15).

Clinical application

The clinical benefits of testosterone gel determined in a range of recent studies were found to apply as much to the older age group as to the younger men studied, and there were no differences in the hormone levels achieved between the groups. Benefits recorded in further studies by Wang and colleagues[68–70] included improved sexual desire, performance and enjoyment, together with improved erectile function and satisfaction. Psychological improvements included an increase in positive moods, and decrease in

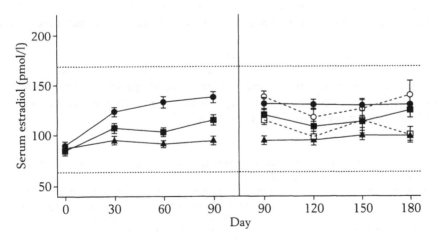

Figure 14 Changes in estradiol in three groups of 75 men (total 227) given testosterone patch (triangle symbol), testosterone gel 5 g (square symbol) or testosterone gel 10 g (circle symbol). Open symbols represent intermediate doses of the gel. Reproduced with permission from reference 65

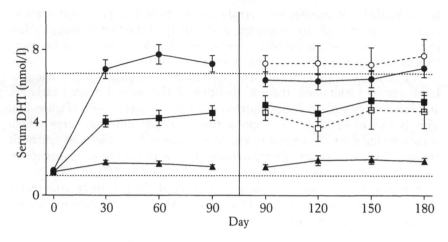

Figure 15 Changes in dihydrotestosterone (DHT) in three groups of 75 men (total 227) given testosterone patch (triangle symbol), testosterone gel 5 g (square symbol) or testosterone gel 10 g (circle symbol). Open symbols represent intermediate doses of the gel. Reproduced with permission from reference 65

negative moods. Muscle strength in leg press exercises, and the arm–chest region, were increased, as was lean body mass. Fat mass and percentage of fat were decreased by the gel, but not by the patch. The increases in lean body mass and decreases in body fat were correlated with changes in average testosterone level obtained after transdermal treatment.

There were the anticipated increases in hematocrit and hemoglobin, but not into the polycythemic range, and no significant changes in the lipid profile. Increases in mean PSA levels were within the normal range, and correlated with serum levels of testosterone, the greatest increases being seen in the 10 g/day testosterone gel group.

Other adverse events were infrequent, and no more common in the group over 60 years of age than in the younger patients below that age (Table 2)[69]. The endocrine patterns, efficacy, and safety were maintained in 163 men given AndroGel® for up to 42 months[70].

Table 2 Treatment-related adverse events in old and young hypogonadal men after AndroGel® treatment for 180 days[69]

Adverse event	Old (≥ 60 years) (n (%))	Young (< 60 years) (n (%))
Skin irritation	2 (6)	9 (8)
Gynecomastia	1 (3)	2 (2)
Prostate disorder	0 (0)	7 (6)
Abnormal laboratory tests	1 (3)	9 (8)

Initial clinical experience with this gel preparation in the London Andropause Clinic has shown a high degree of acceptance and clinical effectiveness.

SUMMARY OF SAFETY DATA FOR ANDROGEN REPLACEMENT THERAPY

A brief résumé of the safety data has been included separately in relation to each testosterone preparation, since their pharmacokinetics and the endocrine patterns they produce are diverse. However, this would seem an appropriate point to provide an overview of the inherent safety of androgen replacement therapy (ART) as seen over the more than 60 years that an increasing range of testosterone preparations have been available.

Prostate safety

This is always mentioned first among the list of possible side-effects of ART. In fact, providing that the precautions of both the ISSAM and Endocrine Society recommendations, of combining a digital rectal examination with PSA measurement before, and 3 months after, starting treatment, are followed and maintained throughout therapy, the risk appears to be minimal. A case could even be made that performing these procedures in a generally high-risk group of men over the age of 50, particularly when combined with transrectal ultrasound and biopsy in cases of concern, is an ideal screening program for the detection of early and eminently treatable prostatic pathology.

In a review article on androgens and the prostate by Frick and associates in 1998, it was concluded that almost all short-term studies of androgen therapy in older men have shown no changes in PSA, prostate size or urine flow rate[71].

Professor Herman Behre in an article on the effects of testosterone on the prostate quoted one cross-sectional, and two longitudinal, studies which showed increases in prostate volume in the first 3 months of treatment from the low norm commonly observed in hypogonadal men, to that seen in untreated healthy men of that age, without any uroflow problems developing. Similarly, these studies showed low PSA values in androgen-deficient men, which rose slightly at the beginning of treatment, but then stabilized at a slightly higher but normal level[72]. This has been the common experience in almost all studies of men with low pretreatment androgen levels, but has been less marked when treatment has been given to men in the low normal or normal range, as in the UKAS (see Appendix 3).

A final authoritative word is given by Professor J. M. Kaufman who, in 2003 in a review of the epidemiological and clinical trial data[73], quoted Eaton and colleagues, who had reviewed the data from eight prospective epidemiological studies and found no large differences in circulating androgens in men who had prostate cancer and men who did not[74]. He also reported that some investigators had found that low levels of serum testosterone predict more aggressive disease, worse prognosis and nonresponsiveness to hormones in patients with metastatic prostate cancer.

In terms of the rarity of androgen therapy unmasking clinically non-apparent tumors, he comments: 'it may be likely that occult foci of well-differentiated prostate adenocarcinoma have limited invasive potential, irrespective of testosterone supplementation'. He adds that the majority of investigators agree that because of the morbidity, prostate biopsies are not justified before ART, provided that the routine screening with DRE and PSA is performed.

Albeit with the usual caveats about the need for long-term placebo-controlled studies, he concludes: 'While a definitive conclusion regarding the long-term safety of androgen supplementation in aging men is not possible, available data support the safety of such treatment in the short term. No evidence of increased risk for clinical prostate cancer or symptomatic BPH has been found in trials lasting up to 3 years.'

Cardiovascular safety

Provided that methyltestosterone is avoided, all the evidence shows that correctly applied androgen therapy is not only safe, but may well be beneficial to the cardiovascular system. Even the very high doses of testosterone enanthate used in the WHO multicenter trial of androgens as a method of male contraception not only caused a marked fall in fibrinogen levels, but also caused no long-term prothrombotic effects[22] or changes in lipid levels[23].

Rises in hemoglobin and hematocrit reported in these and other studies appeared to be related only to high-dosage testosterone treatment with injections of testosterone enanthate or implants, and, as shown in the UKAS, were not a problem with oral or transdermal preparations. Many clinicians regarded the slight increase within the physiological range of these hematological parameters as being beneficial.

Alexandersen and colleagues have outlined some of the range of mechanisms by which testosterone may have an antiatherogenic effect[75]. In a study of men undergoing endocrine therapy for prostate cancer, testosterone suppression was associated with increased aortic stiffness, only partly explained by age and blood pressure. Loss of androgens in men might therefore adversely affect cardiovascular risk[76].

Furthermore, English and coworkers found in an epidemiological study that men with coronary artery disease have significantly lower levels of androgens than do normal controls, challenging the preconception that physiologically high levels of androgens in men account for their increased relative risk of coronary artery disease[77]. They were able to show that low-dose supplemental testosterone treatment with a patch in men with chronic stable angina reduces exercise-induced myocardial ischemia[78], while it has even been proposed that testosterone is 'a natural tonic for the failing heart'[79,80].

Psychosexual safety

Again, the evidence here shows that ART is generally beneficial, with a lessening of irritability, no increase in aggressiveness and a restoration of libido to the normal pre-existing levels for that individual. This is confirmed by the findings of the high-dose male contraception studies[14], which reported results suggesting that sexual awareness and arousability can be increased by supraphysiological levels of testosterone.

However, these changes are not reflected in modifications of overt sexual behavior, which in eugonadal men may be more determined by sexual relationship factors. This contrasts with hypogonadal men, in whom testosterone replacement clearly stimulates sexual behavior. There was no evidence to suggest an alteration in any of the mood states studied, in particular those associated with increased aggression. The authors concluded that supraphysiological levels of testosterone maintained for up to 2 months could promote some aspects of sexual arousability without stimulating sexual activity in eugonadal men within stable heterosexual relationships. Raising testosterone levels did not increase self-reported ratings of aggressive feelings.

SUMMARY

Overall, it appears that ART has a good risk–benefit profile, and is worth a carefully applied and monitored therapeutic trial in men whose symptoms indicate a diagnosis of androgen deficiency.

References

1. Morales A, Lunenfeld B. Investigation, treatment and monitoring of late-onset hypogonadism in males. Official recommendations of ISSAM. International Society for the Study of the Aging Male. *Aging Male* 2002;5:74–86

2. Tremblay RR, Morales AJ. Canadian practice recommendations for screening, monitoring and treating men affected by andropause or partial androgen deficiency. *Aging Male* 1998;1:213–18

3. Morales A, Lunenfeld B. Androgen replacement therapy in aging men with secondary hypogonadism. *Aging Male* 2001;4:151–62

4. Swerdloff RS. Presented at the *First Annual Andropause Consensus 2000 Meeting of the Endocrine Society*, 2000:1–6

5. Cunningham GR, Swerdloff RS. Testosterone replacement strategies: signs, symptoms, potential benefits and potential risks. Presented at the *Second Annual Andropause Consensus Meeting of the Endocrine Society*, 2001

6. Korkia P, Stimson GV. *Anabolic Steroid Use in Great Britain: An Exploratory Investigation.* London: HMSO, 1993

7. Nieschlag E, Wang C, Handelsman DJ, et al. *Guidelines for the Use of Androgens.* Geneva: WHO, 1992

8. Heinemann LAJ, Zimmermann T, Vermeulen A, Thiel C, Hummel W. A new 'Aging Males' Symptoms' (AMS) rating scale. *Aging Male* 1999;2:105–14

9. Curran MJ, Bihrle W III. Dramatic rise in prostate-specific antigen after androgen replacement in a hypogonadal man with occult adenocarcinoma of the prostate. *Urology* 1999;53:423–4

10. Behre HM, von Eckardstein S, Kliesch S, Nieschlag E. Long-term substitution therapy of hypogonadal men with transscrotal testosterone over 7–10 years. *Clin Endocrinol (Oxf)* 1999;50:629–35

11. Behre HM, Bohmeyer J, Nieschlag E. Prostate volume in testosterone-treated and untreated hypogonadal men in comparison to age-matched normal controls. *Clin Endocrinol (Oxf)* 1994;40:341–9

12. Morales A. Androgen replacement therapy and prostate safety. *Eur Urol* 2002;41:113–20

13. Pechersky AV, Mazurov VI, Semiglazov VF, et al. Androgen administration in middle-aged and ageing men: effects of oral testosterone undecanoate on dihydrotestosterone, oestradiol and prostate volume. *Int J Androl* 2002;25:119–25

14. Anderson RA, Bancroft J, Wu FC. The effects of exogenous testosterone on sexuality and mood of normal men. *J Clin Endocrinol Metab* 1992;75:1503–7

15. Behre HM, Wang C, Handelsman DJ, Nieschlag E. Pharmacology of testosterone preparations. In Nieschlag E, Behre HM, eds. *Testosterone: Action, Deficiency, Substitution.* Cambridge: Cambridge University Press, 2004:405–44

16. Werner AA. The male climacteric. *J Am Med Assoc* 1939;112:1441–3

17. Werner AA. The male climacteric: report of two hundred and seventy-three cases. *J Am Med Assoc* 1946;132:188–94

18. Heller CG, Myers GB. The male climacteric: its symptomatology, diagnosis and treatment. *J Am Med Assoc* 1944;126:472–7

19. Behre HM, Nieschlag E. Comparative pharmacokinetics of testosterone esters. In Neischlag E, Behre HM, eds. *Testosterone: Action, Deficiency, Substitution.* Heidelberg: Springer, 1998:329–48

20. von Eckardstein S,.Nieschlag E. Treatment of male hypogonadism with testosterone undecanoate injected at extended intervals of 12 weeks: a phase II study. *J Androl* 2002;23:419–25

21. Anderson RA, Wallace EM, Wu FC. Effect of testosterone enanthate on serum lipoproteins in man. *Contraception* 1995;52:115–19

22. Anderson RA, Ludlam CA, Wu FC. Haemostatic effects of supraphysiological levels of testosterone in normal men. *Thromb Haemost* 1995;74:693–7

23. Wu FC, Farley TM, Peregoudov A, Waites GM. Effects of testosterone enanthate in normal men: experience from a multicenter contraceptive efficacy study. World Health Organization Task Force on Methods for the Regulation of Male Fertility. *Fertil Steril* 1996;65:626–36

24. Ruzicka L, Goldburg MW, Rosenburg HR. Herstellung des 17-Methyl-testosterons undanderer Androsten- und Androstanderivative Zusammen. *Z P* 1935

25. Nieschlag E. [Is methyltestosterone no longer used therapeutically?]. *Dtsch Med Wochenschr* 1981;106: 1123-5

26. Vogel W, Klaiber EL, Broverman DM. A comparison of the antidepressant effects of a synthetic androgen (mesterolone) and amitriptyline in depressed men. *J Clin Psychiatry* 1985;46:6-8

27. Aakvaag A, Stromme SB. The effect of mesterolone administration to normal men on the pituitary-testicular function. *Acta Endocrinol (Copenh)* 1974;77: 380-6

28. Wang C, Burger HG, de Kretser DM, et al. Effect of mesterolone on serum FSH, LH and plasma testosterone in normal men. *Andrologia* 1974;6:111-18

29. Luisi M, Franchi F. Double-blind group comparative study of testosterone undecanoate and mesterolone in hypogonadal male patients. *J Endocrinol Invest* 1980;3:305-8

30. Jockenhovel F, Vogel E, Reinhardt W, Reinwein D. Effects of various modes of androgen substitution therapy on erythropoiesis. *Eur J Med Res* 1997;2:293-8

31. Jockenhovel F, Bullmann C, Schubert M, et al. Influence of various modes of androgen substitution on serum lipids and lipoproteins in hypogonadal men. *Metabolism* 1999;48:590-6

32. Nieschlag E, Mauss J, Coert A, Kicovic P. Plasma androgen levels in men after oral administration of testosterone or testosterone undecanoate. *Acta Endocrinol (Copenh)* 1975;79:366-74

33. Coert A, Geelen J, de Visser J, van der Vies J. The pharmacology and metabolism of testosterone undecanoate (TU), a new orally active androgen. *Acta Endocrinol (Copenh)* 1975;79:789-800

34. Shackleford DM, Faassen WA, Houwing N, et al. The contribution of lymphatically transported testosterone undecanoate to the systemic exposure of testosterone after oral administration of two andriol (r) formulations in conscious lymph duct-cannulated dogs. *J Pharmacol Exp Ther* 2003;306:925-33

35. Bagchus WM, Hust R, Maris F, Schnabel PG, Houwing NS. Important effect of food on the bioavailability of oral testosterone undecanoate. *Pharmacotherapy* 2003;23:319-25

36. Elbers JMH, Bagchus WM, Houwing NS. Characteristics of Andriol® Testocaps®, a new oral testosterone undecanoate formulation for the treatment of testosterone deficiency. *Aging Male* 2002;4:210

37. Schurmeyer T, Wickings EJ, Freischem CW, Nieschlag E. Saliva and serum testosterone following oral testosterone undecanoate administration in normal and hypogonadal men. *Acta Endocrinol (Copenh)* 1983;102:456-62

38. Skakkebaek NE, Bancroft J, Davidson DW, Warner P. Androgen replacement with oral testosterone undecanoate in hypogonadal men: a double blind controlled study. *Clin Endocrinol (Oxf)* 1981;14:49-61

39. Davidson DW, O'Carroll R, Bancroft J. Increasing circulating androgens with oral testosterone undecanoate in eugonadal men. *J Steroid Biochem* 1987;26:713-15

40. Conway AJ, Boylan LM, Howe C, Ross G, Handelsman DJ. Randomized clinical trial of testosterone replacement therapy in hypogonadal men. *Int J Androl* 1988: 247-64

41. Gooren LJ. A ten-year safety study of the oral androgen testosterone undecanoate. *J Androl* 1994;15: 212-15

42. Uyanik BS, Ari Z, Gumus B, Yigi-toglu MR, Arslan T. Beneficial effects of testosterone undecanoate on the lipoprotein profiles in healthy elderly men. A placebo controlled study. *Jpn Heart J* 1997;38:73–82

43. Deansley R, Parkes AS. Further experiments on the administration of hormones by the subcutaneous implantation of tablets. *Lancet* 1938;2:606–8

44. Vest SA, Howard JE. Clinical experiments with androgens. IV. A method of implantation of crystalline testosterone. *J Am Med Assoc* 1939;113:1869–72

45. Bishop PMF, Folley SJ. Implantation of testosterone in cast pellets. *Lancet* 1944;1:434

46. Bishop PMF, Folley SJ. Absorption of hormone implants. *Lancet* 1951; 2:229–32

47. Reiter T. Testosterone implantation: the method of choice for treatment of testosterone deficiency. *J Am Geriatr Soc* 1965;13:1003–12

48. Reiter T. *Reiter's Treatment of Testosterone Deficiency*. Cambridge: Organon Laboratories Ltd, 1965

49. Handelsman DJ. *Testosterone Implants: A Manual of Scientific and Clinical Information*. Sydney: Organon (Australia) Pty Ltd, 1992

50. Handelsman DJ, Conway AJ, Boylan LM. Pharmacokinetics and pharmacodynamics of testosterone pellets in man. *J Clin Endocrinol Metab* 1990;71:216–22

51. Handelsman DJ. Pharmacology of testosterone pellet implants. In Nieschlag E, Behre HM, eds. *Testosterone: Action, Deficiency, Substitution*. Heidelberg: Springer, 1990:136–54

52. Conway AJ, Boylan LM, Howe C, Ross G, Handelsman DJ. Randomized clinical trial of testosterone replacement therapy in hypogonadal men. *Int J Androl* 1988;11:247–64

53. Handelsman DJ, Conway AJ, Boylan LM. Suppression of human spermatogenesis by testosterone implants. *J Clin Endocrinol Metab* 1992;75:1326–32

54. Zhang G-Y, Li G-Z, Wu FW, *et al.* Contraceptive efficacy of testosterone-induced azoospermia in normal men. *Lancet* 1990;336:955–59

55. Handelsman DJ, Mackey M-A, Howe C, Turner L, Conway AJ. An analysis of testosterone implants for androgen replacement therapy. *Clin Endocrinol* 1997;47:311–16

56. Jayle MF. In memoriam. In Mauvais-Jarvis P, Vickers CF, Wepierre J, eds. *Percutaneous Absorption of Steroids*. London: Academic Press, 1980:273–83

57. Delanoe D, Fougeyrollas B, Meyer L, Thonneau P. Androgenisation of female partners of men on medroxy-progesterone acetate/percutaneous testosterone contraception [letter]. *Lancet* 1984;1:276

58. Schaison G, Couzinet B. Percutaneous dihydrotestosterone treatment. In Nieschlag E, Behre HM eds. *Testosterone: Action, Deficiency, Substitution*. Berlin: Springer Verlag, 1998:423–36

59. Goldstat R, Briganti E, Tran J, Wolfe R, Davis SR. Transdermal testosterone therapy improves well-being, mood, and sexual function in premenopausal women. *Menopause* 2003;10:390–8

60. Atkinson LE, Chang Y, Snyder PJ. Long-term experience with testosterone replacement through scrotal skin. In Nieschlag E, Behre HM, eds. *Testosterone: Action, Deficiency, Substitution*. Berlin: Springer Verlag, 1998:365–88

61. Bals-Pratsch M, Knuth UA, Yoon

YD, Nieschlag E. Transdermal testosterone substitution therapy for male hypogonadism. *Lancet* 1986;2:943–6

62. Ahmed SR, Boucher AE, Manni A, Santen RJ, Bartholomew M, Demers LM. Transdermal testosterone therapy in the treatment of male hypogonadism. *J Clin Endocrinol Metab* 1988;66:546–51

63. Feldmann RJ, Maibach HI. Regional variation in percutaneous penetration of 14C cortisol in man. *J Invest Dermatol* 1967;48:181–3

64. Snyder PJ, Peachey H, Berlin JA, et al. Effects of testosterone replacement in hypogonadal men. *J Clin Endocrinol Metab* 2000;85:2670–7

65. Swerdloff RS, Wang C, Cunningham G, et al. Long-term pharmacokinetics of transdermal testosterone gel in hypogonadal men. *J Clin Endocrinol Metab* 2000;85:4500–10

66. Gruenewald DA, Matsumoto AM. Testosterone supplementation therapy for older men: potential benefits and risks. *J Am Geriatr Soc* 2003;51:101–15

67. Arver S, Dobs AS, Meikle AW, et al. Long-term efficacy and safety of a permeation-enhanced testosterone transdermal system in hypogonadal men. *Clin Endocrinol (Oxf)* 1997;47:727–37

68. Wang C, Berman N, Longstreth JA, et al. Pharmacokinetics of transdermal testosterone gel in hypogonadal men: application of gel at one site versus four sites: a General Clinical Research Center Study. *J Clin Endocrinol Metab* 2000;85:964–9

69. Wang C, Swerdloff RS, Iranmanesh A, et al. Transdermal testosterone gel improves sexual function, mood, muscle strength, and body composition parameters in hypogonadal men. Testosterone Gel Study Group. *J Clin Endocrinol Metab* 2000;85:2839–53

70. Wang C, Cunningham G, Dobs A, et al. Long-term testosterone gel (AndroGel) treatment maintains beneficial effects on sexual function and mood, lean and fat mass, and bone mineral density in hypogonadal men. *J Clin Endocrinol Metab* 2004;89:2085–98

71. Frick J, Jungwirth A, Rovan E. Androgens and the prostate. In Nieschlag E, Behre HM, eds. *Testosterone: Action, Deficiency, Substitution*. Heidelberg: Springer, 1998:259–91

72. Behre HM. Testosterone effects on the prostate. *Aging Male* 2000;3:5

73. Kaufman JM. The effect of androgen supplementation on the prostate. *Aging Male* 2003;6:166–74

74. Eaton NE, Reeves GK, Appleby PN, Key TJ. Endogenous sex hormones and prostate cancer: a quantitative review of prospective studies. *Br J Cancer* 1999;80:930–4

75. Alexandersen P, Haarbo J, Byrjalsen I, Lawaetz H, Christiansen C. Natural androgens inhibit male atherosclerosis: a study in castrated, cholesterol-fed rabbits. *Circ Res* 1999;84:813–19

76. Dockery F, Bulpitt CJ, Agarwal S, Rajkumar C. Testosterone suppression in men with prostate cancer is associated with increased arterial stiffness. *Aging Male* 2002;5:216–22

77. English KM, Mandour O, Steeds RP, Diver MJ, Jones TH, Channer KS. Men with coronary artery disease have lower levels of androgens than men with normal coronary angiograms [see Comments]. *Eur Heart J* 2000;21:890–4

78. English KM, Steeds RP, Jones TH, Diver MJ, Channer KS. Low-dose

transdermal testosterone therapy improves angina threshold in men with chronic stable angina: a randomized, double-blind, placebo-controlled study. *Circulation* 2000; 102:1906–11

79. Webb CM, McNeill JG, Hayward CS, de Zeigler D, Collins P. Effects of testosterone on coronary vasomotor regulation in men with coronary heart disease. *Circulation* 1999;100:1690–6

80. Pugh PJ, English KM, Jones TH, Channer KS. Testosterone: a natural tonic for the failing heart. Q *J Med* 2000;93:689–94.

6 Sex steroids and the brain

INTRODUCTION

At no time in life is the brain a rigid, hard-wired structure like a printed circuit, with a fixed number of components repeatedly performing in the same way. It is a continually evolving 'organism', more like a forest of trees, each being shaped by the nourishment of a wide variety of biochemical nutrients, by sex steroids borne in the blood supply, and in some cases locally produced hormones, neurosteroids, fruits of their activity. The 'winds' of thought, training, reflex responses and other neuronal activity play through their branches and develop and strengthen some areas, while causing others to wither and atrophy.

The influence of sex steroids on the brain is often difficult to interpret, both because of uncertainty over which cross the blood–brain barrier and which are produced locally in different parts of the brain, and because of the interactions and conversions between them and other endocrine variables modifying behavior.

SEX STEROIDS AND STEROID RECEPTORS IN THE BRAIN

Exogenous steroids

Transport of steroids into various tissues in the body is dependent on their binding to transport proteins, their rate of dissociation from these proteins, their membrane permeability and their capillary transit time through an organ[1] (Figure 1). Steroids dissociate slowly from their specific binding proteins, and as transit time through the brain is rapid, being less than a second, apart from free testosterone, only the albumin-bound fraction might theoretically make a significant additional contribution to exogenous brain levels.

In practice, however, the concentrations of sex steroids in the cerebrospinal fluid are mainly limited to their free levels in the plasma, as only this fraction can rapidly and easily cross the blood–brain barrier. Of the

Capillary exchange

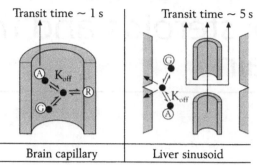

Figure 1 The 'free intermediate' model for the transport of protein-bound substances into tissues depends on transit time, net rate of dissociation (K_{off}) from plasma protein (albumin, A, or globulin, G) and rate of diffusion through membrane. Reproduced with permission from reference 1

total plasma testosterone, 54% is albumin-bound and 44% is bound to sex hormone-binding globulin (SHBG), and this leaves only 2% free to enter the brain. Similar considerations apply to estrogens. Depending partly on whether the blood–brain barrier is intact, and whether the cerebrospinal fluid (CSF) is normal, usually defined as having a total protein level of less than 450 mg/l, the CSF concentrations of testosterone and estradiol are only 10–25% above the plasma unbound concentrations[2]. This is assumed to be due to their fractional release from the weakly bound albumin portion.

These facts are crucial when considering the prevention and treatment of cerebral disorders such as dementia with sex steroids, and whether drugs such as danazol, which greatly raise free hormone levels, should be used as supplementary treatments[3].

This also suggests that, paradoxically, it may be more effective to raise estrogen levels in the brain by giving postmenopausal women testosterone rather than estrogen. For example, increasing plasma testosterone from 1000 pmol/l to 2000 pmol/l, both within the physiological range for women, and easily achieved with a variety of low-dosage testosterone treatments such as 50–100-mg pellet implants 6-monthly, would raise the level of testosterone in the CSF from 14 to 28 pmol/l, assuming an SHBG level of 50 nmol/l (Figure 2). By contrast, using a highly estrogenic form of hormone replacement therapy (HRT), to raise a woman's estrogen level from 100 to 500 pmol/l, would double the SHBG to 100 nmol/l and only raise the CSF estrogen from about 1.5 to 4 pmol/l.

Such increases in SHBG with the more estrogenic HRT preparations may also partly explain the phenomenon of tachyphylaxis, where, especially with estradiol pellet implants, severe menopausal symptoms may recur even at very high estrogen levels. Furthermore, as discussed later in this

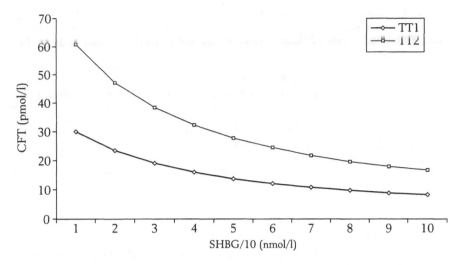

Figure 2 Effect on plasma calculated free testosterone (CFT) of raising a woman's total testosterone from 1 nmol/l (TT1) to 2 nmol/l (TT2) at various levels of sex hormone-binding globulin (SHBG)

chapter, it can suggest reasons for the inability of some equine estrogen preparations to prevent Alzheimer's disease.

Also, such SHBG increases suggest that clinical and research studies which attempt to link steroid levels with symptoms such as libido, behavior patterns such as aggression and cognitive function should therefore focus on the free hormone fractions rather than their total or so-called bioavailable levels.

These SHBG increases may explain why symptoms of androgen deficiency such as memory loss, depression and irritability have been found to be more highly correlated with free than with total testosterone. Also, behavioral patterns such as dominance have generally been more associated with the free testosterone levels represented by salivary testosterone estimations, than with total testosterone[4].

Hormonal effects on the brain can be broadly categorized into 'organizational' and 'activational'. The organizational effects are those produced during neuronal differentiation, growth and development. The activational are reversible effects produced by hormones to modify pre-established patterns of brain function.

In the nervous system, neurons and astrocytes, however, contain the enzyme aromatase, which can convert circulating testosterone to estrogen, and an estrogen precursor, androstenedione, to estrone. Apart from the importance of estrogen in reproductive activity, throughout life estrogenic steroids play a crucial part in the formation, maintenance and remodeling of neuronal circuits in the brain.

Table 1 Relative concentrations of testosterone (T) and estrogen (E$_2$) in men and women at different ages, showing total and free testosterone and estrogen levels, and theoretical levels of 'brain estradiol', assuming 100% conversion from free testosterone in the brain

	Total T (pmol/l)	Free T (pmol/l)	Total E$_2$ (pmol/l)	Free E$_2$ (pmol/l)	Brain E$_2$ (pmol/l)
Young male	20 000	400	100	2	402
Andropausal male	10 000	200	100	2	202
Young female	2000	40	500	10	50
Menopausal female	1000	20	50	1	21

In the male, total and free testosterone levels exceed those of the corresponding estrogen fractions by a factor of 100 or more (Table 1).

These calculations highlight the fact that even in the female, in overall terms, both total and free testosterone levels exceed those of estrogen by a factor of approximately four in the premenopause, and a factor of ten in the untreated postmenopause. However, the more estrogenic HRT preparations cause a greater rise in SHBG, and while the free estrogen levels are maintained, free testosterone falls.

Endogenous steroids: neurosteroids

So-called neurosteroids[5] are synthesized in the central and peripheral nervous system from cholesterol or steroidal precursors imported from peripheral sources. They include compounds such as pregnenolone (PREG) and dehydroepiandrosterone (DHEA). It is thought that these compounds might act as allosteric modulators of neurotransmitter receptors, such as γ-aminobutyric acid A (GABA-A), N-methyl-D-aspartate (NMDA) and sigma receptors[6].

Progesterone (PROG) is also a neurosteroid, and a progesterone receptor (PROG-R) has been identified in peripheral and central glial cells. Progesterone affects the brain directly, and in the hypothalamus it raises the set point for body temperature, which could be of interest in relation to the disturbances of temperature regulation experienced by women, and to a lesser extent men, in the menopause. It affects sexual behaviors and gonadotropin secretion synergistically with other steroids.

The relative production capability of these cells (Figure 3) can be summarized as follows: astrocytes are the major producers of PROG, DHEA and androgens, oligodendrocytes are the predominant source of PREG and neurons are the main source of estrogens[7].

At different places in the brain, neurosteroid concentrations vary according to environmental and behavioral circumstances, such as stress, sex recognition and aggressiveness. A physiological function of neurosteroids in

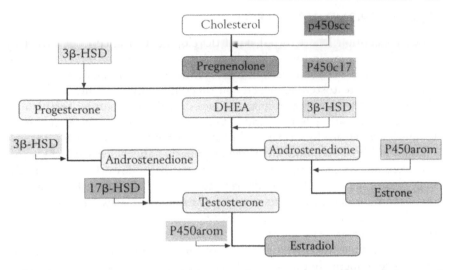

Figure 3 Sex steroid synthesis in the central nervous system. Major products and enzymes involved are shown: astrocyte products; ■ oligodendrocytes; ■ neurons. HSD, hydroxysteroid dehydrogenase; DHEA, dehydroepiandrosterone. Reproduced with permission from reference 7

the central nervous system is strongly suggested by the role of hippocampal PREG with respect to memory, as observed in aging rats.

TESTOSTERONE AND REPRODUCTION

Testosterone affects every aspect of our development, behavior and personality, and to a considerable extent decides our sexual, social and medical history.

Conception itself is largely determined by the father's attractiveness to the female, including his physique, voice, erotic drive, potency and fertility. In the choice of a partner, women are also influenced by male dominance, success and possibly even by the sweet smell of success in the form of pheromones, also derived from testosterone.

Two of the main symptoms of androgen deficiency in the adult male are lack of libido and erectile dysfunction, both often made worse by the other hallmark symptoms of the andropause, depression, irritability and general lack of vitality. These symptoms illustrate the important ways in which testosterone influences our mental well-being and behavior patterns.

Many conditions which damage the testis and affect fertility, from non-descent to mumps, can also affect the production or action of testosterone. There is currently concern about environmental influences on fertility, particularly in relation to xenoestrogens[8] and antiandrogens[9]. We need to consider the evidence in relation to the impact of such 'hormonal havoc' on the psyche, as well as reproductive processes[10].

TESTOSTERONE IN THE FETUS

Once conception has occurred, fetal development is notably governed by the Y chromosome in the male, which dictates testicular development and function. From the sixth week of intrauterine life, the interstitial cells start producing the testosterone, which will shape not only the genitalia, but also the brain and the pattern of behavior laid down[11]. The natural template of the body and brain is female, and it takes testosterone to change it. Levels of this hormone are four times higher at this time than at any other stage of infancy and boyhood, until the surge at puberty. This is perhaps why xeno-estrogens and antiandrogens may have a particularly powerful effect on the male fetus, and cause lifelong damage to form and function. For example, testosterone is necessary to develop the scrotum, and draw the testes down into it. Nondescent can lead to infertility and failure to produce sufficient testosterone to drive the boy through puberty.

At the cellular level, testosterone appears to affect three main areas of brain development. In the cerebral cortex, testosterone causes thickening of the right side, while the left is thicker in the female, as is the corpus callosum. In the hypothalamus, there are gender-specific differences in brain nuclei and the neuronal paths linking them. There are also differences in the hippocampal region, the preoptic septal region and the limbic system, especially the amygdala[12]. Sex is hard-wired into us from this early stage, although our wires may become crossed later on in life.

TESTOSTERONE AND BEHAVIOR

The baby boy is different from the baby girl in much more than anatomy. He is much less sensitive to touch and sound, and less easily comforted by soft words and singing. He is also less interested in communicating, which begins a lifelong pattern of lesser verbal fluency, but is more active and wakeful. These differences are reinforced by parental behavior towards them, with rough-and-tumble and visual stimulation for the boys, and cuddling and soothing talk for the girls.

The male toddler retains his interest in things and spatial coordination skills, while the girl develops her interest in people, relationships and language, and interpersonal skills. By the age of 4 the boys and girls often play apart, and favor different types of activities to suit their skills. At school the boy tends to prefer active pastimes using spatial coordination and physical strength, using up a larger play-space, while the girls, who talk more and fight less, form more social, less competitive groups. Sexual stereotyping occurs early on in life, more or less regardless of attempts at equal treatment and political correctness.

At puberty, under the drive of the sex steroids, the mental as well as the physical differences in the sexes become even more obvious. While testosterone is shaping the male body, causing the voice to break, and embarrassing erections and testosterone volcanoes in the form of acne, this is also a turning point in male psychology.

As well as the surging libido, the influence of testosterone in determining the drive to succeed, whether in physical or intellectual pastimes or both, becomes much more apparent at this time, especially in the 'high-testosterone male'. It is what distinguishes the men from the boys.

THE HIGH-TESTOSTERONE MALE

Testosterone has been called 'the hormone of kings – the king of hormones'[13]. To justify this statement it is necessary to look at both ancient history and recent research.

Dominance amongst men has throughout recorded history been decided by a combination of predominantly testosterone-related physical and mental attributes. The anabolic action of testosterone, particularly combined with the physical activity of sports, hunting or fighting, builds the muscular physique, but in large amounts may limit height by causing early closure of the epiphyses.

Sexual dominance was also highly prized among leaders, and its loss often signaled the end of power for that potentate. Towards the end of his reign, the Bible records how King David lost his sexual vigor, and the young Adonijah then declared his intention to take over his throne. The Graeco-Roman physician Aretaeus, who gave the first detailed description of diabetes, wrote:

For it is the semen, when possessed of vitality, which makes us to be men, hot, well braced in limbs, well voiced, spirited, strong to think and act[14].

Drive, energy and dominant behavior have generally also been shown to be testosterone linked. The earliest observations, ushering in the dawn of endocrinology, according to the American writer Paul de Kruif in his historic book *The Male Hormone* published in 1945, were related to the effects of castration in animals and men[15]. This simple operation would tame the wildest horse and the wildest of men. Boys castrated before puberty would turn into tall, asthenic men, less competitive and aggressive than their intact peers. In the Byzantine Empire, for over 1000 years such eunuchs were highly prized as ideal administrators, posing no threat to those in power or vying for it. Recent research, and clinical evidence from studies of testosterone treatment, have reinforced this view of the primacy arising from testicular drive.

The very informative journal *Hormones and Behavior* recently quoted evidence relating testosterone, endurance and Darwinian fitness to three forms of American side-blotched lizards[16]. Orange-throated males were aggressive and ultradominant and actively defended a very large territory with many females. Blue-throated males defended smaller territories with fewer females. Yellow-throated 'sneaker' males did not defend a territory, but ranged widely, having secretive sex with any unguarded females, and themselves mimicking female behavior if confronted by territory-holding males of the other varieties. Testosterone levels, endurance and range size were all 50% higher in the orange-throated lizards. The downside to this dominance was that their survival from one breeding season to another was much lower, probably because they were involved in more fights. A blind controlled trial of testosterone–silastic implants given to the other two varieties produced a change to the sexual activity, endurance and territorial behavior of the orange-throated form.

Turning to American lounge-suited legal lizards, the Massachusetts Male Aging Study showed that the high testosterone male 'attempts to influence and control other people ... expresses his opinion forcibly and his anger freely, and ... dominates social interactions'[17].

Having high levels of testosterone seems to make these men hard-driving, competitive and sometimes more successful. If educational, financial and social backing is lacking, this can lead to their becoming violent criminals, another proven high-testosterone group[18]. Still, they are more likely to get away with their crimes if defended by characteristically high-testosterone lawyers, trial advocates showing the greatest levels of this hormone.

According to further important work by Dabbs and colleagues, using salivary measurements of free testosterone, this hormonal gradient applies to other occupations, actors, entertainers and even doctors having higher levels than clergymen[4]. It could be argued that, rather like the riches produced by the aggressive, competitive behavior associated with it, high testosterone levels may throw up obstacles to entering the kingdom of heaven. The psychodynamic disturbances arising from unsatisfied libidinous urges, or 'ecclesiogenic syndrome'[19], in young priests are recognized by psychotherapists working with celibate orders as one of the main reasons for giving up their ministry. This becomes less of a problem with age as their hormone levels subside, and perhaps ecumenical politics becomes a channel for sublimation of competitive urges. Also, strict vegetarian diets, as followed by some Hindu and Buddhist sects, have been shown to lower testosterone levels by 14%, which may make testosterone-generated desires less of a block to spiritual progress[20].

The short-term effects of experimental infusions of testosterone in men reinforce these observations. Compared with a control group having infusions of saline, a hormonally treated group showed less deterioration in repetitive mental performance tasks, especially in those with less endogenous testosterone[21].

Similar benefits have been reported by hypogonadal men undergoing androgen treatment for the andropause, including not only restoration of libido and potency, but also relief of depression and irritability, which are part of the pattern of symptoms which characterizes this condition.

Improvements are also reported in a range of activities from crossword puzzles to golf.

These considerations led to the idea that each man may have his own 'reference range' for several endocrine variables including testosterone. As well as postural, diurnal and possibly seasonal[22] variations, clinical experience suggests that genetic[23] and behavioral patterns can play a major role in deciding at what level an individual feels he is functioning best in terms of general and sexual drive, energy, enthusiasm and physical activity. Certainly, 10 years' clinical experience with a range of captains of industry, tycoons, politicians and men who are sometimes called 'movers and shakers' shows that they need higher doses of testosterone to restore their competitive edge than the less ambitious.

TESTOSTERONE AND STRESS

There is a wealth of evidence from both primate and human research that a male's testosterone level changes when his status changes, rising when he achieves or defends a dominant position, and falling when he is dominated. Mazur and Lamb reported three experiments confirming this in men[24].

In the first experiment, subjects played in doubles tennis matches in which winners received $100 apiece. Most winners of the matches who had decisive victories showed subsequent rises in testosterone, relative to the losers of these matches; however, the winners of one very close match, in which there was no clear-cut triumph, did not show testosterone rises.

In the second experiment, subjects won $100 prizes, or not, depending on the random draw of a lottery. Winners in this situation, where their fortune came without any effort of their own, did not show subsequent testosterone rises, compared with the losers.

The third experiment used the natural setting of a medical school graduation. Rises in testosterone were observed among new recipients of the M.D. degree 1 and 2 days after the ceremony. In these experiments, changes in testosterone showed some relationship to subjects' moods. These results suggest that when a man achieves a rise in status through his own efforts and has an elation of mood over the achievement, he is likely to have a rise in testosterone.

However, even fans supporting winning teams of basketball or football players can have a rise in testosterone, while supporters of losing teams showed a fall[25].

Successful love matches can also cause rises in testosterone in both players[26]. Salivary testosterone concentrations were measured in male and female members of four heterosexual couples on a total of 11 evenings before and after sexual intercourse, and 11 evenings on which there was no intercourse. Testosterone increased during the evening when there was intercourse and decreased when there was none. The pattern was the same for males and females. Early evening measurements did not differ on the two kinds of days, suggesting that sexual activity affects testosterone more than initial testosterone affects sexual activity.

Both excessive and unpleasant physical and mental stress can activate the hypothalamic–pituitary–adrenal axis and reduce either the amount or the activity of androgens. A review by Christiansen in 1998[12] of the effects of various types of stress included a variety of mental and physical stressors. Extreme endurance training in military cadets, involving psychic stress and deprivation of food and sleep, resulted in a marked drop in testosterone levels, as have intensive on-duty periods in resident physicians.

Less acute psychological stress, such as financial problems, serious quarrels and loss of close friends or relatives, has also been shown to lower androgen levels. Serious physical illnesses ranging from life-threatening trauma and liver disease[27] to leprosy[28] have been related to reduced testosterone levels, although it is always difficult to establish which came first.

STRESS DAMAGE IN THE BRAIN

Professor Bruce McEwen has documented in great detail the many ways in which stress and consequent high levels of corticosteroids and reduction in testosterone can damage the brain, especially the hippocampus, and how sex steroids, particularly estrogens, can protect it[29].

He emphasizes that hormones and neurotransmitters play a vital role in protecting the brain from stress and in helping the nervous system to recover from it. In earlier life, this system can be extremely effective where stress is neither extreme nor excessively long-term. In later life, a number of factors can undermine this antistress system of the brain.

Memories of danger and threat

Memories of situations that are potentially threatening to life or to well-being need to be well remembered. Learning about the nature of danger and threat, and how these situations are best dealt with, is essential for survival in all animals. It is not surprising, therefore, that mechanisms are in place to ensure that traumatic memories are strongly and rapidly learned and assimilated into experience. The amygdala and the hippocampus work together to achieve this.

The amygdala records emotional content[30], i.e. fear, panic and distress, whereas the hippocampus records the contextual memories of when, what, where and how. The contextual memories are necessary for us to learn to avoid, escape or cope with dangers, but the emotional learning is necessary for the event to be well remembered. If beta-blockers are used to hinder formation of the emotional content[31], then the memory is not recalled so effectively.

Epinephrine helps further to develop and strengthen the *emotional* aspects of the memory, while cortisol helps to solidify the fear and link the shock with the circumstances of the trauma. Hence, cortisol governs the *contextual* aspects of the memory. Unlike epinephrine, cortisol, which is raised during prolonged periods of stress, is able to enter the brain, and the hippocampus has a multitude of receptors for cortisol. In these ways, stress hormones and neurotransmitters act on the synapses to mediate the development of adaptive fear memories.

Damaging effects of stress

If stressful experiences are not too intense or too long in duration, a feedback mechanism enables the synapses to return to normal after the event, and the fear learning fulfills a positive function. A feedback loop of hypothalamus, pituitary, adrenals and hippocampus reins in the production of neurotransmitters and the system is restored to a normal state of balance.

However, when the stress levels exceed a threshold level or continue for long periods of time, the system loses its effectiveness and the hormones are not turned off quickly or effectively enough. In animals suffering frequent stress, the feedback loop becomes weakened, but this also seems to happen in some older animals, purely as a result of aging. The effect of this is to expose the brain to frequent and excessive levels of glucocorticoids which can damage the hippocampus. This effect has been termed the *glucocorticoid cascade hypothesis*[32]. In Cushing's syndrome, the high levels of glucocorticoids produced caused hypertension, diabetes, immune system problems, memory problems and shrinkage of the hippocampus.

In these ways, normal levels of stress hormones promote the necessary storage of painful memories, but elevated levels over long periods can impair memory.

Stress and the hippocampus

People suffering stress in earlier life show a reduction in the size of the hippocampus. This is also true of people who have suffered post-traumatic stress disorder (PTSD) and childhood sexual abuse. In 1996, Sheline and colleagues[33] found the same pattern in patients suffering from chronic depression. Many depressed patients have high levels of glucocorticoids. Even when they were not depressed at the time of the study, but had been depressed earlier in life, these changes in the hippocampus were present. The degree of damage is proportional to the duration of the depression.

In PTSD, the traumatic event is heavily engraved in the brain, often obliterating more recent and less significant events. PTSD affects about 15% of those experiencing extreme trauma, and half of this group will develop shrinkage of the hippocampus and possible cognitive impairment in later life.

The cause of this shrinkage produced by cortisol is thought to be due to two processes occurring at the synapses. First, neurogenesis is reduced.

Normally, new nerve cells are being produced in the brain in response to learning. For example, it has been shown that London taxicab drivers who have to pass exams on 'the knowledge', so they can work out the quickest routes from one place to another in the city, show a hippocampus which is larger than average, and this may increase with time spent in the job[29]. During extreme stress, the process of neurogenesis is put on hold to a large degree. Second, synaptic remodeling takes place. The axons and dendrites of the neurons become shorter. This is known as plasticity.

It is believed that these two processes of reduced neurogenesis and plasticity help to protect the hippocampus from permanent damage from severe or prolonged stress, but they also result in memory problems while in operation. These transient and relatively mild memory problems, in response to less severe and reversible stress, may reflect the 'benign memory deficit' complained of by so many older people but whose existence is not always recognized by memory experts and clinicians.

Interestingly, it has also been suggested that while disrupting more mundane memory formation, the remodeling and lowered neurogenesis may actually benefit the formation of adaptive stress memories. With fewer new cells being produced, it is thought that these may be specifically dedicated to the formation of memory of the particular ongoing stress event which has brought about the hippocampal changes[29]. It is also possible that these new cells may survive longer[34]. This could result in a much stronger memory that is also much longer-lasting.

If the danger is real, as when young children have to learn to live among minefields, the memory will need to be strong and long-lasting. When the danger is not real, the effect on quality of life may be devastating.

Recovery from stress

If the level and duration of stress do not exceed what one might term the 'traumatic' thresholds, the hippocampus can make use of the feedback loop to switch off production of catabolic stress hormones, such as cortisol and epinephrine, and gradually return to normal with the help of anabolic hormones such as testosterone and estrogen, which can be of great importance in encouraging neurogenesis and dendritic regrowth. This recovery tends to be reduced in older people by the reduced availability of sex steroids, and should be helped by appropriate hormone replacement.

Benign memory deficit

In young people, stress and distress can affect the hippocampus to cause mild and transient memory disorder that will dissipate and normalize once the stress is past.

In aging people, where factors conspire to hinder or impair recovery, memory difficulties may be more severe and longer-lasting, manifesting as the phenomenon described as 'benign memory deficit'. The existence of this condition has been frequently denied, and is considered by many to be an early manifestation of dementia. If animal studies are shown to be correct, and irreversible stress changes can lead eventually to cell atrophy in the hippocampus, the latter view may unfortunately be true.

However, recognition and treatment of benign memory deficit in its early stages with suitable HRT may mean that in some cases true dementia could be avoided.

TESTOSTERONE AND THE AGING BRAIN

We have already seen the various ways in which testosterone can shape the developing brain, and the question arises how gonadal steroids may affect the aging brain. There is considerable evidence that maintenance of adequate levels of testosterone and estrogens can reduce our mental as well as physical rate of decline, and these endocrine effects are increasingly being counted in the cost–benefit analyses underlying the argument for hormone replacement therapy in both sexes.

MOOD

A decrease in testosterone levels has been associated with depression in aging men, with clinical improvement occurring after replacement therapy, together with enhanced verbal ability and spatial memory function in the large majority of investigations where these have been studied.

For example, Barrett-Connor and coworkers[35] carried out a cross-sectional population-based study examining the association between endogenous sex hormones and depressed mood in community-dwelling older men. Participants included 856 men, aged 50–89 years, who attended a clinic visit between 1984 and 1987. The authors reported that levels of bioavailable testosterone and bioavailable estradiol decreased with age, but total testosterone, DHT and total estradiol did not. Beck Depression Inventory (BDI) scores increased with age. Low bioavailable testosterone levels and high BDI scores were associated with weight loss and lack of physical activity, but not with cigarette smoking or alcohol intake. By linear regression or quartile analysis, the BDI score was significantly and inversely associated with bioavailable testosterone (both $p = 0.007$), independent of age, weight change and physical activity; similar associations were seen for DHT ($p = 0.048$ and $p = 0.09$, respectively). Bioavailable testosterone levels were 17% lower for the 25 men with categorically defined depression than levels observed in all other men ($p = 0.01$). Neither total nor bioavailable estradiol was associated with depressed mood. They suggested a trial of testosterone treatment in depressed men with low bioavailable testosterone.

Such a trial was carried out by Alexander and associates[36]. They studied mood and response to auditory sexual stimuli in 33 hypogonadal men receiving testosterone (T) replacement therapy, ten eugonadal men receiving T in a male contraceptive clinical trial and 19 eugonadal men not administered T. Prior to and after 6 weeks of hormone administration, men completed a mood questionnaire, rated sexual arousal to and sexual enjoyment of auditory sexual stimuli, and performed a dichotic listening task measuring selective attention for sexual stimuli.

Mood questionnaire results suggested that T has positive effects on mood in hypogonadal men when hormone levels are well below the normal male range of values, but does not have any effects on mood when hormone levels are within or above the normal range. However, increased sexual arousal and sexual enjoyment were associated with T administration regardless of gonadal status.

Eugonadal men administered T also increased in the bias to attend to sexual stimuli. In contrast, the comparison group of eugonadal men not administered T showed no mood or sexual behavior changes across the two test sessions. These data were taken to support a positive relationship between T and sexual interest, sexual arousal and sexual enjoyment in men.

Similarly, Wang and colleagues in 2000[37] reported the effects of 180 days of treatment with 1% T gel preparation (50 or 100mg/day, contained in 5 or 10g gel, respectively) compared with those of a permeation-enhanced T patch (5mg/day) on defined efficacy parameters in 227 hypogonadal men. In the T gel groups, the T dose was adjusted up or down to 75mg/day (contained in 7.5g gel) on day 90 if serum T concentrations were below or above the normal male range. No dose adjustment was made with the T patch group. Sexual function and mood changes were monitored by questionnaire, body composition was determined by dual energy X-ray absorptiometry and muscle strength was measured by the one repetitive maximum technique on bench and leg press exercises. Sexual function and mood improved maximally on day 30 of treatment, without differences across groups, and showed no further improvement with continuation of treatment. They concluded that T gel replacement improved sexual function and mood, increased lean mass and muscle strength (principally in the legs), and decreased fat mass in hypogonadal men with less skin irritation and discontinuation compared with the recommended dose of the permeation-enhanced T patch.

Almeida and Barclay in a review of sex hormones and their impact on dementia and depression as reported in the scientific literature between 1990 and 2000[38] concluded that estrogen had a positive effect in preventing, but not treating, Alzheimer's disease (AD), and that preliminary reports on the use of testosterone and DHEA suggest that they may improve depressed mood.

Some of the most conclusive work, however, has been carried out by Seidman and his group at Columbia University in New York, who in 1998[39] reported that testosterone replacement therapy is an effective treatment of some depressive symptoms in hypogonadal men, and may be an effective augmentation treatment for selective serotonin reuptake inhibitor (SSRI)-refractory major depression in such men. They treated five depressed men who had low testosterone levels, and had not responded to an adequate SSRI trial, with 400 mg testosterone replacement biweekly for 8 weeks. Patients were assessed at baseline and biweekly thereafter using the Hamilton Depression Rating Scale (HAM-D) and the Endicott Quality of Life Enjoyment and Satisfaction Scale (Q-LES-Q). In these patients, whose mean age was 40 years and mean testosterone level 277 ng/dl, all had a rapid and dramatic recovery from major depression following testosterone augmentation. The mean 21-item HAM-D decreased from 19.2 to 7.2 by week 2, and to 4.0 by week 8, and the mean Q-LES-Q increased from 45 to 68%. Three of four subjects who underwent discontinuation of testosterone under single-blind placebo treatment began to relapse.

In a key article in 2002[40], the same group reviewed data from studies assessing testosterone secretion in depressed men, the psychiatric effects of testosterone replacement and the efficacy of androgen treatment for depression. They emphasize that dysregulation of the hypothalamic–pituitary–adrenal (HPA) axis in depression is one of the oldest and most consistent findings in biological psychiatry. It is suggested that depression arises in the context of disturbed HPA feedback mechanisms. Such a theory can explain many observations, including the link between depression and adverse life experiences or chronic stress.

Hypothalamic–pituitary–gonadal (HPG) axis dysregulation may be particularly important in depression in middle-aged and elderly men, where testosterone levels are declining. Psychiatric symptoms of testosterone deficiency (e.g. dysphoria, fatigue, irritability and low libido) are also symptoms of depression, and appear to be variably expressed. These authors admit, however, that currently the relationship between the HPG axis and male depressive illness is poorly understood. Similarly, the role of exogenous testosterone in antidepressant treatment is unclear, particularly with regard to age-associated hypogonadism.

However, in uncontrolled studies of treatment of andropausal symptoms with a wide range of testosterone preparations carried out over the past 60 years, an improvement in mood has also been routinely reported.

Certainly in the UK Andropause Study reported in Appendix 3, relief of the symptom of depression, which was present prior to treatment in 62%, was a consistent feature of testosterone therapy, and a high proportion of patients could be weaned off antidepressants within the first 3 months of treatment.

DEMENTIA

Dementia is defined as 'the loss of mental, or cognitive, abilities severe enough to interfere substantially with one's usual daily activities'[41]. With an aging population around the world, it is a dreaded companion for the end of

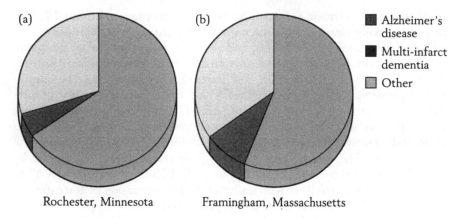

Figure 4 Causes of dementia: incidence rates from Rochester, Minnesota (a) and prevalence rates from Framingham, Massachusetts (b). Reproduced with permission from referernce 41

life in more and more people. Because of its frequency, current lack of effective treatment and ability to create total dependency, it also is an escalating humanitarian and financial threat to civilized societies.

In most studies, Alzheimer's disease (AD) accounts for one-half to two-thirds of cases, and cerebrovascular dementia for less than one-tenth (Figure 4). The incidence of AD increases exponentially with advancing age, doubling every 5 years between ages 65 to 90, rising from 1% to 50% over that time span (Figure 5). Although most studies report up to a three times higher frequency of this form of dementia in women, the picture is obscured by their greater life expectancy than that of men. However, along with other forms of arterial degeneration, men may narrow the gap in terms of cerebrovascular dementia.

Also, studies of AD patients show that women tend to lose their memory and capacity to manipulate objects in space sooner than men. These abilities are controlled by the hippocampus at the base of the brain and the parietal lobes at the back, two areas particularly rich in aromatase enzymes.

Women's life expectancy in many countries rose from 65 in 1950 (1% AD) to 80 years by the millennium (10% AD), and is projected to rise to 90 in another 50 years (50% AD). The likely consequent increase in dementia is not a pleasing prospect, and adds urgency to research into finding causes and effective remedies for what is at present a virtually untreatable condition.

The economic implications of this rise in the incidence of dementia is underlined by a recent report form the London School of Economics for the AD Research Trust in the UK on 'Cognitive impairment in older people: its implications for future demand for services and costs'[42]. The consequences

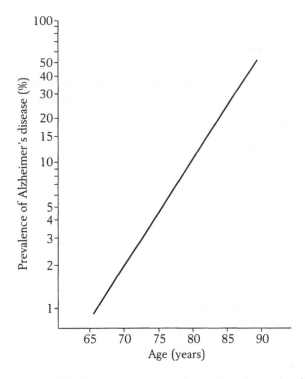

Figure 5 Prevalence of Alzheimer's disease with age (note log scale of prevalence). Reproduced with permission from reference 41

of these projections in financial terms are spelt out in the 'Introduction' to this book.

It has recently been shown that magnetic resonance imaging scans can give volumetric measures of the hippocampus which may be useful in identifying nondemented individuals who satisfy neuropathological criteria for AD, as well as pathological stages of AD that may be present decades before initial clinical expression[43]. If this information is to be other than a delayed death sentence, we urgently need to know whether interventions such as HRT in either men or women can postpone or prevent dementia.

SEX STEROIDS AND ALZHEIMER'S DISEASE: THEORY

AD is characterized histologically by intraneuronal neurofibrillary tangles of hyperphosphorylated tau protein, and deposition of large globular neuritic plaques composed of β-amyloid peptide aggregates between neurons in vulnerable regions of the brain. The tau protein is most clearly seen in the pyramidal neurons in the cerebral cortex, which undergo a progressive loss of dendritic branches at the same time that a neurofibrillary tangle develops within the cell body. Neuritic plaques by contrast show evidence of an inflammatory reaction to the accumulation of β-amyloid, a core of this proteinaceous waste product and reactive microglia being surrounded by a ring of reactive astrocytes.

Given that there is a high concentration of aromatase in many regions of the brain, and that testosterone is the most abundant sex steroid in both men and women after age 50, there are many potentially beneficial actions of estrogens, which may to some extent be extrapolated to testosterone, as listed in Table 2 (partially derived from Henderson's excellent book on *Hormone Therapy and the Brain*[41]).

Some of the equally varied ways in which testosterone could have a beneficial action in AD have been demonstrated in experimental animals. First, Gouras and colleagues showed in neuronal culture that treatment with testosterone increases the secretion of nonamyloidogenic, and decreases amyloidogenic, peptides in rat cerebrocortical neurons[45]. They suggest that: 'These results raise the possibility that testosterone supplementation in elderly men may be protective in the treatment of AD.'

Also in relation to the formation of β-amyloid peptide, it has been shown by Gandy and coworkers that in men being treated for prostate cancer[46] by testosterone suppression, plasma β-amyloid levels doubled, and then stabilized at the higher level for at least 6 months. The conclusions drawn were that: 'These data support the hypothesis that levels of circulating Aβ may be under the control of gonadal hormones and suggest that gonadal hormone replacement therapy might prevent or delay AD in post-andropausal men.'

Other mechanisms have also been shown by which testosterone might be of benefit in AD. Papasozomenos and Shanavas[47] found in rats that testosterone prevents the hyperphosphorylation of tau protein by inhibiting the heat shock-induced overactivation of an enzyme called glycogen synthase kinase-3β. Again it was suggested by these workers that androgens given to aging men, or, in combination with estrogens, to postmenopausal women, could prevent or delay AD.

Table 2 Actions of androgens and estrogens on the brain[7,41]

Improved neuronal growth, regeneration and synaptic plasticity
Modulation of neurotrophin action
Effects on transmitter systems e.g. ACh, Nor-Ep, 5-HT, Dopamine, GABA, NMDA, GLU
Reduced programmed cell death (apoptosis)
Increased Apo-E
Induction of Tau protein
Reduced formation of beta amyloid
Reduced inflammation and astroglial response to injury
Improved cerebral and ? basal ganglia bloodflow
Improved cerebral metabolism
Neuroprotective antioxidant properties

In the human brain a marked decrease in total cell number and vasopressin cell number has been observed in senescence in the suprachiasmatic nucleus, the hypothalamic nucleus regulating circadian rhythms. This degeneration was even more pronounced in AD, and might be related to disturbances in the sleep–wake cycle and endocrine rhythms that occur in this condition.

Goudsmit[48] has shown that vasopressin-producing neurons, the maintenance of which was previously shown to depend on plasma levels of sex steroids, could be restored in a number of brain structures by subcutaneous testosterone administration to senescent male rats for 1 month. He suggested that this reversibility of changes in vasopressin cell innervation in the senescent rat brain through peripheral testosterone supplementation might open new possibilities for the development of therapeutic strategies in age-related disorders of the central nervous system[48].

SEX STEROIDS AND ALZHEIMER'S DISEASE: CLINICAL PRACTICE

In women, there is encouraging evidence that HRT with estrogens may prevent dementia, due to AD[49,50], although other studies have not been able to show benefit[51]. Interestingly, in general the more recent studies appear to show greater protective effects, averaging a 50% reduction in AD, considerably larger than in earlier ones, perhaps due to the trend to more frequent use of estradiol in preference to equine estrogen preparations such as Premarin®[52,53].

A recent review in the *Journal of the American Medical Association* of the benefits and harms of postmenopausal HRT[54] confirmed previous more detailed reports derived from the analysis of randomized control trials and cohort studies[55] that women with menopausal symptoms had improvements in verbal memory, vigilance, reasoning and motor speed with HRT, but no enhancement of other cognitive functions. Generally, no benefits were observed in asymptomatic women. A meta-analysis of observational studies suggested that HRT was associated with a decreased risk of dementia (summary odds ratio 0.66, 95% confidence interval 0.53–0.82)[55]. However, possible biases and lack of control for potential confounding variables limited interpretation of these studies. The studies did not contain enough information to assess adequately the effects of progestin use, various estrogen preparations or doses, or duration of therapy.

Another meta-analysis by Hogervorst and colleagues[52] covering both epidemiological and experimental studies showed greater benefit from HRT in the former, again suggesting that it protects against the development of clinically diagnosed AD. Both healthy and demented women of low education seemed to benefit most from HRT.

Also, it has been shown that estrogens may potentiate the actions of other treatments. For example, drugs that inhibit cholinesterase increase brain levels of acetylcholine, improving the action of cholinergic neurons, although with limited benefit when used alone in patients with AD. However, in a multicenter trial, women with AD using HRT, and later randomized to receive the anticholesterase drug tacrine, performed significantly better in tests of cognitive performance than women on placebo[56].

Furthermore, a group at Oxford University[53] have suggested that the lack of effect of estrogen replacement therapy (ERT) in some studies is due to insufficient conversion of estrone to estradiol because of a lack of folic acid to catalyze this process. They found in women diagnosed with AD and normal controls that a high ratio of estradiol to total estrogens is associated with AD, but, in subjects with a high ratio, the dementia severity was lower in those with high serum folate levels. They conclude that if this association is causal, then supplementation with folic acid might be considered in future studies of ERT in the prevention and treatment of AD.

In this context it should be noted that some ERT preparations, especially the cheapest, and therefore most commonly and longest used, are based on conjugated equine estrogens, containing about 50–65% estrone[57], which may be insufficiently converted to estradiol in folate deficient women, especially on a restricted diet later in life. This could explain much of the evidence of a negative effect on both AD and strokes coming from the Women's Health Initiative (WHI) study[58,59].

As a further example of the complex interactions between different steroid hormones in the treatment of AD, because progesterone can downregulate as well as potentiate the neurotropic effects of estrogen, it has been suggested that the usual combination of the two may reduce their potential beneficial effects[60].

Obviously, not all ERT preparations are the same, especially when combined with various forms of synthetic progestogens, and we should learn from the previous experiences of the different side-effects of various oral contraceptives. In analyzing the protective effects of ERT in different studies, it would seem necessary to go into further detailed examination of types of preparations used and duration of treatment.

The same conditions apply to studies of testosterone replacement, but, largely because of the relatively much fewer men receiving this therapy, studies of the effectiveness of testosterone treatment in preventing or treating AD are small in number. However, the same Oxford group[61] have shown that men with diseases of AD type (DAT) ($n = 39$) had lower levels ($p = 0.005$) of total serum testosterone ($TT = 14 \pm 5$ nmol/l) than controls ($n = 41$, $TT = 18 \pm 6$ nmol/l). Lower TT was more likely in men with DAT, independent of potential confounding factors (odds ratio = 0.78, 95% confidence interval ≥ 0.68–0.91). In women there was no difference in TT levels between cases ($n = 44$) and controls ($n = 62$). They concluded that low TT may be a comorbid feature of DAT in men. However, low TT levels could also exacerbate the disease, so prospective longitudinal studies should investigate whether low TT levels precede or follow the onset of DAT.

However, in a nursing-home-based study of the relationship of sex hormone levels to dependence in activities of daily living in the frail elderly[62], higher testosterone levels were associated with better levels of activity, lower dependency and greater mobility.

More directly, Tan[63] has documented the high frequency of memory loss in andropausal patients, as evidence of the importance of testosterone in maintaining cognitive function, especially in diabetics where androgen deficiency[64], ischemia and hypoglycemic attacks add to the cumulative metabolic brain damage. He has also reviewed a range of early studies which show improvement in cognitive function in dementia treated with testosterone[65,66].

ANDROGENS AND CEREBROVASCULAR DISEASE

Evidence of androgens having a favorable effect on dementia due to cerebrovascular disease is more extensive, and has an equally firm theoretical foundation. Experimentally, testosterone has been found to protect animals against diet-induced atherosclerosis[67]. Androgens in man reduce various coagulation factors in the blood, including fibrinogen[68], and overall have an antithrombotic tendency. They promote hemoglobin synthesis, and nitric oxide synthase (NOS) activity, not just in the penis, but in the cranial vasculature as well, as shown by the facial flushing and occasional headaches experienced when testosterone therapy is combined with sildenafil[3].

It has also been shown that testosterone affects the diameter of male rat cerebral arteries through NOS- and endothelium-dependent mechanisms[69].

Low testosterone levels have been found in men with stroke[70], although, as with the low levels found epidemiologically in association with cardiovascular disease, it is uncertain whether this is cause or effect.

ANDROGENS AND PARKINSON'S DISEASE

There are a number of interesting endocrine correlations between AD and Parkinson's disease (PD). As with AD, epidemiological studies have shown ERT to be associated in women with a reduction in risk of PD[57], and estrogens have been shown to attenuate neuronal death in rodent models of PD. Transdermal estradiol therapy particularly appears to show a slight prodopaminergic, i.e. anti-PD effect, and therefore would appear preferable in this respect. Also, a high incidence of androgen deficiency has been found in male PD patients, and this, like the frequently coexisting depression, responds to testosterone treatment[71]. It has also been reported in epidemiological studies from the Netherlands that a previous history of depression is three times as common in men with PD[72].

A few isolated clinical cases of men responding with dramatic improvement to androgen treatment have been recorded on film: clinical evidence of men with PD showing marked benefit from testosterone was reported by the Polish urologist, Professor Andrez Gomula, at the 4th ISSAM conference in Prague in February 2004[73]. Sixteen men suffering from PD and ADAM (androgen deficiency in the adult male), aged 64–78 years, were studied. The hormonal therapy used was to induce endogenous testosterone synthesis by human chorionic gonadotrophin (hCG). The patients were filmed during follow-up over 1–4 years at different stages of treatment.

The results showed that after treatment, Parkinsonian symptoms greatly improved. Physical symptoms of motor slowness and insufficieny, hand tremor, muscular tremor and rigidity of the legs clearly improved or disappeared, as did standing and walking alone, and ease of movement. Daily activities of living such as eating, dressing, personal hygiene and handwriting were all made easier. Clear improvements in many symptom areas were also documented by the film evidence. Withdrawal of therapy resulted in the return of symptoms at the level prior to the start of treatment. It was concluded that quality of life was hugely better for both the patients and the families when testosterone levels were raised. It is difficult to deny the evidence of one's own eyes of the benefit, which appeared to far exceed any placebo effect, of the therapeutic potential of testosterone treatment in PD. Properly designed therapeutic trials are urgently needed.

What might be the mechanisms by which sex steroids have an influence on the neuropathology of PD? Apart from the androgen and estrogen actions relating to the neuronal degeneration seen in AD listed in Table 2, many of which have also been suggested to be relevant to that seen in PD, there are a number which may be linked indirectly by ceruloplasmin, one of the transport proteins linked to changes in iron and copper metabolism seen in both these conditions.

It was shown as long ago as 1966[74] that oral contraceptives raised copper and ceruloplasmin levels in the blood in proportion to the level of estrogen they contained. Where there is a congenital deficiency of ceruloplasmin (Wilson's disease), excess amounts of free, unbound, copper pass out into many body organs. In the liver this causes a characteristic type of cirrhosis, and in the brain, degeneration of the basal ganglia.

Wilson's disease (WD) patients often present with PD. Furthermore, most patients with PD have reduced ceruloplasmin. WD is an autosomal recessive disease (requires two faulty copies of a gene to produce a homozygote individual) that afflicts one in 1000 people. However, the number of people with one faulty copy (heterozygotes) is much larger, probably about 2% of the population.

It has been suggested[75] that the large number of heterozygotes for WD are at greatly increased risk of idiopathic PD, because these people accumulate free copper in the basal ganglia at a slower rate than homozygotes, which accounts for the fact that PD usually develops after 40 years of age. In addition, the excess copper results in impaired zinc absorption, which would account for the low levels of zinc in the brains of PD patients. Moreover, the high levels of iron found in the substantia nigra of PD patients may perhaps be explained by free copper binding to iron-binding protein-1 (IBP-1), causing it to malfunction and preventing it from detaching itself from the transferrin receptor (TfR) inhibition gene, resulting in expression of TfR even when the cell has plenty of iron.

The gradual accumulation of iron and copper would explain the damage inflicted on the substantia nigra by free radicals catalyzed by these two metals, which is exacerbated by the low levels of CuZnSOD, due to the zinc deficiency mentioned above. It was also proposed that if this hypothesis is correct, then PD could be used to help discover the gene (or genes) responsible for WD and vice versa. Furthermore, idiopathic PD could be prevented by identifying the heterozygote individuals and providing them with zinc supplementation, copper chelation therapy and phlebotomy to eliminate iron.

The higher levels of ceruloplasmin maintained both by estrogens and by testosterone would be likely to reduce the oxidative neuronal damage caused by the accumulation of free radicals, both in heterozygotes for WD, and possibly even in those without this hereditary factor in PD. As confirmed by Cyr and colleagues[76], studies using *in vivo* and *in vitro* models, as well as epidemiological data, suggest that estrogens provide neuroprotection of central nervous system (CNS) cells implicated in the etiology of neurodegenerative disorders such as AD and PD.

Numerous genomic or nongenomic mechanisms of action of estrogens in the brain have been documented that implicate classical nuclear estrogen receptors as well as possible estrogen membrane receptors and the antioxidant activity of steroids, and their effect on fluidity as well as on antiapoptotic proteins and growth factors. Selective estrogen receptor modulators (SERMs) have estrogenic and/or antiestrogenic activity depending on the target tissue. Hence, SERMs have the same beneficial effect as estrogen in the skeleton and cardiovascular system but act as antagonists in the breast and uterus. The finding of beneficial side-effects of SERMs in the CNS might improve their risk–benefit ratio in traditional indications.

Finally, it has been found that a functional polymorphism in the 5' promoter region of heat-shock protein (HSP70–1), which is one of the inhibitory proteins, or 'safety-catch', on the ligand-binding domain of the androgen receptor, may affect susceptibility to PD[77]. This is one more of the many possible ways in which sex steroids, particularly testosterone, may be implicated in the neurodegenerative disorders in both men and women.

CONCLUSION

We have seen some of the many ways in which testosterone creates a hormonal destiny which shapes men's minds as well as their bodies from womb to tomb. To what extent our hormonal individuality is being modified by environmental factors, and can be benefited by HRT with androgens in older men, is an exciting and rapidly expanding field of study.

References

1. Pardridge WM. Transport of protein-bound hormones into tissues *in vivo*. *Endocr Rev* 1981;2:103–23

2. Sodergard R, Backstrom T. Sex-hormone-binding globulin and albumin concentrations in human cerebrospinal fluid. *J Steroid Biochem* 1987;26:557–60

3. Carruthers M. More effective testosterone treatment: combination with sildenafil and danazol. *Aging Male* 2000;3:16

4. Dabbs JM, de La Rue D, Williams PM. Testosterone and occupational choice: actors, ministers, and other men. *J Pers Soc Psychol* 1990;59:1261–5

5. Baulieu EE, Robel P, Schumacher M. Neurosteroids: beginning of the story. *Int Rev Neurobiol* 2001;46:1–32

6. Gago N, Akwa Y, Sananes N, *et al.* Progesterone and the oligoden-droglial lineage: stage-dependent biosynthesis and metabolism. *Glia* 2001;36:295–308

7. Bates KA, Harvey AR, Carruthers M, Martins RN. Androgens, andropause and neurodegeneration. 2004; in press

8. Sharpe RM, Skakkebaek NE. Are oestrogens involved in falling sperm counts and disorders of the male reproductive tract? *Lancet* 1993;341:1392–5

9. Kelce WR, Stone CR, Laws SC, Gray EL, Kemppainen JA, Wilson EM. Persistant DDT metabolite p,p'-DDE is a potent androgen receptor antagonist. *Nature (London)* 1995;375:581–5

10. Colborn T, Dumanoski D, Myers JP. *Our Stolen Future*. London: Abacus, 1997

11. Moir A, Jessel D. *Brain Sex*. London: Michael Joseph, 1989

12. Christiansen K. Behavioural corre-lates of testosterone. In Nieschlag E, Behre HM, eds. *Testosterone: Action, Deficiency, Substitution*. Berlin: Springer-Verlag, 1998:107–42

13. Carruthers M. *Male Menopause: Restoring Vitality and Virility*. London: HarperCollins, 1996

14. Medvei VC. *A History of Endocrinology*. Lancaster, England: MTP Press Ltd, 1982

15. de Kruif P. *The Male Hormone*. New York: Harcourt, Brace and Company, 1945

16. Sinervo B, Miles DB, Frankino WA, Klukowski M, DeNardo DF. Testosterone, endurance, and Dar-winian fitness: natural and sexual selection on the physiological bases of alternative male behaviors in side-blotched lizards. *Horm Behav* 2000;38:222–33

17. Gray A, Jackson DN, McKinlay JB. The relation between dominance, anger, and hormones in normally aging men: results from the Massa-chusetts Male Aging Study. *Psychosom Med* 1991;53:375–85

18. Dabbs JM, Jurkovic GJ, Frady RL. Salivary testosterone and cortisol among late adolescent male offend-ers. *J Abnorm Child Psychol* 1991;19:469–78

19. Luthe W. *Autogenic Therapy: Dynamics of Autogenic Neutraliza-tion*. New York: Grune and Strat-ton, 1970

20. Hamalainen E, Adlercreutz H, Puska P, Pietinen P. Diet and serum hormones in healthy men. *J Steroid Biochem* 1984;20:459–64

21. Klaiber EL, Broverman DM, Gogel W, Abraham GE, Cone FL. Effects of infused testosterone on mental

performances and serum LH. *J Clin Endocrinol Metab* 1971;32:341–9

22. Dabbs JM. Age and seasonal variation in serum testosterone concentration among men. *Chronobiol Int* 1990;7:245–9

23. Meikle AW, Stringham J, Bishop D, West D. Quantitation of genetic and non-genetic factors influencing androgen production and clearance rates in men. *J Clin Endocrinol Metab* 1988;67:104–9

24. Mazur A, Lamb TA. Testosterone, status and mood in human males. *Horm Behav* 1980;14:236–46

25. Bernhardt PC, Dabbs JM, Fielden JA, Lutter CD. Testosterone changes during vicarious experiences of winning and losing among fans at sporting events. *Physiol Behav* 1998;65:59–62

26. Dabbs JM, Mohammed S. Male and female salivary testosterone concentrations before and after sexual activity. *Physiol Behav* 1992;52: 195–7

27. Handelsman DJ. Testicular dysfunction in systemic disease. *Endocrinol Metab Clin North Am* 1994;23:839–56

28. Morley JE, Distiller LA, Sagel J, et al. Hormonal changes associated with testicular atrophy and gynaecomastia in patients with leprosy. *Clin Endocrinol (Oxf)* 1977;6: 299–303

29. McEwen BS. *The End of Stress as We Know It.* Washington, DC: Joseph Henry Press, 2002

30. LeDoux JE. Emotion circuits in the brain. *Annu Rev Neurosci* 2000;23: 155–84

31. Van SA, Everaerd W, Cahill L, McGaugh JL, Gooren LG. Memory for emotional events: differential effects of centrally versus peripherally acting beta-blocking agents. *Psychopharmacology* 1998;138: 305–10

32. Sapolsky RM. Stress, glucocorticoids, and damage to the nervous system: the current state of confusion. *Stress* 1996;1:1–19

33. Sheline YI, Wang PW, Gado MH, Csernansky JG, Vannier MW. Hippocampal atrophy in recurrent major depression. *Proc Natl Acad Sci U S A* 1996;93:3908–13

34. Gould E, McEwen BS. Neuronal birth and death. *Curr Op Neurobiol* 1993;3:676–82

35. Barrett-Connor E, Von Muhlen DG, Kritz-Silverstein D. Bioavailable testosterone and depressed mood in older men: the Rancho Bernardo Study. *J Clin Endocrinol Metab* 1999;84:573–7

36. Alexander GM, Swerdloff RS, Wang C, et al. Androgen–behavior correlations in hypogonadal men and eugonadal men. I. Mood and response to auditory sexual stimuli. *Horm Behav* 1997;31:110–19

37. Wang C, Swedloff RS, Iranmanesh A, et al. Transdermal testosterone gel improves sexual function, mood, muscle strength, and body composition parameters in hypogonadal men. Testosterone Gel Study Group. *J Clin Endocrinol Metab* 2000;85:2839–53

38. Almeida OP, Barclay L. Sex hormones and their impact on dementia and depression: a clinical perspective. *Expert Opin Pharmacother* 2001;2:527–35

39. Seidman SN, Rabkin JG. Testosterone replacement therapy for hypogonadal men with SSRI-refractory depression. *J Affect Disord* 1998;48:157–61

40. Seidman SN. Declining testosterone and depression. *Aging Male* 2002;4:214

41. Henderson VW. *Hormone Therapy and the Brain.* New York: Parthenon Publishing, 2000

42. Comas-Herrera A, Wittenberg R,

Pickard L, Knapp M, and MRC-CFAS. *Cognitive impairment in older people: its implications for future demand for services and costs.* PSSRU 1728. London: Alzheimer's Research Trust, 1–7. 2003

43. Gosche KM, Mortimer JA, Smith CD, Markesbery WR, Snowdon DA. Hippocampal volume as an index of Alzheimer neuropathology: findings from the Nun Study. *Neurology* 2002;58:1476–82

44. Henderson VW. Estrogen, cognition, and a woman's risk of Alzheimer's disease. *Am J Med* 1997;103:11S–8S

45. Gouras GK, Xu H, Gross RS, *et al.* Testosterone reduces neuronal secretion of Alzheimer's β-amyloid peptides. *Proc Natl Acad Sci U S A* 2000;97:1202–5

46. Gandy S, Almeida OP, Fonte J, *et al.* Chemical andropause and amyloid-β peptide. *J Am Med Assoc* 2001;285:2195–6

47. Papasozomenos SC, Shanavas A. Testosterone prevents the heat shock-induced overactivation of glycogen synthase kinase-3 beta but not of cyclin-dependent kinase 5 and c-Jun NH2-terminal kinase and concomitantly abolishes hyperphosphorylation of tau: implications for Alzheimer's disease. *Proc Nat Acad Sci U S A* 2002;99:1140–5

48. Goudsmit E, Filers E, Swaab DF. Changes in vasopressin neurons and fibers in aging and Alzheimer's disease: reversibility in the rat. *Prog Clin Biol Res* 1989;317:1193–1208

49. Tang MX, Jacobs D, Stern Y, *et al.* Effect of oestrogen during menopause on risk and age at onset of Alzheimer's disease. *Lancet* 1996; 348:429–32

50. Kawas C, Resnick S, Morrison A, *et al.* A prospective study of estrogen replacement therapy and the risk of developing Alzheimer's disease: the Baltimore Longitudinal Study of Aging. *Neurology* 1997;48: 1517–21

51. Mulnard RA. Estrogen as a treatment for Alzheimer disease. *J Am Med Assoc* 2000;284:307–8

52. Hogervorst E, Williams J, Budge M, Riedel W, Jolles J. The nature of the effect of female gonadal hormone replacement therapy on cognitive function in postmenopausal women: a meta-analysis. *Neuroscience* 2000;101: 485–512

53. Hogervorst E, Smith D. The interaction of serum folate and estradiol levels in Alzheimer's disease. *Neuroendocrinol Lett* 2002;23:155–60

54. Nelson HD, Humphrey LL, Nygren P, Teutsch SM, Allan JD. Postmenopausal hormone replacement therapy: scientific review. *J Am Med Assoc* 2002;288:872–81

55. LeBlanc ES, Janowsky J, Chan BK, Nelson HD. Hormone replacement therapy and cognition: systematic review and meta-analysis. *J Am Med Assoc* 2001;285:1489–99

56. Schneider LS, Farlow MR, Henderson VW, Pogoda JM. Effects of estrogen replacement therapy on response to tacrine in patients with Alzheimer's disease. *Neurology* 1996;46:1580–4

57. *Management of the Menopause.* BMS Publications Ltd, 2002

58. Rapp SR, Espeland MA, Shumaker SA, *et al.* Effect of estrogen plus progestin on global cognitive function in postmenopausal women: the Women's Health Initiative Memory Study: a randomized controlled trial. *J Am Med Assoc* 2003;289:2663–72

59. Wassertheil-Smoller S, Hendrix SL, Limacher M, *et al.* Effect of estrogen plus progestin on stroke in postmenopausal women: the Women's Health Initiative: a randomized trial. *JAMA* 2003;289:2673–84

60. Henderson VW. Oestrogens and dementia. *Novartis Found Symp* 2000,230.254-05

61. Hogervorst E, Williams J, Budge M, Barnetson L, Combrinck M, Smith AD. Serum total testosterone is lower in men with Alzheimer's disease. *Neuroendocrinol Lett* 2001; 22:163-8

62. Breuer B, Trungold S, Martucci C, et al. Relationships of sex hormone levels to dependence in activities of daily living in the frail elderly. *Maturitas* 2001;39:147-59

63. Tan RS. Memory loss as a reported symptom of andropause. *Arch Androl* 2001;47:185-9

64. Smith KW, Feldman HA, McKinlay JB. Construction and field validation of a self-administered screener for testosterone deficiency (hypogonadism) in ageing men. *Clin Endocrinol (Oxf)* 2000; 53:703-11

65. Tan RS, Pu SJ. The andropause and memory loss: is there a link between androgen decline and dementia in the aging male? *Asian J Androl* 2001;3:169-74

66. Tan RS. Andropause and testosterone supplementation for cognitive loss. *J Androl* 2002;23:45-6

67. Alexandersen P, Haarbo J, Byrjalsen I, Lawaetz H, Christiansen C. Natural androgens inhibit male atherosclerosis: a study in castrated, cholesterol-fed rabbits. *Circ Res* 1999;84:813-19

68. Anderson RA, Ludlam CA, Wu FC. Haemostatic effects of supraphysiological levels of testosterone in normal men. *Thromb Haemost* 1995;74:693-7

69. Geary GG, Krause DN, Duckles SP. Gonadal hormones affect diameter of male rat cerebral arteries through endothelium-dependent mechanisms. *Am J Physiol Heart Circ Physiol* 2000;279:H610-18

70. Fung MM, Barrett-Connor E, Bettencourt RR. Hormone replacement therapy and stroke risk in older women. *J Women's Health* 1999;8:359-64

71. Okun MS, McDonald WM, DeLong MR. Refractory nonmotor symptoms in male patients with Parkinson disease due to testosterone deficiency: a common unrecognized comorbidity. *Arch Neurol* 2002;59:807-11

72. Schuurman AG, van den Akker M, Ensinck KT, et al. Increased risk of Parkinson's disease after depression: a retrospective cohort study. *Neurology* 2002;58:1501-4

73. Gomula A. Successful treatment of Parkinsonism with hCG: preliminary findings. *Aging Male* 2004; 7:31

74. Carruthers ME, Hobbs CB, Warren RL. Raised serum copper and caeruloplasmin levels in subjects taking oral contraceptives. *J Clin Pathol* 1966;19:498-500

75. Johnson S. Is Parkinson's disease the heterozygote form of Wilson's disease: PD = 1/2 WD? *Med Hypotheses* 2001;56:171-3

76. Cyr M, Calon F, Morissette M, Grandbois M, Di Paolo T, Callier S. Drugs with estrogen-like potency and brain activity: potential therapeutic application for the CNS. *Curr Pharm Des* 2000;6: 1287-1312

77. Wu YR, Wang CK, Chen CM, et al. Analysis of heat-shock protein 70 gene polymorphisms and the risk of Parkinson's disease. *Hum Genet* 2004;114:236-41

Appendix 1A. Investigation, treatment and monitoring of late-onset hypogonadism in males: official recommendations of the International Society for the Study of the Aging Male

Reproduced from The Aging Male 2002;5:74–86

Standards, Guidelines and Recommendations
of The International Society for
The Study of the Aging Male (ISSAM)

Investigation, treatment and monitoring of late-onset hypogonadism in males

Official Recommendations of ISSAM

A. Morales and B. Lunenfeld*

*Department of Urology, Queen's University Kingston, Ontario, Canada; *Faculty of Life Sciences Bar-Ilan University, Ramat Gan, Israel*

Key words: AGING, HYPOGONADISM, TESTOSTERONE REPLACEMENT

INTRODUCTION

The field of hormonal alterations in the aging male is attracting increasing interest in the medical community and the public at large. Simultaneously, industry has realized the growing importance and enormous potential of the impact of a rapidly mounting population of males over the age of 50 years. This population will be positioned for special health needs in the first quarter of this century and probably beyond. Among these needs, hormone replacement therapy will find its proper place, as it has for postmenopausal women over the last 25 years.

It is fully recognized that the endocrinological changes associated with male aging are not limited to sex hormones. On the contrary, profound changes occur in other hormones such as growth hormone, dehydroepiandrosterone (DHEA), melatonin and, to a lesser extent, thyroxin. However, androgen decline in the aging male (ADAM), or partial androgen deficiency of the aging male

(PADAM), also widely known as andropause, is a fast-developing field (since there is no consensus on nomenclature, the terms late-onset hypogonadism, PADAM and male climacteric are acceptable and used interchangeably). The understanding of ADAM among large sections of the medical profession dealing with mature men (i.e. primary care, internists, urologists, etc.) has not kept pace with the developments in the field. The International Society for the Study of the Aging Male (ISSAM) believes that it is somewhat premature to provide guidelines for the diagnosis, treatment and monitoring of men diagnosed with or suspected of suffering from ADAM. On the other hand, a great deal of confusion and misunderstanding exists surrounding the same three issues (diagnosis, treatment and monitoring) of the condition. Therefore, ISSAM – in fulfilling its mandate – considers that this is an opportune time to provide factual information on the various

Correspondence: Professor A. Morales, Kingston General Hospital, Kingston, Ontario, Canada, K7L 2V7

STANDARDS, GUIDELINES AND RECOMMENDATIONS

clinical aspects of the andropause in the form of a set of practical recommendations dealing exclusively with ADAM and androgen replacement therapy (ART). It is anticipated that further recommendations and guidelines on other similar areas of competence for ISSAM will be produced in the future.

Opinions on the need for and effects of hormone replacement in aging change frequently and long-held views are now being vigorously challenged. The material in these Recommendations represents recent information on the andropause; however, it may require frequent updates as new and relevant data become available. At the appropriate time, they may also be upgraded to guidelines for the evaluation and treatment of ADAM.

A draft of Society's Recommendations was previously published in this Journal[1] to give the opportunity for discussion at the 2002 biannual meeting of ISSAM. The Recommendations were reviewed by a panel of experts, a number of suggestions were submitted by well-informed physicians as well as representatives of industry and the document was presented and discussed in Berlin during the regular meeting of ISSAM. They were approved in principle. Further opportunity was given to the membership for criticisms. Some were received and incorporated when deemed appropriate by the authors.

DEFINITION

In men, gonadal function is affected in a slow progressive way as part of the normal aging process[2]. This process, leading to hypogonadism is variously known as male climacteric, andropause or, more appropriately, ADAM or PADAM. The terms andropause and male climacteric are biologically wrong and clinically inappropriate, but they adequately convey the concept of emotional and physical changes that, although related to aging in general, are also associated with significant hormonal alterations. The clinical manifestations of male secondary hypogonadism have been well defined over 50 years[3] but ART was not widely accepted, in part due to unrealistic expectations and adverse effects due to improper management

of early androgen preparations. The diagnostic criteria are presently better understood. For instance, recently, a couple of validated questionnaires[4,5] have been proposed for either screening, diagnosing and/or assessing response to therapy[5]. More sophisticated diagnostic and monitoring questionnaires are in development. Although they may prove useful for screening and diagnosis of ADAM, all require further, wider experience, particularly in their transcultural applicability.

RECOMMENDATION 1

Definition: A biochemical syndrome associated with advancing age and characterized by a deficiency in serum androgen levels with or without a decreased genomic sensitivity to androgens. It may result in significant alterations in the quality of life and adversely affect the function of multiple organ systems.

DIAGNOSIS

Clinical

The clinical picture is described in the definition below. It should be remembered that there is significant interindividual variability in the onset, velocity and depth of the androgen decline associated with age, and no factors have emerged that predict the characteristics or effects of the age-related hypogonadism. As a rule of thumb, the mean serum testosterone level decreases after the age of 50 years at a rate of approximately 1% per year. This is by no means a constant phenomenon: biochemical hypogonadism is detected in only about 7% of the age group less than 60 years old but increases to 20% in those over 60 years of age[6]. It may be argued, therefore, that only a minority of individuals develop ADAM. This may not be the case. Associated with advancing age, there is also an increase in the levels of sex hormone binding globulin (SHBG) which translates into a further decrease in bioavailable testosterone (free plus albumin-bound fractions). When the diagnosis is based on the measurement of bioavailable testosterone, up to 70% of men over the age of 60 were found to be hypogonadal[4]. To compound the difficulties in establishing biochemical and clinical correlates, there are three important areas that require further elucidation:

(1) It is not yet known what level of serum testosterone defines deficiency in an older man, although it is generally accepted that 2 standard deviations below normal values for young men is conclusively abnormal (11 nmol/l total testosterone or 0.255 nmol/l free testosterone when using methods described by Vermeulen and colleagues[7]. For bioavailable testosterone the value of 3.8 nmol/l has been recommended. A tool for calculating free and bioavailable testosterone can be found on the ISSAM website at www.issam.ch). Since normal ranges vary significantly from laboratory to laboratory, the results from each patient should be compared with the normal ranges established by each laboratory.

(2) In older men, there may be variable responses by the target organs (brain, bone, prostate, muscle, etc.) to the levels of androgens.

(3) The response by target organs may be influenced by a variety of endocrine disruptors, the nature of which is only beginning to be explored in men.

The combination of these three uncertainties is important: deficiency may become clinically apparent at different points within an individual or a population, depending on the marker used (e.g. androgen levels, bone mineral density).

RECOMMENDATION 2

ADAM or the andropause is a syndrome characterized primarily by:

(1) The easily recognized features of diminished sexual desire and erectile quality, particularly nocturnal erections[8];

(2) Changes in mood with concomitant decreases in intellectual activity, spatial orientation ability, fatigue, depressed mood and irritability[9];

(3) Decrease in lean body mass with associated diminution in muscle volume and strength[10,11];

(4) Decrease in body hair and skin alterations[12];

(5) Decreased bone mineral density resulting in osteopenia and osteoporosis[13];

(6) Increase in visceral fat.

(These manifestations need not all be present to identify the syndrome. In addition, the severity of one or more of them does not necessarily match the severity of the others, nor do we yet understand the uneven appearance of these manifestations. Moreover, the clinical picture may or may not be associated with low testosterone. Therefore, the clinical diagnosis should be supported by biochemical tests confirming the presence of hypogonadism).

Biochemistry

Establishing the presence of slight hypogonadism on a purely clinical basis is, in most cases, difficult and unreliable. Only the more severe cases lead to clinical suspicion. Despite this, there is some controversy as to the need for hormonal evaluation of the aging man. For instance, hormonal evaluation in men with erectile dysfunction has been questioned on the basis that it is not cost-effective[14]. Although this scepticism is not shared by others[15,16], there are several reasons to justify, at least, basic hormonal assessment of men with erectile dysfunction. It is commonly accepted that the combination of low sexual desire and erectile difficulties may be the result of serious hormonal abnormalities. The reality is not as simple or clear-cut as that. Not only may hypogonadal men be capable of adequate sexual erections but hormonal supplementation resulting in normal testosterone values does not always result in restoration of libido and improvement in the quality of erectile function[17].

In men at risk, or suspected of having hypogonadism, the ideal test would be the measurement of free testosterone by the equilibrium dialysis method. This method, however, is difficult to perform, not automated and largely inaccessible to most clinicians. Measurement of 'free testosterone' by radioimmunoassay is widely available but should be discouraged due to its unreliability. Determination of bioavailable testosterone is attainable in some parts of the world but it is expensive and not readily accessible. Measurement of total testosterone is readily available but the results need to be interpreted with caution, particularly in the elderly and the obese in whom elevations of SHBG may result in a factual hypogonadism that is not disclosed by the results of a total testosterone determination.

The calculated free testosterone is an adequate compromise when only determinations of total testosterone and SHBG are available[7]. The formula for calculated free testosterone is available from the Society's web page. Calculated free testosterone is an indirect but reliable method. 'The evaluation of aged men's androgenicity should rely on at least one of these assessments' (bioavailable testosterone or calculated free testosterone)[18].

It should be remembered, however, that the methodology for assessment of SHBG is not standardized and that the results of calculated free testosterone may vary among different areas of the world.

RECOMMENDATION 3
In patients at risk or suspected of hypogonadism the following biochemical investigations should be done:

(1) Serum sample for testosterone determination between 08.00 and 11.00. The most reliable and widely acceptable parameter to establish the presence of hypogonadism is the measurement of bioavailable testosterone or, alternatively a calculated free testosterone.

(2) If testosterone levels are below or at the lower limit of the accepted normal values, it is prudent to confirm the results with a second determination together with assessment of follicle stimulating hormone (FSH), luteinizing hormone (LH) and prolactin.

OTHER ENDOCRINOLOGICAL ALTERATIONS ASSOCIATED WITH ADVANCING AGE

It is important to dispel the concept that endocrinopathies of elderly men are narrowly focused on testosterone. Although hypotestosteronemia is the most widely recognized and investigated hormonal alteration associated with the aging process, the production of several other hormones is also profoundly affected by age. Increasing attention is being paid to these hormones because changes in their levels can be responsible for some of the manifestations previously attributed exclusively to testosterone deficiency.

DHEA and DHEA-S

The decline in both DHEA and its sulfate DHEA-S is a more constant feature of advancing age than hypogonadism. By the fifth decade, the levels of DHEA decrease to less than 30% of those in men under the age of 30 years[19]. There is a widespread belief that declining levels of DHEA run in parallel with a decrease in well-being and that supplemental exogenous DHEA results in an improvement in quality-of-life parameters[20]. More recently, a study in healthy aging men found no beneficial effect of DHEA over placebo[21].

DHEA and DHEA-S are weak androgens secreted primarily by the adrenal glands. Their role in the maintenance of an adequate androgen milieu is not known with certainty but appears to be limited. Limited trials[22] have shown that exogenous DHEA does not have a detrimental effect on prostate-specific antigen (PSA) values; however, only properly controlled long-term studies will provide a clear picture on the effectiveness and safety of adrenal androgens in the treatment of global androgen deficiency states. Behavioral correlates of DHEA and DHEA-S in the male are inconsistent[23] and consensus on their usefulness does not exist[24].

Growth hormone

The production of growth hormone (GH), after puberty, also decreases with age, about 14% per decade[25,26]. Since the production of circulating insulin-like growth factor-I (IGF-I) is controlled by GH levels, both decline together. This reduction is associated with changes in lean muscle mass, bone density, hair distribution and the pattern of obesity also described in hypogonadal states[27,28]. Administration of GH can reverse these alterations[29] and does so more efficiently in eugonadal men than in their hypogonadal counterparts[30]. Whether the possible clinical improvement after GH administration will be outweighed by undesirable side-effects and whether the improvements would be sufficient to justify the financial burden, deserve further inquiry. The same applies to the use of the newer, orally active GH-releasing peptides and related non-peptide secretagogues.

Melatonin

Melatonin secretion by the pineal gland in response to hypoglycemia and darkness also decreases with age regardless of these stimuli[31]. The physiological role of the pineal gland is not completely understood but it is involved in gonadal function and regulation of biorhythms[32]. Other physiological effects ranging from analgesic and antioxidative[33] to immunomodulating[34] properties have been attributed to melatonin. Olcese presented evidence indicating that administration of melatonin slows the growth of cancer cells in rodents[35]. However, the large popular enthusiasm around the hormone has a precarious scientific basis. It is likely that administration of melatonin may improve the significant sleep disorders frequently seen in the elderly. As mentioned before, profound hypogonadism is associated with alterations in melatonin production[11], therefore making difficult the attribution of some symptoms (sleep disturbances) exclusively to deficits of one or the other hormone. Evidence is emerging of a wide range of direct and indirect activities of melatonin on many human organ systems[36].

Thyroxin

With aging, there is an increase in serum thyroid stimulating hormone (TSH) levels and a decrease in thyroxin, although TSH levels in the elderly who have hypothyroidism are lower than in younger patients with the same disease. Hypothyroidism should be suspected if there are occurrences of unexplained high levels of cholesterol and creatinine phosphokinase, severe constipation, congestive heart failure with cardiomyopathy and unexplained macrocytic anemia. In the elderly there may be overt and subclinical thyroid deficiency. The diagnosis may not be clinically evident, and only an index of suspicion supported by biochemical evidence confirms the diagnosis. Symptoms of hypothyroidism may mask those of hypogonadism[37].

Leptin

The production of corticosteroids and estradiol in males, remains fairly constant throughout life. In contrast, leptin, a relatively recently described hormone from adipocytes, is altered in hypogonadism which explains, in part, some the changes in fat distribution observed in these men[38]. Levels of leptin can be brought down by androgen supplementation[39] that usually results in a decrease in the degree of obesity[40].

The following recommendation is put forward regarding other endocrine alterations associated with aging:

RECOMMENDATION 4

It is recognized that significant alterations in other endocrine systems occur in association with aging but the significance of these changes is not well understood. In general terms, determinations of DHEA, DHEA-S, melatonin, GH and IGF-I are not indicated in the uncomplicated evaluation of ADAM. Under special circumstances, or for well-defined clinical research, assessment of these and other hormones may be warranted.

TREATMENT

Indications

It is common clinical wisdom that a firm diagnosis is desirable prior to embarking on any therapeutic plan. This also applies to the treatment of the hypogonadal man. The goals of treatment most commonly include the restoration of sexual functioning as well as libido and sense of well-being. Equally important, androgen replacement can prevent or improve already established osteoporosis and optimize bone density, restore muscle strength and improve mental acuity and normalize GH levels, especially in elderly males[32,41]. Testosterone replacement therapy should maintain not only physiological levels of serum testosterone but also the metabolites of testosterone including estradiol, to optimize maintenance of bone and muscle mass, libido, virilization and sexual function. Since some of the manifestations of ADAM are shared with other conditions independent of a man's androgenic status, appropriate biochemical confirmation of hypogonadism should be sought out prior to initiation of treatment.

This recommendation is considered mandatory before consideration of ART:

RECOMMENDATION 5
A clear indication (a clinical picture together with biochemical support) should exist prior to initiation of androgen therapy.

Age

As mentioned previously, aging of the pituitary–gonadal axis is progressive. Hence, age more likely correlates with the severity of the biochemical changes and clinical manifestations. These aging men, however, because of associated infirmities and other socioeconomic reasons, are less likely to be considered for treatment. Therefore, the following recommendation applies:

RECOMMENDATION 6
In the absence of defined contraindications, age is not a limiting factor to initiate ART in aged men with hypgonadism.

Preparations

Current, generally available treatment options include buccal and oral tablets and capsules, intramuscular preparations, both long- and short-acting, implantable long-acting slow-release pellets and transdermal scrotal and non-scrotal patches and gels. Neither injectable preparations nor slow-release pellets reproduce the circadian pattern

of testosterone production by the testes. This is accomplished best by the transdermal preparations, although oral testosterone may also approximate a circadian rhythm by dose adjustments. The relevance of reproducing a circadian rythmicity during ART remains unknown. Common testosterone preparations and their recommended doses are shown in Table 1.

Oral preparations

Oral androgen preparations have become popular because of their convenience aspects (such as dose flexibility, possibility of immediate discontinuation, self-administration). However, they demand special consideration because they undergo rapid hepatic and intestinal metabolism. Therefore, special precautions may be necessary in order to achieve adequate serum androgen levels.

An oral preparation that is widely used throughout the world (and which is currently in clinical development in the USA) is testosterone undecanoate. As the only effective and safe oral testosterone ester, it circumvents the first passage through the liver, it is free of liver toxicity and brings serum testosterone levels within the physiological range. It is liposoluble and for this reason it must be taken with meals. Studies have shown that oral testosterone undecanoate

Table 1 Most frequently used testosterone preparations

	Generic name	Trade name	Dose
Injectable	testosterone cypionate	Depo-testosterone cypionate	200–400 mg every 3–4 weeks i.m.
	testosterone enanthate	Delatestryl	200–400 mg every 2–4 weeks i.m.
		Testoviron, Testosterone depot	
	mixed testosterone esters	Sustanon 250	250 mg every 3 weeks i.m.
Oral	fluoxymesterone*	Halotestin	5–20 mg daily
	methyltestosterone*	Metandren	10–30 mg daily
	testosterone undecanoate	Andriol	120–200 mg daily
	mesterolone	Proviron	25–75 mg daily
		Vistinon, Vistimon	
Subcutaneous	testosterone implants	—	1200 mg every 6 months
Transdermal	testosterone patches	Androderm	2.5–7.5 mg daily
		Testoderm	10–15 mg/day
	testosterone gel	Androgel	5–10 g

*17α-alkylated testosterone preparations fluoxymesterone and methyltestosterone are both associated with serious liver toxicity; i.m., intramuscularly

improves libido, erectile function and general well-being, increases bone mineral density and improves body composition[42,43].

In order to prevent the rapid metabolic breakdown in the liver, some oral agents available in some countries (particularly in the USA) are chemically modified. These alkylated androgens generally provide erratic androgenic activity and exhibit a potential for significant liver toxicity which includes hepatocellular adenomas and carcinomas, cholestatic jaundice and hemorrhagic liver cysts[44].

Finally, the oral dihydrotestosterone (DHT) derivative mesterolone is available in some countries. The compound is not aromatizable and cannot therefore be biotransformed into estradiol. As a consequence, it only exerts a partial androgenic effect, making it a suboptimal treatment option.

None of the oral medications results in a faithful reflection of the circadian level variations. However, careful selection of the timing and amount of the dosing may ameliorate this problem.

Parenteral preparations

Injectable esters of testosterone have been available for the longest time and their effects are well recognized. They are inexpensive and safe but their use carries several major drawbacks which include:

(1) The need for periodic (every 2–3 weeks) deep intramuscular injections.

(2) Wide swings in serum levels, initially (in about 72 h), result in supraphysiological levels of serum testosterone followed by a steady decline over the next 10–14 days[45].

(3) The steady decline frequently results in a very low nadir immediately before the next injection. This phenomenon translates in wide swings in mood and well-being – the rollercoaster effect – which is disconcerting and upsetting to both patients and their partners.

(4) Parenteral androgens do not provide the normal circadian patterns of serum testosterone and the intermittent supraphysiological levels that they produce may result in the development of breast tenderness and gynecomastia.

The most widely used parenteral preparations are the 17β-hydroxyl esters of testosterone which include the short-acting propionate and the longer-acting enanthate and cypionate. The propionate is rarely used because its short half-life requires administration every other day. The enanthate and cypionate esters of testosterone, on the other hand, can be administered at the dose of 200–400 mg every 10–21 days to maintain normal average testosterone levels[46]. Higher doses will not maintain testosterone levels in the normal range beyond the 3-week limit. Another option is a preparation containing a mixture of four testosterone esters (propionate, phenylpropionate, isocaproate and decanoate), each with a different elimination half-life, which is claimed to prolong the duration of action.

Appropriate treatment of hypogonadism with injectable esters of testosterone has been shown to improve libido, sexual function, energy levels, mood and bone density if they are caused by an androgen deficiency[47]. Persistent supraphysiological levels of serum testosterone may result in infertility due to suppression of LH and FSH production[48]. Although concern exists about the psychosexual effects of markedly elevated levels of testosterone in serum, evidence has been presented indicating that, even in eugonadal men, amounts up to five times the physiological replacement doses of testosterone cypionate have only minimal psychosexual effects[49].

Transdermal preparations

Transdermal testosterone therapy (TTT) offers a close reflection on the variable levels in testosterone production manifested in normal men over the 24-h circadian cycle. TTT is available in both scrotal and non-scrotal patches and in a gel form. The scrotal TTT lost its appeal due to inconveniences such as the inability to remain in place and the need for frequent shaving of the scrotal skin. In addition, due to the high concentrations of 5α-reductase in the scrotal skin, they produce abnormally high levels of DHT[50]. Transdermal non-scrotal patches produce normal levels of estradiol but, as opposed to the scrotal ones, result in normal levels of DHT[51]. In addition, to producing physiologically appropriate serum levels of testosterone, they lower levels of SHBG, promote virilization and increase bone mineral density[52].

Also, the testosterone patches, as compared to injectable forms, minimize excessive erythropoiesis and suppression of gonadotropins[53]. Most common side-effects of the body patches are related to the need to use enhancers to facilitate absorption; this frequently results in various degrees of skin reactions, occasionally reaching significant chemical burns. This may be prevented with the use of triamcinolone. The testosterone gel offers all the advantages of the patches[54], without the frequent skin reactions. Its only drawbacks reside in the potential for contamination of others and the lack of long-term studies with its use. The efficacy of transdermal DHT therapy has been reported recently[55,56].

Regarding the widely available forms of therapy, the following two recommendations are included:

RECOMMENDATION 7
Currently available preparations of testosterone (with the exception of the alkylated ones) are safe and effective. The treating physician should have sufficient knowledge and adequate understanding of the advantages and drawbacks of each preparation.

RECOMMENDATION 8
The purpose of ART is to bring and maintain serum testosterone levels within the physiological range. Supraphysiological levels are to be avoided.

ADVERSE EFFECTS

Like most medications, androgens have a potential for undesirable side-effects. These concerns are, primarily in regard to the liver, the prostate, lipid profile and cardiovascular system, hematological changes, sleep patterns and social behavior and emotional state.

Liver

Reports of liver toxicity manifested by jaundice and alteration of liver function, as well as the development of hepatic tumors, have been limited almost exclusively to cases in which the alkylated forms of testosterone have been used. Invariably, inserts of commercial preparations mention the potential for liver toxicity. Therefore, regardless of the form of ART employed, this recommendation is proposed:

RECOMMENDATION 9
Liver function studies are advisable prior to onset of therapy, quarterly during the first year and on a yearly basis thereafter during treatment.

Lipid and cardiovascular safety

The relationship between hypogonadism and alterations of the lipid profile remains to be completely resolved. Evidence is emerging supporting the concept that hypogonadism is associated with potentially unfavorable changes in triglycerides and high-density lipoprotein cholesterol and that such abnormalities can be corrected by restoring a physiological androgen milieu[57]. Other studies support the view that low testosterone is a significant risk factor for coronary artery disease[58–60]. Although most recent evidence continues to support the concept of a beneficial effect of androgens in coronary artery disease[61], the relationships between androgens and cardiovascular risk factors are complex and still understood only imperfectly. Similarly, the relationships between androgen levels in the serum and other lipoprotein sub-fractions have not been fully investigated[62]. Therefore, caution is advisable when supplementing androgens in men with significant risk factors for cardiovascular disease. The picture is further blurred by the fluid retention associated with androgen administration; this may add to any possible adverse effect of androgen therapy to the cardiovascular system.

This recommendation was approved on the issue of lipid alterations:

RECOMMENDATION 10
A fasting lipid profile prior to initiation of treatment and at regular intervals (no longer than 1 year) during treatment is recommended.

Prostate safety

It is well established that, in the absence of sufficient androgens the prostate gland fails to develop. Most studies, however, have shown no significant increases in PSA or prostate volume following administration of androgens to hypogonadal men[63]. Evidence from placebo-controlled studies of men receiving androgen supplementation indicate that the differences between the men on hormones and those on placebo were insignificant in regard to prostate volume, PSA or obstructive symptoms[64,65]. Although testosterone has not been implicated in the development of benign prostate hypertrophy (BPH), nevertheless, in the presence of severe lower urinary tract obstructive symptoms (LUTOS), the administration of testosterone may result in the development of urinary retention. Whether testosterone promotes the development of prostate cancer remains to be elucidated. Current evidence indicates that serum levels of sex hormones bear no relation to the development of prostate cancer and there is either no change or only a modest increase in PSA levels after testosterone administration[66]. The suspicion of prostate cancer is, however, an absolute contra-indication for androgen therapy. On the other hand, prostatic biopsies prior to onset of ART in the absence of an abnormal digital rectal examination (DRE) or PSA level are not indicated. However, a rapid increase in PSA or the appearance of abnormalities in the DRE are clear indications for a thorough evaluation of the prostate to rule out the presence of carcinoma. In this situation the administration of testosterone may have served as an early warning to the presence of an occult prostatic malignancy[67].

The issue of prostate safety and exogenous androgens is, perhaps, the gravest concern. The topic was recently reviewed[68]. The following three separate recommendations were considered and approved:

RECOMMENDATION 11
Digital rectal examination (DRE) and determination of serum prostate-specific antigen (PSA) are mandatory in men over the age of 40 years as baseline measurements of prostate health prior to therapy with androgens, at quarterly intervals for the first 12 months and yearly thereafter. Transrectal ultrasound-guided biopsies of the prostate are indicated only if the DRE or the PSA are abnormal.

RECOMMENDATION 12
Androgen administration is absolutely contraindicated in men suspected of having carcinoma of the prostate or breast cancer.

RECOMMENDATION 13
Androgen supplementation is contraindicated in men with severe bladder outlet obstruction due to an enlarged, clinically benign prostate. Moderate obstruction represents a partial contraindication to ART. Once the urinary

obstruction has been successfully treated, these men are candidates for androgen supplementation.

Mood and behavior

The consequences of testosterone deficiency in mood regulation are widely accepted[69,70] to the point that, recently, a hypothesis has been advanced suggesting that perinatal androgen deficiency promotes deficient cognitive development[71]. However, concerns exist regarding the promotion of sexually aggressive behavior following testosterone administration. Significant behavioral changes can be observed with supraphysiological levels of androgens. Proper treatment, aimed at maintenance of physiological plasma levels, makes this a rare occurrence and certainly not a sufficient cause to withhold treatment[72].

RECOMMENDATION 14
ART normally results in improvements in mood and well-being. The development of negative behavioral patterns during treatment calls for dose modifications or discontinuation of therapy.

Hematology

The stimulatory effect of testosterone administration on bone marrow has long been recognized even in the presence of advanced malignant disease[73]. Testosterone therapy in older men often can result in a significant increase in red blood cell mass and hemoglobin levels[74]. In younger, healthier individuals, such as those receiving androgens for sexual dysfunction, the effects can also be marked[75]. Therefore, dose adjustments or phlebotomies may be necessary. Rarely, ART has to be discontinued due to polycythemia.

RECOMMENDATION 15
Polycythemia occasionally develops during ART. Periodic hematological assessment is indicated. Dose adjustments may be necessary.

Sleep apnea

Other possible effects of testosterone treatment include exacerbation of sleep apnea[76] although hypotestosteronemia has been cited as a cause of the condition[77].

RECOMMENDATION 16

There is insufficient evidence for a recommendation regarding safety of ART in men with sleep apnea. It is suggested, therefore, that good clinical judgement and caution be employed in this situation.

MONITORING PATIENTS ON ART

Hormonal replacement may be initiated for a variety of indications but treatment is normally for life. Monitoring of these patients is also a lifetime commitment that cannot be taken lightly. Monitoring, of course requires to be tailored to the indications and the individual needs of the patient. For instance, if the indication is osteoporosis, serial bone mineral density determinations are the method for monitoring therapeutic response. In this regard, the studies by Behre and colleagues[78] provide an elegant and graphic illustration on the effectiveness of chronic testosterone supplementation in increasing bone mineral density and in moving older men out of the range of high fracture risk. Another common indication for testosterone administration is for treatment of sexual dysfunction. In this situation, a simple and effective rule of monitoring is that, frequently, the patient's report is the most reliable indicator of treatment effectiveness[59]. In addition to the specific areas of interest, long-term monitoring of these patients centers on six domains in which concerns have existed for possible serious adverse events: the liver, lipid profile and cardiovascular disease, erythopoiesis, the prostate, sleep disorders and social behavior and emotional state.

RECOMMENDATION 17

Monitoring during ART is a shared responsibility. The physician must emphasize to the patient the need for periodic evaluations and the patient must agree to comply with these requirements. Since ART is normally for life, monitoring is also a lifetime mutual duty.

CONCLUSIONS

There is clear evidence that advancing age is associated with a decline in the production of several hormones. The most prominent alterations are related to the sex steroids but other hormones such as growth hormone and melatonin are also profoundly affected. The clinical syndrome of ADAM or andropause has been described but a direct causality between its manifestations and the alterations in a specific hormone are not yet fully established. There is, however, a growing body of literature supporting the concept of a clinical picture associated with hypogonadism in aging men that impacts significantly on the quality of life. Equally, there is sufficient evidence to support the concept that appropriate treatment of these men results in alleviation of some of the manifestations of the andropause. It behoves a variety of medical specialties to be familiar with the consequences of this condition, its investigation, treatment and monitoring.

Our understanding of ADAM is still incomplete and there exist a number of controversial issues in regard to hormonal replacement in elderly men. Standards or guidelines on the subject are, therefore, premature. Recommendations, however, are justified with the present state of knowledge. Recommendations[79] and guidelines[80–82] in the area of ART require frequent updates as further information emerges. We provide this set of Recommendations for physicians interested in the diagnosis and treatment of aging men with symptoms of hypogonadism. Recommendations, guidelines and standards are, normally, work in progress. They will be discussed again at the biannual meeting of ISSAM in Prague, February 2004.

References

1. Morales A, Lunenfeld B. Androgen replacement therapy in aging men with secondary hypogonadism. Draft recommendations for endorsement by ISSAM. *Aging Male* 2001;4:151–62
2. Kaufman JM. Hypothalamic–pituitary–gonadal funtion in aging men. *Aging Male* 1999;2:157
3. Werner AA. The male climacteric. *J Am Med Assoc* 1946;132:188
4. Morley JE, Charlton E, Patrick P, *et al.* Validation of a screening questionnaire for androgen deficiency in aging males. *Metabolism* 2000;49:1239

5. Heinemann LAJ, Saad F, Thiele K, Wood-Duphenee S. The Aging Males' Symptom rating scale: cultural and linguistic validation into English. *Aging Male* 2001;4:14–22

6. Vermeulen A, Kaufman JM. Aging of the hypothalamo–pituitary–testicular axis in men. *Horm Res* 1995;43:25

7. Vermeulen A, Verdonck L, Kaufman JL. A critical evaluation of simple methods for the estimation of free hormones in serum. *J Clin Endocrinol Metab* 1999;84:3666

8. Morales A, Heaton JPW. Hormonal erectile dysfunction: evaluation and management. *Urol Clin NA* 2001;28:279

9. Alexander GM, Swerdloff RS, Wang C, Davidson T, McDonald V, Steiner B, *et al.* Androgen behavior correlations in hypogonadal and eugonadal men: cognitive abilities. *Horm Behav* 1998;33:85

10. Urban RJ, Bodenburg YH, Gilkison C, Fowworth J, Coggan AR, Wolfe RR. Testosterone administration to elderly men increases skeletal muscle strength and protein synthesis. *Am J Physiol* 1995;269:820

11. Tenover JS. Androgen administration to aging men. *Endocrinol Metab Clin NA* 1994;23:877

12. Hibberts NA, Howell AE, Randall VA. Balding hair follicle dermal papilla cells contain higher levels of androgen receptors than those from non-balding scalp. *J Endocrinol* 1998;156:59

13. Behre HM, Kliesch S, Leifke E, Link TM, Nieschlag E. Long term effect of testosterone therapy on bone mineral density in hypogonadal men. *J Clin Endocrinol Metab* 1997;82:2386

14. Kropman RF, Verdijk RM, Lyklama AAB, Nijeholt A, Roelfsma F. Routine endocrine screening in impotence: significance and cost-effectiveness. *Int J Impotence Res* 1991;3:87

15. Vermeulen A. Routine endocrine screening in impotence: significance and cost effectiveness. [Editorial]. *Int J Impotence Res* 1991;3:85

16. Buvat J, Lemaire A. Endocrine screening in 1022 men with erectile dysfunction: clinical significance and cost-effective strategy. *J Urol* 1997;158:1764

17. Morales A, Johnston B, Heaton JWP, Lundie M. Testosterone supplementation in hypogonadal impotence: assessment of biochemical measurements and therapeutic outcomes. *J Urol* 1997;157:849

18. Tremblay RR. Practical consequences of the validation of a mathematical model in assessment of partial androgen deficiency in the aging male using bioavailable testosterone. *Aging Male* 2001;4:23–9

19. Herbert J. The age of dehydroepiandrosterone. *Lancet* 1995;345:1193

20. Morales AJ, Nolan JJ, Nelson JC, *et al.* Effects of replacement dose of dehydroepiandrosterone in men and women of advancing age. *J Clin Endocrinol Metab* 1994;78:1360

21. Arlt W, Callies F, Koehler L, *et al.* Dehydroepiandrosterone supplementation in healthy men with an age related decline of dehydroepiandrosterone secretion. *J Clin Endocrinol Metab* 2001;86:4686

22. Vaughn ED, Cox DS. Chronic administration of dehydroepiandrosterone (DHEA) does not increase serum testosterone or prostatic specific antigen (PSA) in normal men. *J Urol* 1998;159:27(abstr 280)

23. Christiansen KH. Behavioral correlates of dehydroepiandrosterone and dehydroepiandrosterone sulfate. *Aging Male* 1998;1:103–12

24. Weksler ME. Hormone replacement for men – not enough evidence to recommend routine treatment with dehydroepiandrosterone. *Br Med J* 1996;312:859

25. deBoer H, Block GJ, van der Veen EA. Clinical aspects of growth hormone deficiency in adults. *Endocrinol Rev* 1995;16:63

26. Veldhuis JD. Elements in the pathophysiology of diminished growth hormone (GH) secretion in aging humans *Endocrinology* 1996;7:41

27. Holmes SJ, Economou G, Whitehouse RW, Adams JE, Shalet SM. Reduced bone mineral density in patients with adult onset growth hormone deficiency. *J Clin Endocrinol Metab* 1994;78:669

28. Block GJ, de Boer H, Gooren LJG, van der Veen EA. Growth hormone substitution in adult growth-hormone deficient men augments androgen effect on the skin. *Clin Endocrinol* 1997;47:29

29. Baum HB, Biller BMK, Finkelstein JS, Cannistraro KB, Oppenheim DS, Schonfeld DA, *et al.* Effects of physiologic growth hormone therapy on bone density and body composition in patients with adult-onset growth hormone deficiency. A randomized placebo controlled trial. *Ann Intern Med* 1996;125:883

30. Lesee GP, Frase WD, Farqhuarson R, Hipkin L, Vora JI. Gonadal status is an important determinant of bone density in acromegaly. *Clin Endocrinol* 1998;48:59

31. Liu R-Y, Zhou J-N, van Heerikhuize J, Hofman MA, Swaab DF. Decreased melatonin levels in post-mortem cerebro-spinal fluid in relation to ageing, Alzheimer's disease and apolipoprotein E-ε4/4 genotype. *J Clin Endocrinol Metab* 1999;84:323

32. Dittgen M, Hoffmann H. New dosage form for pulsatile delivery of melatonin: development and

testing in animal and human subjects. *Aging Male* 1998;1:141–8

33. Sewerynek E, Melchirri D, Reiter RJ, Ortiz GG, Lewinski A. Lipopolysaccharide-induced hepatotoxicity is inhibited by the antioxidant melatonin. *Eur J Pharmacol* 1995;293:327

34. Maestroni GJM. The immunoneuroendocrine role of melatonin. *J Pineal Res* 1993;14:1

35. Olcese J. Melatonin and the aging male. *Aging Male* 1998;1(Suppl 1):9

36. Olcese J. Cellular and molecular mechanisms mediating melatonin action. *Aging Male* 1998;1: 113–28

37. Samuels H, Pekary AE, Hershman JM. Hypothalamic–pituitary–thyroid axis in aging. In Morley JE, van den Berg L, eds. *Endocrinology of Aging*. Totowa, NJ: Humana Press, 2000:41–62

38. Bray GA, York DA. Leptin and clinical medicine: a new piece in the puzzle of obesity. *J Clin Endocrinol Metab* 1997;82:2771

39. Luukkaa V, Personen U, Huhtaniemi I, Lehtonen A, Tilvis R, Tuomilehto J, *et al*. Inverse correlation between serum testosterone and leptin in men. *J Clin Endocrinol Metab* 1998;83:3243

40. Behre HM, Simoni M, Nieschlag E. Strong association between leptin and testosterone. *Clin Endocrinol* 1997;47:237

41. Finkelstein JS, Kilbanski A, Neer RM, Doppelt SH, Rosenthal DI, Segre GV, *et al*. Increases in bone density during treatment of men with idiopathic hypogonadotrophic hypogonadism. *J Clin Endocrinol Metab* 1989;69:776

42. Gooren LJG. Long-term safety of the oral androgen testosterone undecanoate. *Int J Androl* 1986;9:21

43. Gooren LJG. Long term safety of the oral androgen testosterone undecanoate. *J Androl* 1994;15:212

44. Bagatell CJ, Bremner WJ. Drug therapy: androgens in men – uses and abuses. *New Engl J Med* 1996;334: 707–11

45. Sokol RZ, Palacios A, Campfield LA. Comparison of the kinetics of injectable testosterone in eugonadal and hypogonadal men. *Fertil Steril* 1982; 37:425–30

46. Bhasin S. Androgen treatment of hypogonadal men. *J Clin Endocrinol Metab* 1992;74:1221–4

47. Morales A, Heaton JWP, Carson CC III. Andropause: a misnomer for a true clinical entity. *J Urol* 2000;163:705–12

48. Bhasin S, Bremner WJ. Emerging issues in androgen replacement therapy. *J Clin Endocrinol Metab* 1997;82:3–7

49. Yates WR, Perry PJ, MacIndoe J, Holman T, Ellingrod V. Psychosexual effects of 3 doses of testosterone cycling in normal men. *Biol Psychiatr* 1999;45:254-60

50. Bradwin SW, Swerdloff RS, Santen RJ. Androgens: risks and benefits. *J Clin Endocrinol Metab* 1991;73:4–7

51. Arver S, Meikle AW, Dobbs AS, *et al*. Permeation enhanced testosterone transdermal systems in the treatment of male hypogonadism: long term effects. *J Endocrinol* 1996;148:254–9

52. De Sanctis V, Vullo C, Urso L, *et al*. Clinical experience using Androderm testosterone transdermal system in hypogonadal adolescents and young men with beta-thalassemia major. *J Pediatr Endocrinol Metab* 1999;11(Suppl 3):891–900

53. Dobbs AS, Meikle AW, Arver S, *et al*. Pharmacokinetics, efficacy and safety of permeation-enhanced testosterone transdermal system in comparison with bi-weekly injections of testosterone enanthate for the treatment of hypogonadal men, *J Clin Endocrinol Metab* 1999;84:3469–78

54. Wang C, Swerdloff RS, Iranmanesh A, Dobbs A, Snyder PJ, Gunningham G, *et al*. Transdermal testosterone gel improves sexual function, mood, muscle strength and body composition parameters in hypogonadal men. *J Clin Endocrinol Metab* 2000; 85:2839

55. Ly LP, Jimenez M, Zhuang TN, Celermajer DS, Conway AJ, Handelsman DJ. A double-blind, placebo-controlled, randomized clinical trial of transdermal dihydrotestosterone gel on muscular strength, mobility, and quality of life in older men with partial androgen deficiency. *J Clin Endocrinol Metab* 2001;86:4078–88

56. Kunelius P, Lukkarinen O, Hannuksela ML, Itkonen O, Tapanainen JS. The effects of transdermal dihydrotestosterone in the aging male: a prospective, randomized, double blind study. *J Clin Endocrinol Metab* 2002;87:1467–72

57. Zmuda JM, Cauley JA, Kriska A. Longitudinal relation between endogenous testosterone and cardiovascular disease risk factors in middle age men. A 13 year follow-up of former risk factor intervention trial participants. *Am J Epidemiol* 1997; 146:609–15

58. Phillips GB. The association of hypotestosteronemia with coronary artery disease in men. *Arterioscler Thromb* 1994;14:701–5

59. Uyanik BS, Ari Z, Gumus B, *et al*. Beneficial effects of testosterone undecanoate on the lipoprotein profiles in healthy elderly men. *Jpn Heart J* 1997; 38:73–7

60. Crook D. Androgens and the risk of cardiovascular disease. *Aging Male* 2000;3:190–5

61. Gooren LJG. Visceral obesity, androgens and the risk of cardiovascular disease and diabetes mellitus. *Aging Male* 2001;4:30–8

62. Tenover JL. Testosterone and the aging male. *J Androl* 1997;18:103–6

63. Behre HM. Prostate volume in treated and untreated hypogonadal men in comparison to age matched controls. *Clin Endocrinol* 1994;40:341–6
64. Cooper CS, Perry PJ, Sparks AE, *et al.* Effects of exogenous testosterone on prostate volume, serum and semen prostate specific antigen levels in healthy young men. *J Urol* 1998;159:441–3
65. Holmäng S, Marin P, Lindtstedt G, *et al.* Effect of long term oral testosterone undecanoate treatment on prostate volume and serum prostate specific antigen in eugonadal middle-aged men. *Prostate* 1993;23:99–106
66. Nomura A, Heilrunn LK, Stemmermann GN, *et al.* Prediagnostic serum hormones and the risk of prostate cancer. *Cancer Res* 1998;48:3515–20
67. Curran MJ, Bihrle W. Dramatic raise in prostate specific antigen after androgen replacement in a hypogonadal man with occult adenocarcinoma of the prostate. *Urology* 1999;53:423–4
68. Morales A. Androgen replacement therapy and prostate safety *Eur Androl* 2002;37:1
69. Wang C, Alexander G, Berman N, *et al.* Testosterone replacement therapy improves mood in hypogonadal men – a clinical research center study. *J Clin Endocrinol Metab* 1996;81:3587–93
70. Ehrenreich H, Halaris A, Ruether E, *et al.* Psychoendocrine sequelae of chronic testosterone deficiency. *J Psychiatr Res* 1999;33:379–87
71. Ozata M, Odabasi Z, Caglayan S, *et al.* Event related male potentials in male hypogonadism. *J Endocrinol Invest* 1999;22:508–13
72. Sternbach H. Age associated testosterone decline in men: clinical issues for psychiatry. *Am J Psychiatr* 1998;155:1310–14
73. Morales A, Connolly J, Burr R, *et al.* The use of radioactive phosphorus to treat bone pain in metastatic carcinoma of the prostate. *Can Med Assoc J* 1970;103:372–3

74. Tennover L. Androgen deficiency in the aging male. Presented at *Postgraduate Course, American Urological Association,* May, 2000
75. Krauss DJ, Taub HA, Lantiga LJ. Risk of blood volume changes in hypogonadal men treated with testosterone enanthate for erectile impotence. *J Urol* 1991;146:1566–70
76. Sandbloom RA, Matsumoto AM, Schoene RB, *et al.* Obstructive sleep apnea syndrome induced by testosterone administration. *N Engl J Med* 1983; 308:508–10
77. Santamaria JD, Prior JC, Fleetham JA. Reversible reproductive dysfunction in men with sleep apnea. *Clin Endocrinol (Oxf)* 1988;28:461–70
78. Behre HM, Kliesch S, Leifke E, Link TM, Nieschlag E. Long-term effect of testosterone therapy on bone mineral density in hypogonadal men. *J Clin Endocrinol Metab* 1997;82:2386
79. Morales A, Bain J, Ruijs A, Chapdelaine A, Tremblay RR. Clinical practice guidelines for screening and monitoring male patients receiving testosterone supplementation therapy. *Int J Impotence Res* 1996;8:95
80. Tremblay RR, Morales A. Canadian practice recommendations for screening, monitoring and treating men affected by andropause or partial androgen deficiency. *Aging Male* 1998;1: 213–18
81. Morales A. Canadian practice recommendations for screening, treatment and monitoring of aging men with androgen deficiency. *Aging Male* 2001; 4(Suppl 1):35–7
82. Kim YC. Hormonal replacement therapy in men: Korean practical recommendations on testosterone supplementation in the aging male. *Aging Male* 2001;4(Suppl 1):30–4

Appendix 1B. Summary from the Second Annual Andropause Consensus Meeting

SUMMARY
FROM THE SECOND ANNUAL ANDROPAUSE
CONSENSUS MEETING

THE ENDOCRINE SOCIETY®

INTRODUCTION

The Second Annual Andropause Consensus 2001 Meeting brought together a multidisciplinary group of practitioners and researchers. Joining the original panel of nine endocrinologists (including three gerontologists) were two urologists, a psychiatrist, and a primary care physician, whose expertise and perspectives further enriched the discussion.

A major goal of the Second Annual Andropause Consensus 2001 Meeting was to develop recommendations for testosterone replacement therapy (TRT) that could be used in a clinical setting.

The need for recommendations that are based upon available data and expert opinion comes from the growing awareness in the medical and lay communities of the potential benefits and risks of testosterone replacement therapy. The preliminary nature of these recommendations is due to the lack of critical data from large clinical trials that would provide more authoritative answers. Until more definitive data are available, the recommendations offered by the Consensus Conference are intended to provide guidance to assist the practitioner.

TESTOSTERONE REPLACEMENT STRATEGIES: SIGNS, SYMPTOMS, POTENTIAL BENEFITS AND POTENTIAL RISKS

For many years, gonadal hormone replacement strategies focused primarily on the treatment of menopausal women. However, the use of TRT to prevent or to treat aspects of male andropause has gained interest among researchers and clinicians. This coincides with a shift in the demographics of aging in the United States that shows an increase in the percentage of older men—a percentage that continues to rise.

The signs and symptoms of low testosterone in adult men may include loss of libido, erectile dysfunction, depression, lethargy, osteoporosis, loss of muscle mass and strength, and some regression of secondary sexual characteristics, such as loss of pubic hair. Alterations in behavior, such as inability to concentrate, diminished interest in activities, sleep disturbance, irritability and depressed mood may also be noted. A definition of andropause (clinically significant androgen deficiency in the elderly male) should include some or all of these symptoms and signs plus a low serum testosterone (T). It is important to keep in mind that some symptoms, because of their nonspecific nature, may not be recognized as a manifestation of androgen deficiency. Some clinicians may attribute an older man's symptoms to the normal aging process—and send him on his way without considering a blood testosterone measurement and, if abnormally low (compared to young male standards), TRT.

The members of the Consensus Conference were aware that data are limited or lacking on the long-term benefits and risks of TRT in older men. Much of the considerations of the panel members were based on projections from studies on hypogonadal younger men (ages 18-65) and data generated in relatively short-term and often underpowered investigations in older men. Because it will be 8-10 years before data on long-term risks are available, we think that preliminary recommendations based upon available data and expert opinion can be useful to clinicians.

There are several potential benefits of TRT. These include improvements in libido, energy level, lean body mass, strength, and bone mineral density (BMD). There also may be an improved mood, sense of well-being, and erectile function. These benefits have been demonstrated in hypogonadal young and middle-aged men, but there are insufficient data at this time to convincingly demonstrate these particular benefits in an older age group. Contraindications to TRT include documented prostate cancer, existing or prior history of breast cancer, and sensitivity to ingredients in T formulations. Relative contraindications include polycythemia (hematocrit ≥52%), untreated sleep apnea, severe obstructive symptoms of benign prostatic hyperplasia (BPH), and advanced congestive heart failure. Potential risks include polycythemia and possibly thrombosis, induction or worsening of sleep apnea, an increase in bladder outlet obstructive symptoms, conversion of an occult prostate cancer into a clinical prostate cancer and an increase in cardiovascular events. A wide array of testosterone formulations are currently available—with more options on the horizon.

These recommendations have been independently reviewed and approved by the Clinical Affairs Committee of The Endocrine Society

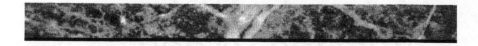

These recommendations have been independently reviewed and approved
by the Clinical Affairs Committee of The Endocrine Society

THE
ENDOCRINE
SOCIETY®

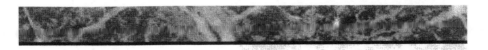

LETTER FROM THE CO-CHAIRS

Dear Colleagues:

We are pleased to present the Summary of the Consensus Session from the Second Annual Andropause Consensus 2001 Meeting. This conference was sponsored by The Endocrine Society and was funded by an unrestricted educational grant from Solvay Pharmaceuticals, Inc. to an independent medical education company. The opinions expressed herein represent only those of the participants.

We especially wish to thank our colleagues in this venture. Their expertise and candid participation have made it a rewarding experience. Please share your comments.

Sincerely,

Glenn R. Cunningham, MD
Conference Co-Chair

Ronald S. Swerdloff, MD
Conference Co-Chair

These recommendations have been independently reviewed and approved by the Clinical Affairs Committee of The Endocrine Society

FACULTY CO-CHAIRS

Glenn R. Cunningham, MD
Professor of Medicine
Professor of Molecular and Cell Biology
Vice Chairman for Research
Department of Medicine
Baylor College of Medicine
Executive, Research Service Line
VA Medical Center
Houston, Texas

Ronald S. Swerdloff, MD
Professor of Medicine
Chief, Division of Endocrinology,
  Metabolism, and Nutrition
Associate Chair, Department of Medicine
Harbor-UCLA Medical Center
UCLA School of Medicine
Torrance, California

FACULTY

Shalender Bhasin, MD
Professor of Medicine
UCLA School of Medicine
Chief, Division of Endocrinology,
  Metabolism, and Molecular Medicine
Associate Chair for Academic Affairs,
  Department of Medicine
Charles R. Drew University of Medicine
  and Science
Los Angeles, California

Marc R. Blackman, MD
Clinical Director
Chief, Laboratory of Clinical
  Investigation
National Center for Complementary
  and Alternative Medicine
National Institutes of Health
Bethesda, Maryland
Professor of Medicine
The Johns Hopkins University
  School of Medicine
Baltimore, Maryland

Adrian S. Dobs, MD, MHS
Professor of Medicine
Division of Endocrinology and
  Metabolism
Vice Chair, Department of Medicine
Director of Clinical Trials Unit
The Johns Hopkins University
  School of Medicine
Baltimore, Maryland

Alvin M. Matsumoto, MD
Professor, Department of Medicine
Division of Gerontology and
  Geriatric Medicine
University of Washington
  School of Medicine
Associate Director, Geriatric Research,
  Education, and Clinical Center
Director, Clinical Research Unit
VA Puget Sound Health Care System
Seattle, Washington

Abraham Morgentaler, MD
Director, Men's Health Boston
Associate Clinical Professor of Surgery
  (Urology)
Harvard Medical School
Boston, Massachusetts

John E. Morley, MB, BCh
Dammert Professor of Gerontology
Director, Division of Geriatric Medicine
Saint Louis University Medical Center
Director, Geriatric Research,
  Education, and Clinical Center
St. Louis Veterans Affairs Medical Center
St. Louis, Missouri

William Rosner, MD
Professor of Medicine
Columbia University
Director, Institute of Health Sciences
St. Luke's/Roosevelt Hospital Center
New York, New York

Robert T. Rubin, MD, PhD
Director, Center for Neurosciences
  Research
Highmark Blue Cross Blue Shield
  Professor of Neurosciences and
  Professor of Psychiatry
MCP Hahnemann University School
  of Medicine
Allegheny General Hospital
Pittsburgh, Pennsylvania

Ridwan Shabsigh, MD
Associate Professor of Urology
Columbia University
Director, New York Center for
  Human Sexuality
New York Presbyterian Hospital
New York, New York

Eugene Shippen, MD
Shillington Diagnostic Center
Shillington, Pennsylvania

Christina Wang, MD
Program Director
General Clinical Research Center
Harbor-UCLA Medical Center
Professor of Medicine
UCLA School of Medicine
Torrance, California

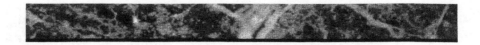

DISCLOSURES

Shalender Bhasin, MD, has received grant/research support from ALZA Corporation, GTx, TheraTech, and Solvay Pharmaceuticals, Inc. He serves on the Speakers' Bureaus for ALZA Corporation and Solvay Pharmaceuticals, Inc. Dr. Bhasin is also a consultant for Cellegy Pharmaceuticals Inc. and TAP Pharmaceutical Products Inc.

Marc R. Blackman, MD, serves on the Speakers' Bureau for Solvay Pharmaceuticals, Inc.

Glenn R. Cunningham, MD, has received grant/research support from, is a consultant for, and is a member of the Speakers' Bureau for ALZA Corporation and Solvay Pharmaceuticals, Inc. Dr. Cunningham has also received grant/research support from Columbia Laboratories.

Adrian S. Dobs, MD, MHS, has received grant/research support from and is a member of the Speakers' Bureau for Solvay Pharmaceuticals, Inc.

Alvin M. Matsumoto, MD, has received grant/research support from and is a consultant for Solvay Pharmaceuticals, Inc. and Columbia Laboratories.

Abraham Morgentaler, MD, is a member of the Speakers' Bureau for Pfizer Inc. and Solvay Pharmaceuticals, Inc.

John E. Morley, MB, BCh, has received grant/research support from and is a member of the Speakers' Bureau for Organon Pharmaceuticals and Solvay Pharmaceuticals, Inc. He is a consultant for Organon Pharmaceuticals and VetPharma.

William Rosner, MD, has no significant relationships to disclose.

Robert T. Rubin, MD, has no significant relationships to disclose.

Ridwan Shabsigh, MD, has received grant/research support from, is a consultant and a member of the Speakers' Bureau for Lily ICOS LLC. He has also received grant/research support from and is a consultant for NexMed and Solvay Pharmaceuticals, Inc. Dr. Shabsigh also serves as a consultant for Pharmacia, where he is also a member of the Speakers' Bureau; has received grant/research support from Boehringer Ingelheim and Vivus, Inc.; and is a member of the Speakers' Bureau for Bayer.

Eugene Shippen, MD, serves on the Speakers' Bureau for Solvay Pharmaceuticals, Inc.

Ronald S. Swerdloff, MD, has received grant/research support from, and has served as a consultant for Solvay Pharmaceuticals, Inc., where he also serves on the Speakers' Bureau. Dr. Swerdloff also serves as a consultant for BioSante Pharmaceuticals, Inc.; GlaxoSmithKline; Ligand Pharmaceuticals; Schering AG; and Solvay Pharma Inc. (Canada).

Christina Wang, MD, has received grant/research support from Columbia Laboratories. She is a consultant for GlaxoSmithKline. Dr. Wang has also received other financial or material support from Organon Pharmaceuticals and Schering AG.

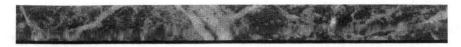

CONSENSUS STATEMENT

When should one suspect testosterone deficiency?

A clinician must consider signs and symptoms and laboratory values when evaluating whether an individual patient is testosterone deficient and if TRT should be initiated.

The normal range for serum total testosterone levels in early morning hours in healthy, young men, 20 to 40 years of age, is approximately 300 ng/dL to 1000 ng/dL. The recommendations of this Consensus panel were predicated on this range for normal serum testosterone. Assuming that a patient has signs or symptoms consistent with androgen deficiency and no contraindications exist, men who fall below the lower limit of this range would likely benefit from treatment independent of age.

Total testosterone levels <200 ng/dL clearly indicate hypogonadism and in most instances, indicate that benefits may be derived from TRT. Total T levels between 200 ng/dL and 400 ng/dL should be repeated and followed up by calculation of free testosterone from total testosterone and sex-hormone binding globulin (SHBG) concentrations, or by measurement of free testosterone levels by the dialysis method, or bioavailable T by the ammonium sulfate precipitation method. If a healthy man has a serum testosterone level >400 ng/dL, it is unlikely he is testosterone deficient, and therefore, clinical judgment should guide the next steps, even if he has symptoms suggestive of testosterone deficiency.

What are the health risks of testosterone deficiency?

In the aging male, the health risks associated with testosterone deficiency include decreases in muscle strength, lean body mass, and sexual function, as well as an increase in body fat, and undesirable alterations in mood and neuropsychological function. Older hypogonadal men are at increased risk for osteoporosis and fracture. In epidemiological studies, low testosterone levels are often associated with central obesity, insulin resistance, and an increased risk of diabetes and cardiovascular disorders.

What general medical disorders are associated with hypogonadism?

A number of systemic disorders may suppress testosterone levels, including hepatic cirrhosis, chronic renal failure, sickle cell anemia, thalassemia, hemochromatosis, human immuno-deficiency virus, amyloidosis, chronic obstructive pulmonary disease (COPD), rheumatoid arthritis, chronic infections, and inflammatory or debilitating conditions. Hypogonadism may be central (hypothalamic or pituitary) or testicular in origin. Many men over age 50 and most men ≥65 years of age with low testosterone levels have functional abnormalities at multiple levels of the hypothalamic-pituitary-testicular axis and may present with low testosterone and low or low-normal luteinizing hormone (LH) levels.

Should all older men with low testosterone levels be evaluated for hypothalamic-pituitary disorders?

After a low T level has been determined and calculated free or bioavailable T levels have been confirmed, serum LH and prolactin levels should be measured. Men with a total T <150 ng/dL, a subnormal or inappropriately normal serum LH, or elevated prolactin levels should be further evaluated with a magnetic resonance imaging (MRI) of the sella turcica area (with and without contrast) to visualize both the hypothalamus and pituitary gland.

Are there any drugs associated with testosterone deficiency?

A number of drugs may affect testosterone levels. Drugs that are known to decrease testosterone levels include GnRH agonists and antagonists, estrogens, progestins, glucocorticoids, ketoconazole, aldactone, thiazide diuretics, opiates, anabolic steroids, amiodarone, and a number of psychotropic agents. Agents that impair testosterone action at the receptor level include aldactone, cimetidine, flutamide, and other androgen antagonists.

How is testosterone deficiency diagnosed in older men? What percentage of men are testosterone deficient at ages 55, 65, 75, and 85?

The signs and/or symptoms of andropause are an important part of the diagnostic complex. Testosterone deficiency is often underdiagnosed and dismissed as physiologic changes consistent with "old age" because symptoms in older men are often nonspecific.

The prevalence of hypogonadism based on total testosterone levels increases with age, beginning at age 20. If free or bioavailable T levels are measured, the percentage of hypogonadal men (hormone levels below the normal range for young healthy adult men) increases even more.

PERCENTAGE OF MEN WITH LOW TESTOSTERONE LEVELS

Age	Testosterone*	T/SHBG†	Bioavailable T‡
20-29	5	0	-
30-39	2	0	-
40-49	8	2	7
50-59	12	9	30
60-69	19	34	44
70-79	28	68	70
80+	49	91	

* <325 ng/dL
† <153 nmol/L less than two standard deviations below the mean for men 21-45 years of age) (Harman et al, 2001)
‡ <70 ng/dL (lowest value observed in normal men 20-45 years of age) (Morley et al, 2000)

2

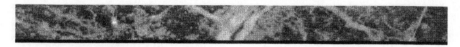

Should men ≥50 years of age be screened regularly for testosterone deficiency?

The majority of panel members suggested that screening for testosterone deficiency should begin at age 50 or 55 and be repeated every 5 years, or more frequently if symptoms are present. One approach is to screen the patient by using a validated questionnaire. Positive responders to the questionnaire should be evaluated further by the measurement of the serum testosterone level.

There are currently three validated questionnaires addressing symptoms and findings related to Andropause. They include the ADAM (Androgen Deficiency in Aging Men) Questionnaire (developed at Saint Louis University), findings from MMAS (Massachusetts Male Aging Study), and a questionnaire that was developed in Germany to assess symptoms associated with aging in men and subsequently validated in an English version (Heinemann LAJ, 1999, 2001). Each questionnaire has unique features and some deficiencies.

Positive responders to one of the questionnaires or to specific questions related to androgen deficiency should then be evaluated further for biochemical verification of androgen deficiency.

What are the absolute and relative contraindications to TRT?

Absolute contraindications include: 1) documented prostate cancer; 2) existing or prior history of breast cancer; 3) sensitivity to ingredients in T formulations; and 4) hematocrit ≥55%.*

Relative contraindications to TRT are: 1) hematocrit ≥52%; 2) untreated sleep apnea; 3) severe obstructive symptoms of BPH; and 4) advanced congestive heart failure (CHF).
* some members of the panel would lower the threshold to ≥52%.

What are the treatment options for andropause?

A variety of T formulations are available for TRT, including injectable T esters, transdermal T patches and gel, trocar-introduced T pellets, and oral testosterone undecanoate capsules (an approved drug in Europe and Canada but not currently available in the United States). The goal is to attain blood levels of testosterone as close to that of the young men's as possible, avoiding the peaks and valleys seen with some preparations. Some formulations and injection schedules provide more physiological levels than others; however, multiple factors must be considered when selecting a specific treatment for an individual patient.

What factors should be used in selecting T formulations and delivery systems to treat patients with andropause?

Many factors influence selection of a delivery system for a given patient: pharmacokinetics (eg, peak and valley, constant levels, and diurnal pattern); preparation-specific adverse effects (eg, skin irritability); adherence (specifically, in the case of testosterone patches); frequency of administration; flexibility of dosing; reversibility in case of adverse effects; patient preference; and cost. While costs associated with treatment is a concern, the optimal choice of therapy should be based primarily on the clinical diagnosis and needs of the patient. Cost of each treatment option may vary according to region, dosage, route of application (ie, office visit vs. self-application), and availability of generic agents. At the present time, the descending order of cost is: gel>patches>injectables.

At this time there is little information comparing efficacy and side effects using different delivery systems in the same patients.

What are the goals in treating andropause?

Treatment goals include: 1) restoring metabolic parameters to the eugonadal state; 2) increasing muscle mass, strength, and function; 3) maintaining BMD and reducing fracture risk; 4) improving neuropsychological function (cognition and mood); 5) improving psychosexual function; and 6) enhancing quality of life.

Are sufficient data available to state that these goals of TRT in andropause will be attained?

To date, small-scale (<108 subjects), short-term (less than 3-year) studies have provided evidence that TRT improves body composition, muscle strength and power, BMD, and cognition in testosterone-deficient men. Several studies of older, hypogonadal men have confirmed that TRT is also associated with improvements in lean body mass, grip strength, BMD, and reductions in fat mass. However, the effects of TRT on fracture rates, physical function, mood and affect, psychosexual function, quality of life, and cardiovascular event rates and atherosclerosis progression are not known. No clinical trials have evaluated the effects of TRT on fracture rates. Epidemiological data suggest that men with low testosterone levels may have a higher prevalence of coronary artery disease than those with normal testosterone levels. Short-term studies indicate that T may decrease angina; however, long-term data from controlled clinical trials evaluating the effects of TRT on cardiovascular disease and atherosclerosis progression are lacking.

What are the risks of TRT in andropause?

The risks of TRT in aging men include gynecomastia, acne, an increase in hematocrit (>55%*), and sleep apnea. It has also been speculated that TRT may cause an occult adenocarcinoma of the prostate to become clinically apparent. In addition, TRT might lead to growth of the prostate and lead to clinical worsening of signs and symptoms of BPH. While potential concerns of the medical community, neither of these drug-related adverse events on the prostate gland has been objectively demonstrated in controlled clinical trials. While TRT may prove to be cardioprotective (see above), testosterone in large doses may lower HDLC levels and adversely affect thrombosis or thrombolysis; thus, TRT could increase cardiovascular risk.
* some members of the panel would lower the threshold to ≥52%.

What is the risk/benefit ratio of TRT in andropause?

Data for both long-term risks and benefits are limited. Long-term data on outcomes and adverse effects are required to adequately assess the risk/benefit ratio.

What is the correct dose of testosterone?

The panel reached consensus on the following: 1) dosage depends on the preparation and its individual pharmacokinetics; and 2) the ideal level of hormone replacement is unknown since different target organs exhibit different dose-response characteristics in terms of benefits and risks. The physician should aim to achieve serum testosterone levels in the

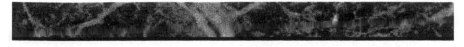

midnormal range for healthy, young men, and select the lowest dose that gives positive effects on desired end points.

How, and with what frequency, should andropause patients be monitored?

Since the goal is to maintain testosterone levels in the mid-normal range, a combination of clinical and biochemical measures should be monitored 6 to12 weeks after initiating TRT. For most patients, a serum total T is adequate, but if the clinical or biochemical responses are inconsistent, a calculated or measured serum free T or bioavailable T should be determined. No "absolute level" of testosterone can be cited as a target until more comprehensive data about risk/benefit relationships become available. Mid-normal range testosterone levels should be obtained at 7 days if a patient is receiving an injection of testosterone enanthate or cypionate every 2 weeks, at 3 to10 hours after application of a testosterone patch (q 24 hours), and at any time after applying transdermal gel (q 24 hours).

- Dosage adjustments should be made between 6 weeks and 3 months after starting treatment.
- Patients using transdermal preparations should be queried about skin irritation or other reactions.
- Serum prostate specific antigen (PSA) and digital rectal examination (DRE) of the prostate should be performed before treatment, at 3 and 6 months after initiating treatment, and then annually.
- If an increase in PSA of ≥1.5 ng/mL/year is verified on repeat testing, if there is an average annual increase of ≥0.75 ng/mL over a minimum of 2 years, or if the PSA is greater than 4.0 ng/mL, urological consultation should be obtained.
- Hematocrit should be checked at the same frequency as serum PSA.

CONCLUSION

Age-related decline in serum T is associated with loss of muscle mass and strength, an increase in fat mass, a decrease in BMD, an increase in the incidence of osteoporosis, loss of libido, erectile dysfunction, impairment of neuropsychological function, and some regression of secondary sexual characteristics. The potential benefits of TRT are improvements in body composition, muscle mass, strength and function, BMD with a reduction of fracture, neuropsychological function (cognition and mood), psychosexual function, and quality of life. The potential risks of TRT in aging men include gynecomastia, acne, an elevated hematocrit, and an increase in the incidence of sleep apnea. There also is concern that TRT may cause an occult prostate cancer to become a clinical prostate cancer or that there will be an increased need for invasive treatment of BPH. There is some reason to think that pharmacological doses of TRT may increase cardio-vascular risk.

An increase in our aging population may result in greater attention paid to the physiological and psychological effects of hypogonadism and other age-related health problems. More clinical trials are needed to assess the long-term benefits and risks of TRT in aging men.

REVIEWS

Bhasin S, Buckwalter JG. Testosterone supplementation in older men: a rational idea whose time has not yet come. *J Androl.* 2001;22:718-731.

Kandeel FR, Koussa VKT, Swerdloff RS. Male sexual function and its disorders: physiology, pathophysiology, clinical investigation, and treatment. *Endocr Rev.* 2001;22:342-388.

Matsumoto AM. Andropause: clinical implications of the decline in serum testosterone levels with aging in men. *J Gerontol A Biol Sci Med Sci.* 2002;57:M76-M99.

Vermeulen A. Androgen replacement therapy in the aging male—a critical evaluation. *J Clin Endocrinol Metab.* 2001;86:2380-2390.

TESTOSTERONE ASSAYS

Rosner W. Errors in the measurement of plasma free testosterone. *J Clin Endocrinol Metab.* 1997;82:2014-2015.

Vermeulen A, Verdonck L, Kaufman JM. A critical evaluation of simple methods for the estimation of free testosterone in serum. *J Clin Endocrinol Metab.* 1999;84:3666-3672.

Winters SJ, Kelley DE, Goodpaster B. The analog free testosterone assay: are the results in men clinically useful? *Clin Chem.* 1998; 44:2178-2182.

EFFECT OF AGE ON SERUM T AND FREQUENCY OF TESTOSTERONE DEFICIENCY IN AGING MEN

Feldman HA, Longcope C, Derby CA, et al. Age trends in the level of serum testosterone and other hormones in middle-aged men: longitudinal results from the Massachusetts male aging study. *J Clin Endocrinol Metab.* 2002;87:589-598.

Gray A, Berlin JA, McKinlay JB, Longcope C. An examination of research design effects on the association of testosterone and male aging: results of a meta-analysis. *J Clin Epidemiol.* 1991; 44:671-684.

Gray A, Feldman HA, McKinlay JB, Longcope C. Age, disease, and changing sex hormone levels in middle-aged men: results of the Massachusetts Male Aging Study. *J Clin Endocrinol Metab.* 1991; 73:1016-1025.

Harman SM, Metter EJ, Tobin JD, Pearson J, Blackman MR. Longitudinal effects of aging on serum total and free testosterone levels in healthy men. Baltimore Longitudinal Study of Aging. *J Clin Endocrinol Metab.* 2001;86:724-731.

Heinemann LA, Zimmermann T, Vermeulen A, Thiel C, Hummel W. A new 'aging males' symptoms' rating scale. *The Aging Male.* 1999; 2:105-114.

Heinemann LA, Saad F, Thiele K, Wood-Dauphinee S. The Aging Males' Symptoms rating scale: cultural and linguistic validation into English. *The Aging Male.* 2001;4:14-22.

Morley JE, Charlton E, Patrick P, et al. Validation of a screening questionnaire for androgen deficiency in aging males. *Metab.* 2000;49:1239-1242.

Morley JE, Kaiser FE, Perry HM 3ʳᵈ, et al. Longitudinal changes in testosterone, luteinizing hormone, and follicle-stimulating hormone in healthy older men. *Metab.* 1997;46:410-413.

HEALTH CONSEQUENCES OF AGING AND TESTOSTERONE DEFICIENCY

Alexandersen P, Haarbo J, Christiansen C. The relationship of natural androgens to coronary heart disease in males: a review. *Atherosclerosis.* 1996;125:1-13.

Barrett-Connor E, Khaw KT. Endogenous sex hormones and cardiovascular disease in men. A prospective population-based study. *Circ.* 1988;78:539-545.

Barrett-Connor E, von Mühlen DG, Kritz-Silverstein D. Bioavailable testosterone and depressed mood in older men: the Rancho Bernardo Study. *J Clin Endocrinol Metab.* 1999;84:573-577.

Baumgartner RN, Koehler KM, Gallagher D, et al. Epidemiology of sarcopenia among the elderly in New Mexico. *Am J Epidemiol.* 1998;147:755-763.

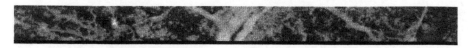

Cooper C, Atkinson EJ, O'Fallon WM, Melton LJ 3ʳᵈ. Incidence of clinically diagnosed vertebral fractures: A population-based study in Rochester, Minnesota, 1985-1989. *J Bone Miner Res.* 1992;7:221-227.

Forbes GB, Reina JC. Adult lean body mass declines with age: some longitudinal observations. *Metab.* 1970;19:653-663.

Frontera WR, Hughes VA, Fielding RA, Fiatarone MA, Evans WJ, Roubenoff R. Aging of skeletal muscle: a 12-year longitudinal study. *J Appl Physiol.* 2000;88:1321-1326.

Gallagher D, Ruts E, Visser M, et al. Weight stability masks sarcopenia in elderly men and women. *Am J Physiol Endocrinol Metab.* 2000; 279:E366-E375.

Gallagher D, Visser M, De Meersman RE, et al. Appendicular skeletal muscle mass: effects of age, gender, and ethnicity. *J Appl Physiol.* 1997;83:229-239.

Khosla S, Melton LJ 3ʳᵈ, Atkinson EJ, O'Fallon WM, Klee GG, Riggs RL. Relationship of serum sex steroid levels and bone turnover markers with bone mineral density in men and women: a key role for bioavailable estrogen. *J Clin Endocrinol Metab.* 1998;83:2266-2274.

Marin P, Holmang S, Gustafsson C, et al. Androgen treatment of abdominally obese men. *Obes Res.* 1993;1:245-251.

TESTOSTERONE FORMULATIONS AND DELIVERY SYSTEMS

Bhasin S, Swerdloff RS, Steiner B, et al. A biodegradable testosterone microcapsule formulation provides uniform eugonadal levels of testosterone for 10-11 weeks in hypogonadal men. *J Clin Endocrinol Metab.* 1992;74:75-83.

Cunningham GR, Cordero E, Thornby JI. Testosterone replacement with transdermal therapeutic systems. Physiological serum testosterone and elevated dihydrotestosterone levels. *JAMA.* 1989;261:2525-2530.

Gooren LJ. A ten-year safety study of the oral androgen testosterone undecanoate. *J Androl.* 1994;15:212-215.

Handelsman DJ, Conway AJ, Boylan LM. Pharmacokinetics and pharmacodynamics of testosterone pellets in man. *J Clin Endocrinol Metab.* 1990;71:216-222.

Meikle AW, Mazer NA, Moellmer JF, et al. Enhanced transdermal delivery of testosterone across nonscrotal skin produces physiological concentrations of testosterone and its metabolites in hypogonadal men. *J Clin Endocrinol Metab.* 1992;74:623-628.

Nieschlag E, Mauss J, Coert A, Kicovic P. Plasma androgen levels in men after oral administration of testosterone or testosterone undecanoate. *Acta Endocrinol (Copenh).* 1975;79:366-374.

Salehian B, Wang C, Alexander G, et al. Pharmacokinetics, bioefficacy, and safety of sublingual testosterone cyclodextrin in hypogonadal men: comparison to testosterone enanthate—a clinical research center study. *J Clin Endocrinol Metab.* 1995;80:3567-3575.

Swerdloff RS, Wang C, Cunningham G, et al. Long-term pharmacokinetics of transdermal testosterone gel in hypogonadal men. The Testosterone Gel Study Group. *J Clin Endocrinol Metab.* 2000;85:4500-4510.

Wang C, Eyre DR, Clark R, et al. Sublingual testosterone replacement improves muscle mass and strength, decreases bone resorption and increases bone formation markers in hypogonadal men—a clinical research center study. *J Clin Endocrinol Metab.* 1996;81:3654-3662.

Wang C, Iranmanesh A, Berman N, et al. Comparative pharmacokinetics of three doses of percutaneous dihydrotestosterone gel in healthy elderly men—a clinical research center study. *J Clin Endocrinol Metab.* 1998;83:2749-2757.

Wang C, Swerdloff RS, Iranmanesh A, et al. Effects of transdermal testosterone gel on bone turnover markers and bone mineral density in hypogonadal men. *Clin Endocrinol (Oxf).* 2001;54:739-750.

Wang C, Swerdloff RS, Iranmanesh A, et al. Transdermal testosterone gel improves sexual function, mood, muscle strength, and body composition parameters in hypogonadal men. The Testosterone Study Group. *J Clin Endocrinol Metab.* 2000;85:2839-2853.

CLINICAL TRIALS WITH TRT IN AGING MEN

de Lignieres B. Transdermal dihydrotestosterone treatment of 'andropause'. *Ann Med.* 1993;25:235-241.

Kenny AM, Prestwood KM, Gruman CA, Marcello KM, Raisz LG. Effects of transdermal testosterone on bone and muscle in older men with low bioavailable testosterone levels. *J Gerontol A Biol Sci Med Sci.* 2001; 56:M266-M272.

Ly LP, Jimenez M, Zhuang TN, Celermajer DS, Conway AJ, Handelsman DJ. A double-blind, placebo-controlled, randomized clinical trial of transdermal dihydrotestosterone gel on muscular strength, mobility, and quality of life in older men with partial androgen deficiency. *J Clin Endocrinol Metab.* 2001;86:4078-4088.

Münzer T, Harman SM, Hees P, et al. Effects of GH and/or sex steroid administration on abdominal subcutaneous and visceral fat in healthy aged women and men. *J Clin Endocrinol Metab.* 2001;86:3604-3610.

Sih R, Morley JE, Kaiser FE, Perry HM, Patrick P, Ross C. Testosterone replacement in older hypogonadal men: a 12-month randomized controlled trial. *J Clin Endocrinol Metab.* 1997;82:1661-1667.

Snyder PJ, Peachey H, Hannoush P, et al. Effect of testosterone treatment on body composition and muscle strength in men over 65 years of age. *J Clin Endocrinol Metab.* 1999;84:2647-2653.

Snyder PJ, Peachey H, Hannoush P, et al. Effect of testosterone treatment on bone mineral density in men over 65 years of age. *J Clin Endocrinol Metab.* 1999;84:1966-1972.

Tenover JS. Effects of testosterone supplementation in the aging male. *J Clin Endocrinol Metab.* 1992;75:1092-1098.

ADDITIONAL READING

Bakhshi V, Elliott M, Gentili A, Godschalk M, Mulligan T. Testosterone improves rehabilitation outcomes in ill older men. *J Am Geriatr Soc.* 2000;48:550-553.

Barrett-Connor E, von Mühlen DG, Kritz-Silverstein D. Bioavailable testosterone and depressed mood in older men: the Rancho Bernardo Study. *J Clin Endocrinol Metab.* 1999;84:573-577.

Bhasin S, Storer TW, Berman N, et al. Testosterone replacement increases fat-free mass and muscle size in hypogonadal men. *J Clin Endocrinol Metab.* 1997;82:407-413.

Bhasin S, Woodhouse L, Casaburi R, et al. Testosterone dose-response relationships in healthy, young men. *Am J Physiol Endocrinol Metab.* 2001;281:E1172-E1181.

Christiansen K. Behavioural correlates of testosterone. In: Nieschlag E, Behre HM, eds. *Testosterone: action deficiency, substitution.* Berlin: Springer Verlag; 1998;107-142.

Forest G, Ruzza G, Mioni R, et al. Osteoporosis and decline of gonadal function in the elderly male. *Horm Res.* 1984;19:18-22.

Larsson L. Histochemical characteristics of human skeletal muscle during aging. *Acta Physiol Scand.* 1983;117:469-471.

Mills TM, Reilly CM, Lewis RW. Androgens and penile erection: a review. *J Androl.* 1996;17:633-638.

Orwoll ES, Klein RF. Osteoporosis in men. *Endocr Rev.* 1995;16:87-116.

Rabijewski M, Adamkiewica M, Zgliczynski S. The influence of testosterone replacement therapy on well-being, bone mineral density and lipids in elderly men. In: Abstracts of the Second World Congress on the Aging Male; February 2000; Geneva, Switzerland. Abstract 099.

Seidell JC, Bjorntorp P, Sjostrom L, Kvist H, Sannerstadt R. Visceral fat accumulation in men is positively associated with insulin, glucose, and C-peptide levels, but negatively with testosterone levels. *Metab.* 1990;39:897-901.

Swerdloff RS, Wang C. The testis and male sexual function. In: *Cecil Textbook of Medicine.* 21ˢᵗ ed. Philadelphia, PA: WB Saunders; 1999;1307-1317.

Tchernof A, Labrie F, Belanger A, et al. Relationships between endogenous steroid hormone, sex hormone-binding globulin and lipoprotein levels in men: contribution of visceral obesity, insulin levels and other metabolic variables. *Atherosclerosis.* 1997;133:235-244.

Tenover JS. Risks and benefits of testosterone in older men. In: VII International Congress of Andrology, 2001.

Vermeulen A, Goemaere S, Kaufman JM. Sex hormones, body composition and aging. *The Aging Male.* 1999;2:8-15.

MANAGEMENT RECOMMENDATIONS FOR ANDROGEN REPLACEMENT THERAPY IN ELDERLY MEN

1. Testosterone deficiency is a condition that occurs frequently in men over age 50.

2. Men over the age of 50 should be screened for androgen deficiency.

3. Initiate screening for testosterone deficiency by administering a questionnaire or by asking about relevant symptoms.

4. If responses to the questionnaire or questions suggest testosterone deficiency, measure an early morning serum testosterone level.

5. If the serum total testosterone concentration is <200 ng/dL, the diagnosis of androgen deficiency is confirmed. Rule out serious hypothalamic or pituitary disease in men with hypogonadotropic hypogonadism. First, measure serum LH and prolactin. If LH is subnormal or prolactin is elevated and the total testosterone is <150 ng/dL, an MRI with and without enhancement should be performed or the patient should be referred for endocrinological evaluation.

6. If the serum testosterone level is >200 and <400 ng/dL, calculate free testosterone from total testosterone and SHBG concentrations, or measure an early morning free testosterone by the dialysis method or bioavailable testosterone by ammonium sulfate precipitation.

7. If the serum testosterone is low compared with healthy, young men ages 20-40 years, look for diseases, drugs, and lifestyle factors associated with low testosterone levels. If possible, provide specific treatment for the underlying condition.

8. The following steps are required before initiating treatment:

   A. Exclusion of absolute contraindications (prostate cancer, breast cancer, hematocrit ≥55%, sensitivity to ingredients in T formulations)
   B. Consideration of relative contraindications (hematocrit ≥52%, severe obstructive sleep apnea, severe congestive heart failure, severe obstructive symptoms of BPH)

9. If there are no contraindications, obtain baseline measurements of:
   A. Hematocrit
   B. Prostate specific antigen (PSA), and
   C. Perform DRE of the prostate

10. If symptoms of androgen deficiency exist, and the patient has low testosterone levels with no contraindications, consider initiation of testosterone treatment.

   A. Discuss goals and potential risks of treatment with patients
   B. Provide patient education
   C. Explain to patient that TRT should aim to provide physiological levels of testosterone
   D. In consultation with the patient, choose a delivery system for TRT based upon pharmacokinetics (eg, peak and valley, constant level, and diurnal pattern); preparation-specific adverse effects (eg, skin irritability); adherence characteristics (in the case of testosterone patches); frequency of administration; flexibility of dosing; reversibility in case of adverse effects; patient preference; and cost.
   E. Obtain a baseline measurement of BMD (DEXA scan)

11. Monitoring

   A. Assess efficacy and potential adverse effects of therapy 6 to 12 weeks after initiating TRT, at 6 months, and then annually.
   B. Assess efficacy by evaluating:
      1) Clinical responses (including changes in affect)
      2) Serum testosterone levels with the goal of a mid-normal range level at:
         a. 7 days after injection of testosterone enanthate or cypionate (q 2 weeks)
         b. 3 to10 hours after application of a testosterone patch (q 24 hours)
         c. any time after application of a testosterone gel (q 24 hours)
   C. Assess potential adverse effects by evaluating:
      1) Hematocrit
      2) PSA
      3) DRE (refer to a urologist if there is any change in the prostate examination)
      4) Sleep apnea.

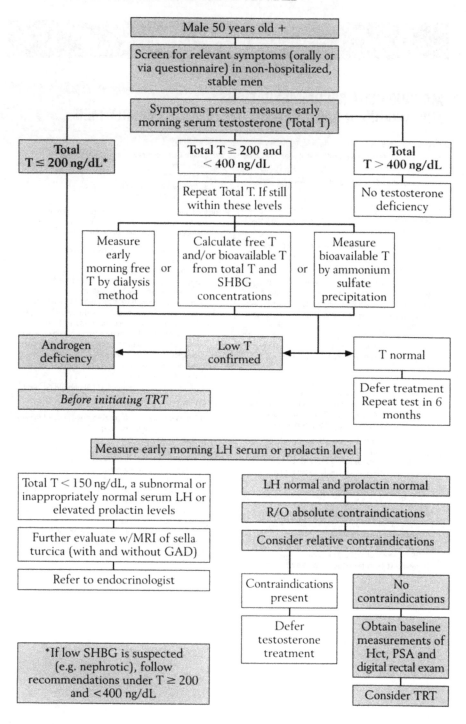

Appendix 1C.
Testosterone pellet implantation

INTRODUCTION

The technique described is based on that of Dr Tiberius Reiter[1], who, in the 1950s and 1960s, treated over 200 patients in his London clinic using the method, with considerable clinical success[2-4]. It has proved reliable in over 1200 implants performed by myself over the past 15 years in the London Andropause Clinic.

PREPARATION OF THE IMPLANT SITE

The site routinely used for testosterone pellet implantation in the male is the buttock. This is preferable to the frequently described lower abdominal wall location[5] because of the greater ease of applying pressure to achieve homeostasis after the procedure, and reduced irritation of articles of clothing such as belts and tight trousers.

After cleaning the skin with an antiseptic routinely used for minor surgical procedures, such as Hibitane®, the track to be used for trochar insertion of the pellets is anesthetized with 5 ml of 2% Xylocaine® (lignocaine), using a hypodermic needle at least 2½–3 in. long, passing from the outer upper quadrant of the buttock diagonally towards the natal cleft to a depth of 1–2 in.

PREPARATION OF THE IMPLANT MATERIALS

The materials required are:

(1) Testosterone pellet implants: experience has shown that 6–10 of the 200-mg pellet implants are required to last the patient 6 months, the generally preferred and most economical implantation interval. These are available from either the local suppliers of Organon pharmaceuticals,

or, in the USA, Food and Drug Administration (FDA)-approved manufacturers such as Bartor Pharmacal Co. Inc. of Rye, New York, who also make an excellent range of implantation trochars.

Organon pellets traditionally come individually packed with cotton wool inside their sterile glass ampoules. This can make the pellet very difficult to extract, and the cotton wool tends to adhere to it, which may account for some of the 'foreign-body' rejections of the pellets which occur weeks or even months later. This cotton-wool 'beard' can be removed by rotating the implant within a fold of gauze held in the sterile gloved hand. Manufacturers who package various multiples of pellets without encasing them in seemingly unnecessary cotton wool would help to save a great deal of time for the doctor and discomfort for the patient when the implants are rejected.

(2) Trochars: unless exceptionally good autoclave sterilization services are available, disposable plastic trochars and cannulae are preferred, such as those provided by Femcare (Urosurgical Ltd., Guildford, Surrey GU4 7WA, UK).

(3) Small basic procedure pack, scalpel and dressings: the disposable pack should have forceps, gauze and cotton-wool swabs inside the plastic tray, which also preferably has a separate compartment into which the pellets can be dropped from their sterile glass ampoules.

The scalpel, or scalpel blade alone, should be small, e.g. size 11, as an incision only large enough to allow the cannula to be inserted is required, and this needs no suture, although small strips of tape can be used to bring the wound edges together.

The dressing applied should be either water-resistant or waterproof, to allow it to remain in place for a week, until the wound has healed.

THE PROCEDURE

After a small incision is made, the trochar with obturator in place is inserted along the anesthetized track in the subcutaneous fat to a distance of 2–3 in. The obturator is then withdrawn and, using the forceps, the pellets, either one or two at a time, are introduced into the trochar, which is supported by a sterile gloved hand held underneath to catch any that may miss the opening, expelled into the fat in a fan-shaped pattern.

Even though successive implant procedures are done in opposite buttocks, especially where there has been previous pellet rejection, there may be considerable scar tissue in the buttock, and an area slightly to one side of the track of previous implants should be chosen.

The number of implants required is kept to the minimum to maintain the patient in a symptom-free state for 5–6 months, although many patients can tolerate a few weeks with minimal symptoms reminding them of their pretreatment state. Others may prefer supplements of oral, transdermal or injected testosterone to tide them over the gap in implant activity, and the 2 weeks it takes after the procedure until testosterone levels are restored.

Firm pressure is applied to the implant site for several minutes after the trochar is withdrawn, and the dressing is then applied. Special care is needed to prevent excessive bleeding at the implant site if patients are on anticoagulants, and regular medication with aspirin may be withdrawn for a week before and after the procedure. The patient is advised to keep the dressing in place for a week, and not to exercise vigorously for 3–4 days after implantation, to minimize the chances of bruising and rejection.

A brief course of antibiotic cover, such as Augmentin®, may be given, with stronger and longer courses of agents such as Ciproxin® given to the few who get recurrent infections.

A detailed instructional film on CD of the testosterone implantation procedure is available on application to the author.

References

1. Reiter T. Testosterone implantation: the method of choice for treatment of testosterone deficiency. *J Am Geriatr Soc* 1965;13:1003–12
2. Reiter T, Horn H, Ben-Uzilio R, Finkelstein M. Plasma levels of testosterone in ageing male patients following implantation of testosterone. *J Am Geriatr Soc* 1964;12:515–16
3. Reiter T. Testosterone implantation: a clinical study of 240 implantations in ageing males. *J Am Geriatr Soc* 1963;11:540–50
4. Reiter T. Treatment of male climacteric by combined implantation. *Practitioner* 1953;170:181
5. Handelsman DJ. Clinical pharmacology of testosterone pellet implants. In Neischlag E, Behre HM, eds. *Testosterone: Action, Deficiency, Substitution.* Heidelberg: Springer, 1998:349–64

Appendix 2A. The Aging Males' Symptoms questionnarie

Aging Males' Symptoms (AMS) questionnaire. Taken from Lunenfeld B, Gooren L, eds. *Textbook of Men's Health*. London: Parthenon Publishing, 2002:34

Which of the following symptoms apply to you at this time? Please, mark the appropriate box for each symptom. For symptoms that do not apply, please mark "none".

	Symptoms				
	none	mild	moderate	severe	extremely severe
Score =	1	2	3	4	5
1. Decline in your feeling of general well-being (general state of health, subjective feeling)	☐	☐	☐	☐	☐
2. Joint pain and muscular ache (lower back pain, joint pain, pain in a limb, general back ache)	☐	☐	☐	☐	☐
3. Excessive sweating (unexpected/sudden episodes of sweating, hot flushes independent of strain)	☐	☐	☐	☐	☐
4. Sleep problems (difficulty in falling asleep, difficulty in sleeping through, waking up early and feeling tired, poor sleep, sleeplessness)	☐	☐	☐	☐	☐
5. Increased need for sleep, often feeling tired	☐	☐	☐	☐	☐
6. Irritability (feeling aggressive, easily upset about little things, moody)	☐	☐	☐	☐	☐
7. Nervousness (inner tension, restlessness, feeling fidgety)	☐	☐	☐	☐	☐
8. Anxiety (feeling panicky)	☐	☐	☐	☐	☐
9. Physical exhaustion / lacking vitality (general decrease in performance, reduced activity, lacking interest in leisure activities, feeling of getting less done, of achieving less, of having to force oneself to undertake activities)	☐	☐	☐	☐	☐
10. Decrease in muscular strength (feeling of weakness)	☐	☐	☐	☐	☐
11. Depressive mood (feeling down, sad, on the verge of tears, lack of drive, mood swings, feeling nothing is of any use)	☐	☐	☐	☐	☐
12. Feeling that you have passed your peak	☐	☐	☐	☐	☐
13. Feeling burnt out, having hit rock-bottom	☐	☐	☐	☐	☐
14. Decrease in beard growth	☐	☐	☐	☐	☐
15. Decrease in ability/frequency to perform sexually	☐	☐	☐	☐	☐
16. Decrease in the number of morning erections	☐	☐	☐	☐	☐
17. Decrease in sexual desire/libido (lacking pleasure in sex, lacking desire for sexual intercourse)	☐	☐	☐	☐	☐

Have you got any other major symptoms? Yes ☐ No ☐
If Yes, please describe: _____

THANK YOU VERY MUCH FOR YOUR COOPERATION

EVALUATION FORM

This form explains how the total score and the scores of the subscales are determined

Question number	Score	Psychological subscale	Somatic subscale	Sexual subscale
1			......	
2			......	
3			......	
4			......	
5			......	
6		......		
7		......		
8		......		
9			......	
10			......	
11		......		
12				......
13		......		
14				......
15				......
16				......
17				......
		....	....	....
Total sum of all subscales = Total score:				

Scores	Severity of complaints
17–26	no
27–36	little
37–49	moderate
≥ 50	severe

Appendix 2B.
Andropause Clinic forms

Including Andropause Check List (ACL) questionnaire (available in Access Database format on application to the author)

PRIVATE AND CONFIDENTIAL

SURNAME:

FIRST NAME:

Personal No: DOB: Initial contact:

Sent Info: GP letter sent: Cancellation date:

Personal Data

Marital State:

Age at introduction:

Occupation:

Phone – home:

Phone – work: Consultant:

Phone – mobile: Source:

Fax: Referral:

Address:

Mailing? ☐

Alt Address:

Mailing? ☐

GP Name:

GP Address:

SURNAME: [   ]   PIN: [   ]

FIRST NAME: [   ]   DOB: [   ]

Presenting Problems (Duration – years)

1. [   ]

2. [   ]

3. [   ]

4. [   ]

5. [   ]

6. [   ]

Other Problems (Years ago)

(BP   CVD   VV   DVT   AN   RH   OA   OP   GF   UTI   DM   JAU   EP   MIG   ANX   DEP)

1. [   ]

2. [   ]

3. [   ]

4. [   ]

5. [   ]

6. [   ]

SURNAME: [ ]   PIN: [ ]

FIRST NAME: [ ]   DOB: [ ]

Testicular Problems	years ago	comments
Nondescent	[ ]	[ ]
Mumps	[ ]	[ ]
Vasectomy	[ ]	[ ]
Trauma	[ ]	[ ]
Hydrocele	[ ]	[ ]
Variocele	[ ]	[ ]
Hernia	[ ]	[ ]
Appendectomy	[ ]	[ ]
Toxic drugs	[ ]	[ ]
Other	[ ]	[ ]

Urinary Problems	severity	comments
Hesitancy	[ ]	[ ]
Poor stream	[ ]	[ ]
Nocturia	[ ]	[ ]
Incontinence	[ ]	[ ]
Urgency	[ ]	[ ]
Hematuria	[ ]	[ ]
Dysuria	[ ]	[ ]
Dribble	[ ]	[ ]

Present Medications	years	comments
Tranquilizers	[ ]	[ ]
Sleeping pills	[ ]	[ ]
Beta-blockers	[ ]	[ ]
Heart or BP		[ ]
Antidepressants		[ ]
Painkillers	[ ]	[ ]
Stomach, Gut	[ ]	[ ]
Antibiotics		[ ]
Other	[ ]	[ ]

Smoking   Stopped for   Started

[ ] per day [ ] years [ ] years ago

Alcohol

present units/week: [ ]

previous max units/week: [ ] [ ] years ago

Exercise

1. Pres mins/week: [ ] – prev mins/week: [ ]

   of [ ]

2. Pres mins/week: [ ] – prev mins/week: [ ]

   of [ ]

3. Pres mins/week: [ ] – prev mins/week: [ ]

   of [ ]

Notes

[ ]

SURNAME: [   ]   PIN: [   ]

FIRST NAME: [   ]   DOB: [   ]

Family History

	Age	Health	Age at Death
Father	[ ]	[ ]	[ ]
Mother	[ ]	[ ]	[ ]

Brothers/Sisters

Sex	Age	Health	Age at Death
[ ]	[ ]	[ ]	[ ]
[ ]	[ ]	[ ]	[ ]
[ ]	[ ]	[ ]	[ ]
[ ]	[ ]	[ ]	[ ]

Marriage/Relationship

Yr. Began	Ended				
[ ]	[ ]	[ ]	[ ]	[ ]	[ ]
[ ]	[ ]	[ ]	[ ]	[ ]	[ ]
[ ]	[ ]	[ ]	[ ]	[ ]	[ ]

Children

Rel. No.				
[ ]	[ ]	[ ]	[ ]	[ ]
[ ]	[ ]	[ ]	[ ]	[ ]
[ ]	[ ]	[ ]	[ ]	[ ]
[ ]	[ ]	[ ]	[ ]	[ ]

Psychosocial History

[   ]

ANDROPAUSE CHECK LIST   SURNAME: [   ]   PIN: [   ]
Severty: 0, none; 1, slight;
     2, moderate; 3, severe; 4, total   FIRST NAME: [   ]   DOB: [   ]

VISIT No.	1	2	3	4	5	6	7	8	9	10
Duration / Medic'n										
Fatigue										
Depression										
Irritability										
Memory										
Skin Cond.										
Sweating										
Vasomotor										
Aches and Pains										
Aging										
Libido Self										
Libido Partner										
Erect. Init										
Erect. Sust										
Erect. a.m.										
Ejac. Prem										
Ejac. Delay										
Orgasm Partner										
Sex. sat. Self										
Sex. sat. Partner										
Gen. Rel. Partner										
Total ACL										
Inter. freq. M										
Inter. freq. D										
Mast. freq. M										
Mast. freq. D										
Total Sex										

BIO and EXAMINATION DATA

Severty: 0, none; 1, slight;
2, moderate:
3, severe; 4, total

SURNAME: [   ]   PIN· [   ]

FIRST NAME: [   ]   DOB: [   ]

BIO DATA	Visit #	1	2	3	4	5	6	7	8	9	10
	weight/kilos										
	height/cm										
	BP1										
	BP2										
	pulse										
	PEF										
	Hip										
	Waist										
	WH/ratio										
EXAM DATA	baldness										
	color										
	beard										
	body										
	axillary										
	pubic										
SKIN:	dryness										
	elasticity										
GYNECOMASTIA											
SCARS											
PENIS:	atrophy										
	foreskin										
SCROTUM:	abnormality										
	development										
TESTES:	R abnorm.										
	R vol.										
	L. abnorm.										
	L. vol.										
PROSTATE:	abnorm.										
	vol.										

VISIT NOTES NAME: [ ] PIN: [ ]

Visit No: [ ] ATTENDANCE DATE: [ ] LAB REF: [ ]

The Physical Examination/Progress showed:

[ ]

The Endocrinology showed:

[ ]

The Biochemistry showed:

[ ]

The Hematology showed:

[ ]

The Urine Chemistry showed:

[ ]

Treatment/Progress:

[ ]

Appendix 3. The UK Andropause Study

INTRODUCTION

The UK Andropause Study (UKAS) is an ongoing analysis of the findings of my clinical work in the Gold Cross Andropause Clinic in Harley Street since it was established in 1989. It is presented to add my personal experience to the work of others, which makes up the main text of the book.

Though the studies reported were not blinded because of the nature of the practice, and the subjective parts of them can be possibly considered as biased, I have tried to make the observations as objective as possible. The laboratory data is given according to the hospital and major independent laboratories reporting them.

The study is a cross-sectional survey of the symptomatology, physiological and psychological findings, and also presents laboratory results of the patients diagnosed as andropausal after full clinical and laboratory profiling during their first visit to the clinic, together with an audit of the responses to different forms of testosterone and other treatment as seen at the follow-up visits. These were usually at 3 months after the first visit, and subsequently at 6-monthly intervals for up to 12 years.

It is appreciated that there are several unavoidable potential sources of bias. Firstly, the findings could be biased towards the cases that respond well clinically, and who therefore wish to continue treatment. However, as far as possible we have followed-up patients who did not originally respond to one form of treatment, and provide them with another that gave them the required results.

Secondly, a holistic approach to treatment was used, with advice and encouragement where needed on stress, alcohol and weight reduction, as well as increasing physical activity and other life-style modifications. However, these were often difficult for the patient to achieve and maintain even with the improved mood and energy induced by testosterone treatment.

Also, where there were other clinical conditions needing intervention, such as hypertension, hyperlipidemia or diabetes, the additional treatment given may have distorted the response attributable to testosterone alone.

Thirdly, the patients did not live in an experimental vacuum, and in the many years of treatment they and their partners could be subject to major life events that may in some cases have influenced their responses to the various interventions. These included relationship break-ups, job-losses, retirement and bereavement. In general however, it was felt that the large number of cases studied evened out these variations in extraneous influences.

Ethical considerations

The retrospective audit of the results of the various treatments was approved by the St Mary's Hospital Local Research Ethics Committee (LREC). Patients gave informed consent to the anonymous use of their data, and where a new product such as Viagra® was concerned, gave written informed consent while it was off-license and being used on a named-patients-only basis.

None of the research was sponsored by grants from any pharmaceutical company and other than being a director of the company owning the clinic, which also was in the process of obtaining a usage patent on danazol, there were no conflicts of interest.

METHODS AND STATISTICS

As far as is possible over the 15-year period of the study, methodology in the clinic was kept constant. Standardized records were kept in the format given in Appendix 2b. The basic patient notes were filled in by hand on the first and subsequent visits, and later entered into the computerized practice management system in a Microsoft Access database.

Full biographical data was recorded on page 1, including current relationships and details of occupation.

The history of presenting problems on page 2 was taken in the patient's own words, and the duration of each assessed. The previous problems history, on the same page, was taken with special reference to conditions that might contribute to the causation of andropause as listed in Chapter 3. Abbreviations were used to prompt routine questioning about hypertension (BP), cardiovascular disease (CVD), varicose veins (VV), deep vein thrombosis (DVT), rheumatic disease (RH), arthritis (AR), osteoporosis (OP), glandular fever or infectious mononucleosis (GF), urinary tract infection (UTI) including non-specific urethritis and sexually transmitted diseases (STDs), diabetes mellitus (DM), jaundice (JAU), epilepsy (EP), migraine (MIG), anxiety (ANX) and depression (DEP).

The history of conditions that might affect the testis on page 3 included

non or late descent, mumps after the age of ten, vasectomy, trauma, hydrocele, varicocele, inguinal hernia operations, appendectomy, toxic drugs –
either abuse such as cannabis or industrial exposure e.g. agrochemicals or
welding – and any other agents that might influence testicular function.

Present medications, also on page 3, included tranquillizers, sleeping
pills, beta-blockers, drugs for heart or blood-pressure, antidepressants,
painkillers, drugs for the stomach or gut, antibiotics, and any other compounds, such as DHEA or alpha-blocking drugs that might have either a
positive or negative effect on testosterone production or action, or erectile
function.

Present urinary symptoms enquired for symptoms of hesitancy, poor
stream, nocturia, incontinence, urgency, hematuria, dysuria or dribble,
grading each from 0 (no problem) to 4 (extreme).

Smoking in terms of number of cigarettes smoked per day, over what
period of years, enabled a rough calculation of total time spent smoking,
which is considered to be the reduction in life expectancy due to the
smoking habit, and may bear a relationship to ED.

Exercise history past and present was also included.

The family history on page 4 included the age and significant illnesses in
parents, brothers and sisters, partners and children, living and dead. Particular enquiries were made about benign and malignant prostatic disease in
male relatives. A brief psychosocial history was also taken, especially to
assess the sexual history, and partners' reactions to sexual problems, as well
as the general state of the relationship. Quite often the partner attended
the initial interview, but areas that might be difficult to discuss were left
until the patient was alone.

Andropause Check List

The key diagnostic questionnaire, the Andropause Check List (ACL, Carruthers 1998[1]) on page 5 was developed from the list of symptoms given in
various articles quoted in Chapter 4. It has been validated to a large extent
by the work carried out by other clinicians more recently, such as Vermeulen[2] and Morley[3], and by cross-correlation with the Heinemann Aging
Male Symptoms (AMS) scale[2] as reported in Chapter 4.

It was administered by the same clinician (MEC) at the initial and subsequent interviews, asking the patient in a non-leading way to rate the
current severity of each symptom on a five-point scale, from none (0),
slight (1), moderate (2), severe (3) to total (4). The initial score, together
with the duration of symptoms, gave a baseline for assessing the effectiveness of any given treatment, and provided a structured format for the
follow-up interviews as well as group data on the effectiveness of that treatment in relieving andropausal symptoms.

The sexual activity questionnaire at the bottom of the ACL included the
monthly frequency of both intercourse and masturbation at the initial and

subsequent visits, and also the maximum daily frequency of both. These provided some further evaluation of the initial state, and response to treatment. At the first visit, a note was made of the duration in years of the symptom, with times less than 1 year being recorded as 1 year. This could be used to establish the time of onset of the symptoms, and sometimes helped to establish their causes, such as stress, break-up of a relationship or starting a particular medication.

Physical examination

The physical examination (page 6) began with systolic and diastolic blood pressure measurements, together with pulse rate, which were recorded at least twice at each visit, using an Omron automatic inflating sphygmomanometer, and the lowest of each entered on the record sheet.

This was followed by measurement of weight and height on accurate scales (Weymed Ltd, London), from which Body Mass Index (BMI) could be calculated. Where there was a history of loss of height, suggesting osteoporosis, the patient's reported initial height was also recorded. Hip and waist circumference measurements enabled abdominal obesity to be assessed, together with its response to treatment, but were seldom recorded in practice.

The remainder of the physical examination data was recorded in numerical form, for ease of data entry and analysis. The presence or absence of each sign was recorded as normal (0), slight (1), moderate (2), severe (3) or total (4). Where ultrasound measurements of testicular or prostatic volumes were taken, these were also entered on the visit record. Brief descriptions of any salient features such as gynecomastia, abdominal scars or testicular masses were also recorded. The patient was initially examined standing for herniae and testicular abnormalities, especially varicocele. More detailed scrotal and testicular examination was then performed with the patient lying, and finally a digital rectal examination was routinely performed.

Laboratory methodology

To minimize endocrine changes due to diurnal variation, and to clarify changes in metabolites such as glucose and lipids, as far as possible samples were taken at 9–10 am after an overnight fast, with nothing except water and any medication from midnight the previous night. Though oral medications such as testosterone undecanoate had been taken 2–4 hours previously, as the patients were fasting it is unlikely that peak values were measured in these fasting samples because it is normally absorbed in the chylomicrons from fatty food. Similarly, except where initially some 3-month readings were taken, samples taken at the end of each 6-month implant cycle were likely to show trough values.

For the first year of the study, samples were sent to the laboratories of Charing Cross Hospital in London. Later, three major local commercial laboratories were used in succession: Technical Laboratory Services Ltd, UniLabs and for the last 5 years, Quest Diagnostics Limited. The comparability of results, and adherence to national and international quality control procedures, were carefully monitored throughout.

Forms of treatment

Patients were initially put on one of two oral preparations. The more commonly used was testosterone undecanoate (TU – Restandol®) manufactured by Organon as 40 mg capsules. As emphasized in Chapter 5, it was important that this form was taken with taken with food, since absorption of this oily preparation is supposed to occur mainly via chylomicrons passing into the intestinal lymphatic system. This could cause irregular absorption according to the fat content of the meal, and some clinicians recommend that it is taken together with omega-3 fish oil capsules. Also, when testosterone was estimated in blood samples from fasting patients taking this preparation, because of the poor absorption in the absence of fat, artificially low hormone levels could be reported.

Another important detail is that unopened stock bottles of this preparation should be stored in the refrigerator at 4°C, as pharmacists are instructed to do, and several patients reported that capsules kept in a warm bathroom cabinet seemed to lose their efficacy after a month or two. Opened bottles should be kept in a cool place, but not refrigerated, as this is thought to cause separation of the long-chain formulation of testosterone from the oleic acid in which it is suspended, though this re-dissolves after a few hours at room temperature.

The other oral form used was mesterolone (MS – Pro-Viron) manufactured by Schering as 25 mg tablets. These were also given twice daily, but can be stored at room temperature, are water-soluble and are not dependant on the fat content of the meal. However, it was found with both oral preparations that treatment was more effective if given with breakfast and lunch, rather than giving a dose with the evening meal, which could give a restless night's sleep and suppress the natural night-time release of gonadotrophins that causes the endogenous morning surge in testosterone production.

Accordingly, patients were usually started on testosterone undecanoate 80 mg with breakfast and 40 mg with lunch, increasing at monthly intervals as judged from the remission of andropausal symptoms, to 80 mg, or a maximum of 120 mg, twice daily. A similar dosage regimen was used with mesterolone, starting with 50 mg with breakfast and 25 mg with lunch, and increasing to 50 mg, or a maximum of 75 mg, twice daily.

If the patient failed to respond to either oral preparation, or found the oral medication difficult to take, they were offered treatment with implants manufactured as cylinders containing 200 mg of pure fused crystals of testosterone (TI – Organon). The implant was given according to the technique described in Chapter 5. The initial dose was six or seven of the 200 mg pellets i.e. 1200 or 1400 mg, according to the size of the patient. Subsequent implant doses were adjusted at the 6-month visit to give optimum symptom relief over the duration of the implant, so that it was just beginning to wear off prior to the next visit. In this way the dosage of testosterone could be kept to a minimum.

As a supplement to any of the above treatments, over the last 4 years of the study, danazol (D-Danol – Sanofi Winthrop) 100 mg alt mane, or depending on the response, mane daily, was added to the androgen regimen, particularly in cases with a raised SHBG and those who did not respond to any of the testosterone treatments alone.

Statistics

The data was collated using a computerized practice management system called the Global Andrology Assessment and Treatment Tracking program (GAATT), developed specifically for use in the Gold Cross Andrology Clinic by Mr Hugh Welford. This program assembled the information on all patients in a database from which individual or group responses to treatment could be assessed.

Statistical tests were performed using the Statistical Package for the Social Sciences (SPSS) version 11.5 program.

CHARACTERISTICS OF POPULATION STUDIED

Exclusion Criteria

As the intention was to study the diagnosis and treatment of the andropause, certain groups of patients were excluded:
1. Cases with primary hypogonadism due to testicular non-descent or bilateral orchidectomy.
2. Asymptomatic individuals attending for general medical screening or just wishing to keep fit.
3. Young men wishing to have anabolic steroid treatment to improve athletic performance or physique, who were discouraged from attending the clinic.
4. Young men with 'locker room syndrome'.
5. Individuals who had been diagnosed as 'Male Mid-life Crisis'.
6. Patients attending for treatment of severe peripheral vascular disease.
7. Patents where the primary diagnosis was depression.

Social Class

Though there was a wide range of occupations, the majority of patients were social classes 1–2.

Age

The mean age of the 1500 patients in the UKAS was 54.2 (range 31–88), and is shown as a histogram in Figure 1.

Further studies of possible causative factors of the andropause as seen in this population are being carried out.

RESULTS

The ongoing analysis of the safety and effectiveness of these forms of androgen treatment has been presented at international conferences, in journals and books over the last ten years[1,4-17]. More detailed reports are being prepared for publication.

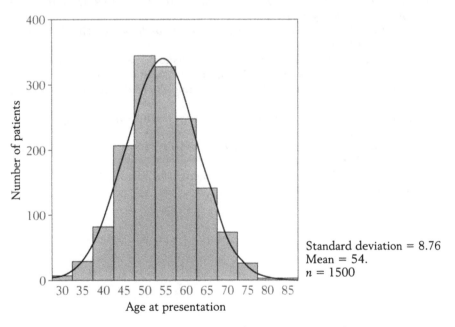

Standard deviation = 8.76
Mean = 54.
n = 1500

Figure 1 Age of presentation of patients in the UKAS. Note andropause symptoms have often been present for 3–5 years prior to attending the clinic for the first time

REFERENCES

1. Carruthers M. HRT for the aging male: a clinical study in 1000 men. *Aging Male* 1998;1:34
2. Heinemann LAJ, Zimmermann T, Vermeulen A, Thiel C, Hummel W. A new 'aging males' symptoms' (AMS) rating scale. *Aging Male* 1999;2:105–14
3. Morley JE, Charlton E, Patrick P, *et al*. Validation of a screening questionnaire for androgen deficiency in aging males. *Metabolism* 2000;49:1239–42
4. Carruthers M. The diagnosis of androgen deficiency. *Aging Male* 2002;4:254
5. Carruthers M. The safety of long-term testosterone treatment. *Aging Male* 2002;4:255
6. Carruthers M. *Medical knowledge management: making specialist advice available on the internet*. Telemedicine 2001 conference, Royal Society of Medicine
7. Carruthers M. *Testosterone Revolution*. London: Thorsons, 2001
8. Carruthers M. A multifactorial approach to understanding andropause. *J Sex Reprod Med* 2001;1:69–74
9. Carruthers M. More effective testosterone treatment: combination with sildenafil and danazol. *Aging Male* 2000;3:16
10. Carruthers M. Androgen defiency in the aging male (ADAM): a multilevel and multinational crisis. *Aging Male* 2000;14:58
11. Carruthers M. *2000: the year of ADAM – the testosterone revolution*. The Andropause Society 6-12-2000
12. Carruthers M. *Diagnosis and treatment of the andropause*. The Andropause Society 6-12-2000
13. Carruthers M. *Beyond Viagra: combining testosterone and sildenafil for the treatment of erectile dysfunction*. Stamford CT: Puglio.P, 1998
14. Carruthers M. *Maximising Manhood: Beating the Male Menopause*. London: HarperCollins, 1997
15. Carruthers M. *Male Menopause: Restoring Vitality and Virility*. London: HarperCollins, 1996
16. Carruthers M. *The case of the caponized farmers: back to nature*. Manchester: British Andrology Society, 1995
17. Carruthers M. Hormone Replacement Therapy for Men. *RCGP Members Reference Book* 1993;283–5

Index

Milton Keynes UK
Ingram Content Group UK Ltd.
UKHW040443071024
449327UK00020B/964

9 780367 393922